100 Ab Workouts

2018

N.Rey | darebee.com

Printed in the United Kingdom. First Printing, 2018.

ISBN 13: 978-1-84481-009-3
ISBN 10: 1-84481-009-7

Warning and Disclaimer
Although every precaution has been taken to verify the accuracy of the information contained herein, the author and publisher assume no responsibility for any errors or omissions. No liability is assumed for damage or injury that may result from the use of information contained within.

Thank you!

Thank you for purchasing **ABS 100 Workouts**, the DAREBEE project print edition. DAREBEE is a non-profit global fitness resource dedicated to making fitness accessible for everyone, no matter the circumstances.

The project is supported exclusively via user donations and paperback royalties.

After printing cost and store fees every book developed by the DAREBEE project makes $1 and it goes directly into our project maintenance and development fund.

Each sale helps us keep the DAREBEE resource growing, maintain it and keep it up.

Thank you for making a difference in its future!

100 workouts

2-Minute Abs
6-Minute Abs
Ab Attack
Ab Builder
Ab Crunch
Ab Master
Ab Mod
Abs & Core
Ab Sculpt
Abs Defined
Abs Fold
Abs of Steel
Abs on Fire
Abs Pro
Abs Unlocked
Abs Upgrade
Active Plank
Anywhere Abs
Armor Abs
Art of Abs
At-Home Abs
Back Up
Beginner Abs
Boxer Abs
Brute Abs
Carver
Chair Abs
Code of Abs
Concrete Core
Core Builder
Core Connect
Core Control
Core Crusher
Core Twister
Crop Top

Crunch Time
Daily Abs
Express Abs
Extreme Abs
Five Minute Plank
Good Morning, Abs
Hardcore
Hello, Abs
Homemade Abs
Ironclad Abs
Killer Abs
Killer Core
Master Pack
Master Plank
Micro Shred
Origami Abs
Shredder Abs
Six Pack
Sofa Abs
Supercut Abs
Superhero Abs
Total Abs
Tough Cookie
Washboard Abs
Ab Decoder
Ab Hub
Anti-Pooch
Beer Belly
Belly Burner
Belly Melt
Bulletproof Abs
Burn Mode
Cardio & Core Express
Cardio & Core

Cardio Crunch
Cardio Sofa
Chisel
Codex
Comeback
Core Burn
Core Forge
Core Fusion
Core Sculpt
Cycle Core
Expedited Delivery
Fab Abs
Flat Stomach
Gut Buster
Hellraiser
Howler
Lean & Mean
Love Handles
Melt Off
Muffin Top
Outcast
Overhaul
Persephone
Pouncer
Power Abs
Rapid Fire
Sizzler
Speedster
Standing Abs
Total Core
Tune Up

Fitness is a journey, not a destination.
Darebee, Project

The Science

The science behind six-pack abs is driven by physiology and biology and there is also a little bit of physics thrown into all this for good measure.

We need to unravel it so we understand what is going and why the things we do, work.

So, first, physiology. The abs, as we think of them, consist of four distinct muscle groups whose scientific names are: rectus abdominis, external obliques, internal obliques and transversus abdominis. To us they are the six-pack, lateral abdominals (internal and external) and the core.

We cannot really think of training the abs without choosing to train all of these muscle groups. Each of them, however, requires specific exercises and, like all muscle groups, they become resistant to change unless they are constantly challenged by mixing the type of exercises they are exposed to and the load each type of exercise applies.

To make things a little more difficult consider that the six pack (rectus abdominis) is treated as one muscle group but is actually a paired muscle running vertically on each side of the anterior wall of the abdomen separated by a midline band of connective tissue called the linea alba. In addition the core abdominals are made up of some twelve complementary muscle groups some of which also belong to the six pack abs (rectus abdominis) and the internal obliques.

All this complexity means that training the abs correctly is not an easy thing to do. Luckily, as we shall see, you have this book in your hands now so you are on the right path to abdominal strength greatness.

Biology also doesn't help. Our bodies evolved to store up fat. The fat percentage of the body is one of the major factors of visibility of the abs (it plays up to an 80% role in terms of importance). This makes diet an important part of acquiring the ripped abs look.

Physics plays a part in terms of energy needs and energy consumption. In some ways the body is an organic machine fashioned to operate in a state of constant equilibrium, homeostasis for the more scientifically minded. This means that the moment the percentage of body fat drops, the hypothalamus kicks in and through a series of biochemical processes, it increases specific hormones in the body called leptin and Ghrelin that reduce the amount of body fat we burn when we diet or exercise. This makes it harder to drop body fat just when we most want to.

Leptin is the hormone of "energy expenditure". It is made predominantly by adipose cells and it helps to regulate the energy balance by inhibiting hunger. Ghrelin is the "hunger hormone", also known as lenomorelin. It regulates appetite and plays a significant role in regulating the distribution and rate of use of energy in the body plus it has stimulatory effects on fat deposition and growth hormone release.

All of this together give us a very clear picture of how to get those rippling abs: exercise to increase abdominal muscle size, exercise to increase energy expenditure and diet to reduce body fat percentage. The juggling of all this is exactly why there is no true shortcut to getting abs. The shredded look requires time, patience, the right diet and a structured approach to exercise. Get it right though and you will be able to have rock-hard abs that you can maintain.

Design Your Regimen

If I need to lose weight

If you are like most people and you carry even a little bit of extra weight - in your midsection for example, doing ab work exclusively will not give you defined abs. Even if you are fairly slim but you have a slight stomach, doing crunches will not reveal your abs simply because our bodies do not burn fat reserves in specific areas of the body through exercise - we lose body fat all over when we reduce our food intake and increase our physical activity levels.

The only way to reduce body fat is to adjust your nutrition and, for faster and better results, also exercise - preferably do high burn and/or high intensity interval training (HIIT) - the workouts you will find in this book in the "Burn & Build" section.

In order for you to have abs you need to build them through ab-centered routines on a regular basis. In order to then see your magnificent abs, you need to reveal them by reducing the cushioning on your stomach through nutritional adjustments and/or additional aerobic exercise. The trick with reducing body fat percentage and building abs is to make sure you burn more energy than you consume. Although not impossible, it's extremely difficult to out-train a bad diet. To see results and see them faster we recommend you combine high intensity cardio training with diet.

To make things easier, the workouts included in the Burn & Build section also include ab-work and we highly recommend that these are the workouts you pick, at least in the beginning of the process until your body fat percentage drops enough for your abdominal muscles to show through. After that, you can refer exclusively to the "Build" section.

To begin, look over the "Burn & Build" section, see what workouts you feel confident you can take on - or just pick at random. They all work your cardiovascular system and abs. We recommend that you do from 3 to 5 workouts per week for maximum results. Rotate workouts so your body doesn't get used to the same routine. If it does you will see diminishing returns for all your hard work. There is a very good rule: if a workout doesn't challenge you it doesn't change you.

In the beginning, you may not feel any difference. If you don't feel the "burn" in your abdominal wall, it's perfectly normal. It takes time to develop muscles there. Be prepared to not feel or see any progress for the first three to four weeks. Eventually, with consistent work, you will begin feeling your muscles tightening up and your abs beginning to burn during and after exercise. It means you are on the right track.

The moment a workout is beginning to feel easy, increase the number of sets or better yet - start picking more challenging workout routines with more complex exercises. Your numbers or difficulty has to continue to go up for you to challenge the muscles you are building. In the beginning simply doing crunches is enough to jump-start the ab-building process but after a while the number of crunches you would have to do will go into thousands if you want to continue seeing results. It's much easier to switch to more complex moves way before that happens to save yourself some time and effort. Your goal is to challenge the muscles every single time you work on your abs.

If I don't need to lose weight

If your body fat is already pretty low the process is a lot more straightforward. All you want to do is build the muscles up enough to make them pop. Go for a minimum of three workouts per week from the "Build" section exclusively and you will see results fairly quickly.

The only thing you should mind is your nutrition. Building muscle requires building materials and most people who are already slim don't have much spare to go around. Apart from ab work you will also need to focus on getting extra quality food to literally feed the process of muscle building. Quality is important here. You need to make sure your daily food intake consists from complex carbs and protein so your body has something to work with. Simple carbs like sugar and bread give you energy but they are not a very good source of building material - they're a better source of energy.

A common mistake in nutrition is to focus exclusively on protein when muscle building but it's exactly the same as having the building materials but not enough workers to build anything. You need both energy and building materials to use, so balance is key.

You will begin to see results almost straight away maybe even as soon as after two weeks of regular, consistent hard work. At first you will see the definition lines of your abs appearing beginning with the central one going from your chest all the way down. Then the individual segments will begin to surface (the six pack). If your nutrition lacks protein and/or complex carbs the segments will remain flat. Increase your food intake slightly making sure you eat quality meals and the segments will begin to fill up as you continue to do your ab workouts.

What if the segments have shown, they even seem to fill up but they haven't yet popped? This means you have to increase the difficulty of your workouts, make them more intense.

Challenge your muscles and watch your body transform itself.

If I do other training

If you do other types of physical activity like running or martial arts or other workouts from elsewhere (that are not included in this collection) then you should pick workouts from the “Build” section straight away.

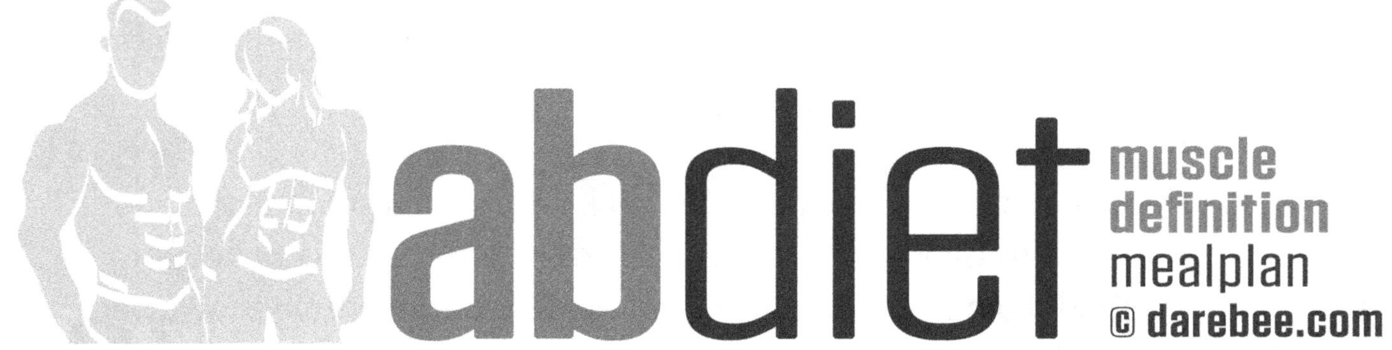

meal 1

1 | bowl of oatmeal with berries
2 | green smoothie
3 | homemade protein or breakfast bar
4 | low fat yogurt with banana or pear
5 | 3-eggs with spinach and mushrooms
6 | 1/2 serving protein pancakes

meal 2 snack

1 | turkey or pork ham with raw veggies
2 | cheese stick with handful of grapes
3 | sliced apple with 1tbs nut butter
4 | cup cantaloupe with almonds
5 | sliced tomato with light mozzarella
6 | pear with walnuts or almonds

meal 3

1 | chicken, green beans and sweet potato
2 | turkey ham whole grain sandwich
3 | sweet potato with cottage cheese
4 | baked salmon with rice and veggies
5 | tuna and lettuce salad with light mayo
6 | chicken breast light Caesar salad

meal 4 snack

1 | low fat Greek Yogurt with honey
2 | handful of almonds, apple or orange
3 | 1/2 homemade protein or breakfast bar
4 | low fat sugar free chocolate milk or shake
5 | sardine bruschetta toast with tomato
6 | cottage cheese with pineapple chunks

meal 5

1 | chicken breast with g.beans or broccoli
2 | meatballs or burger with cucumbers
3 | tuna and lettuce salad with light mayo
4 | lean pork with cauliflower and broccoli
5 | baked ground pork with eggplant
6 | baked salmon with broccoli

meal 6 snack

1 | low fat Greek yogurt with cinnamon
2 | hardboiled egg with 1/2tsp light mayo
3 | turkey or pork ham with cucumbers
4 | low fat sugar free chocolate milk or shake
5 | 1/2 chicken breast strips with garlic yogurt
6 | cubed ham with cottage cheese

six meals a day - six options each

meat | poultry | fish | dairy amounts: up to 6oz [170g] per meal
nuts: a handful a day maximum - can be split between meals
bread: always wholegrain, maximum 1 slice a day or none
meals 2, 4, and 6 are optional / post & pre workout meals

Manual

Each workout has three levels of difficulty: I, II and III.

If you are new to exercise or you haven't done any training in a long while you should start on Level I. You don't have to stay on level I consistently, if you feel that you can do more, you can advance a level. Level III is the hardest level of difficulty and it can be pretty challenging to complete.

All reps, located under every exercise next to its name, are given in total for each side. So "20 flutter kicks", for example, means you do 10 per leg = 20 in total.

If the sets for the workout are located at the top of the poster - the workout is a circuit.You repeat each exercise one after the other until the curcuit is complete, rest and repeat it again (see number of sets for your selected level I, II or III).

If the sets are located underneath each exercise - it's a traditional workout. You complete each exercise individually, do all the sets and then move on to the next exercise.

The workouts are split into two parts **BURN & BUILD and BUILD** and then organized in alphabetical order so you can find the workouts you favor easier and faster.

Before you start:

Look over the workout you chose to do and make sure you understand all of the exercises illustrated so it doesn't slow you down once you have started.

Video Exercise Library:
https://darebee.com/exercises

All of the routines in this collection are suitable for both men and women, no age restrictions apply.

1 2-Minute Abs

If you only have two minutes to spare towards some exercise you can do no better than the 2-Minute Abs workout. Abs are required every time we do something physical and they play a pivotal role in supporting the spine, affecting posture and enhancing physical performance. The 2-Minute Abs program helps you strengthen this critically important muscle group.

2-minute **abs**

DAREBEE WORKOUT © **darebee.com**

20 seconds each exercise | no rest between exercises

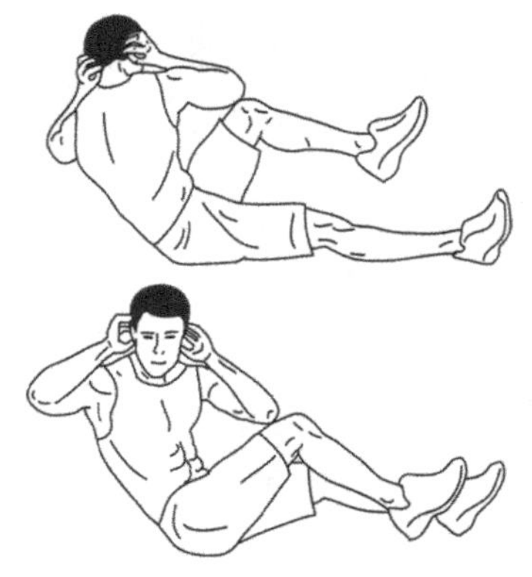

1. knee-to-elbow crunches

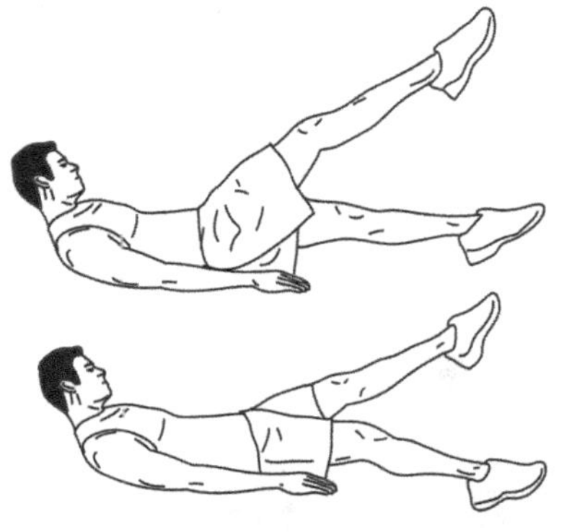

2. flutter kicks

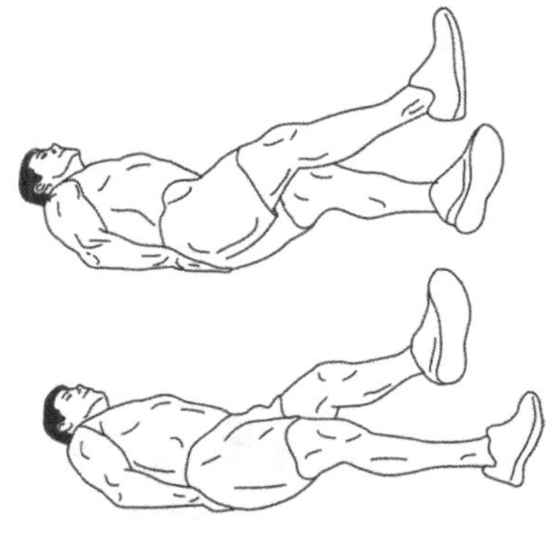

3. scissors

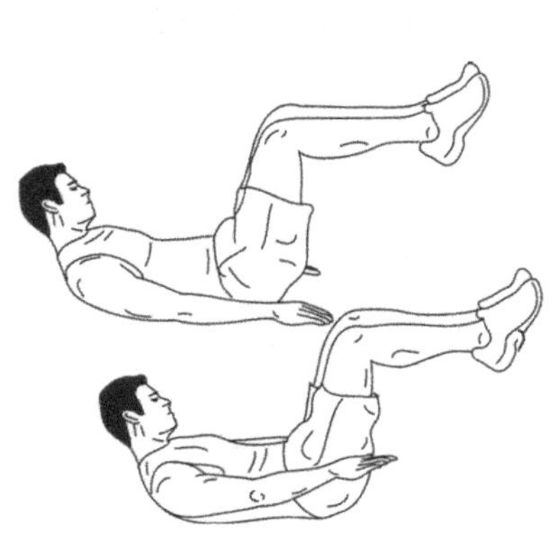

4. hundreds

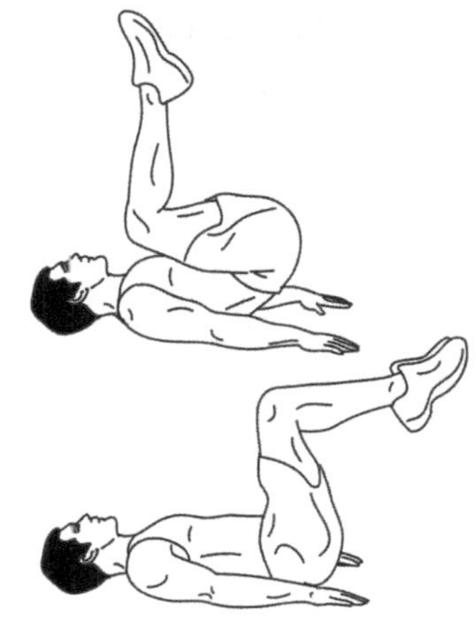

5. reverse crunches

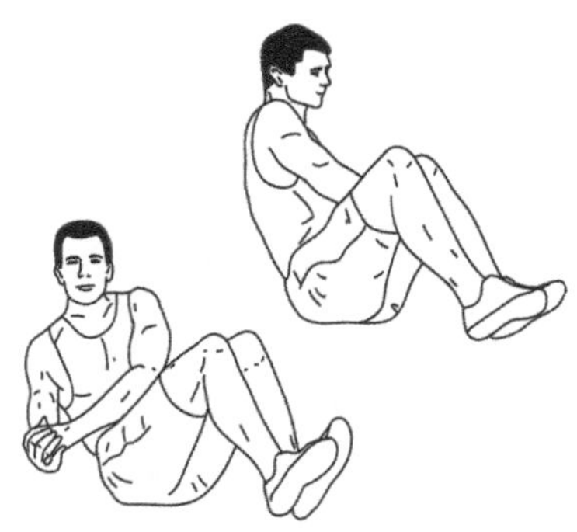

6. sitting twists

2 6-Minute Abs

A strong core and well-trained abdominals provide a solid foundation for most athletic activities. The 6-minute abs workout should be part of your regular abs & core exercise routine. Performed regularly it leads to incremental improvements in overall athletic ability and aids in better posture and coordination. It is perfectly suitable for any level of fitness.

6-minute abs

DAREBEE WORKOUT © darebee.com

Repeat each exercise for exactly one minute with no rest in between.

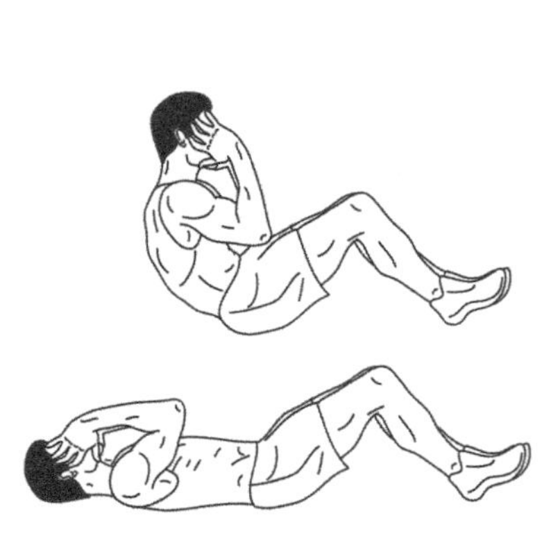

1min sit-ups

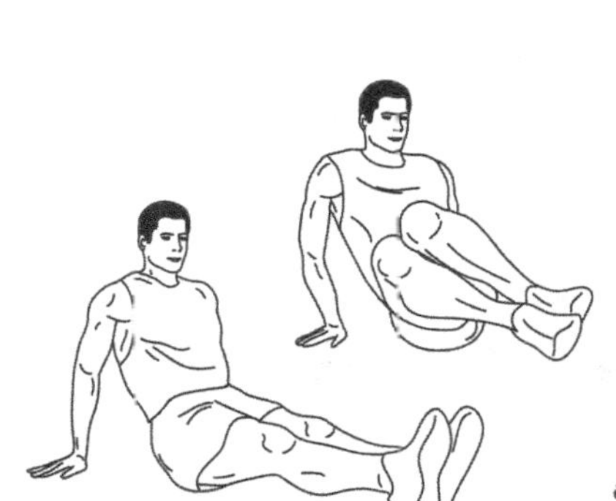

1min knee-in & twist

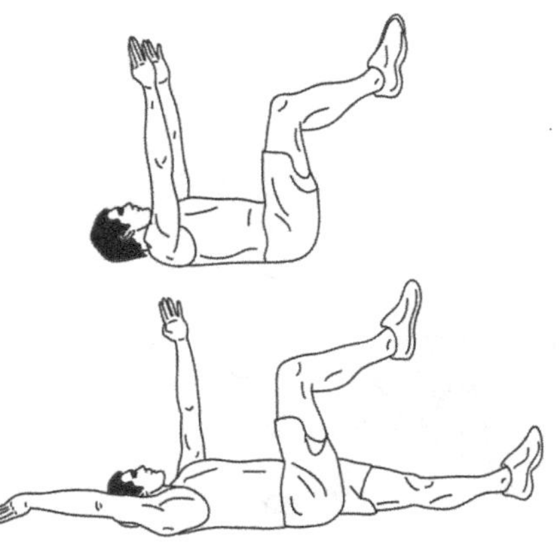

1min dead bug

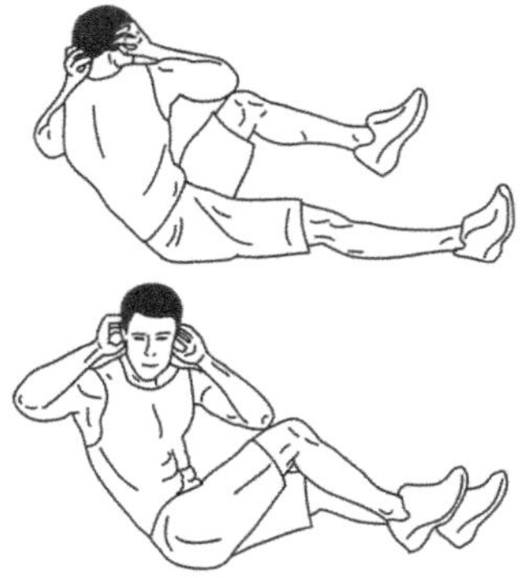

1min knee-to-elbow crunches

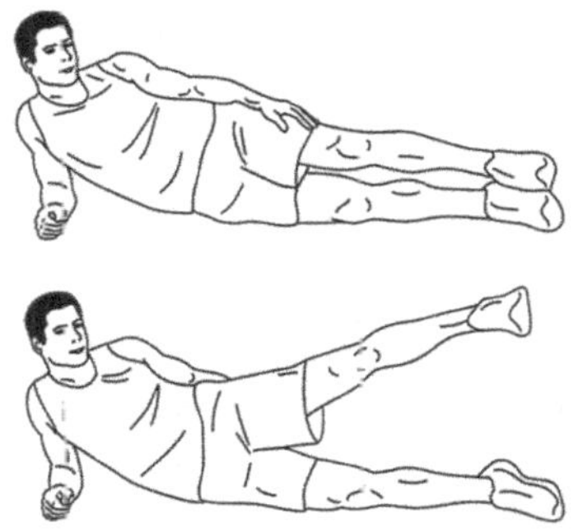

1min side leg raises
30sec per side

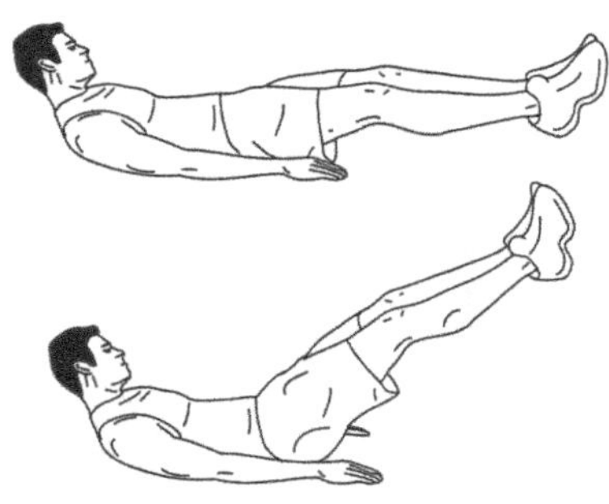

1min leg raises

3 Ab Attack

Be kind to yourself by torturing your abs a little. Abs play such a critical part in physical performance, posture, energy transfer from the lower body to the upper one (like when you punch or sprint) and back again that just doing enough here is simply not enough. So challenge yourself and see if you can do the whole Level III and if yes then add EC for good measure.

ab attack

DARBEE WORKOUT © darebee.com

LEVEL I 3 sets **LEVEL II** 4 sets **LEVEL III** 5 sets **REST** up to 2 minutes

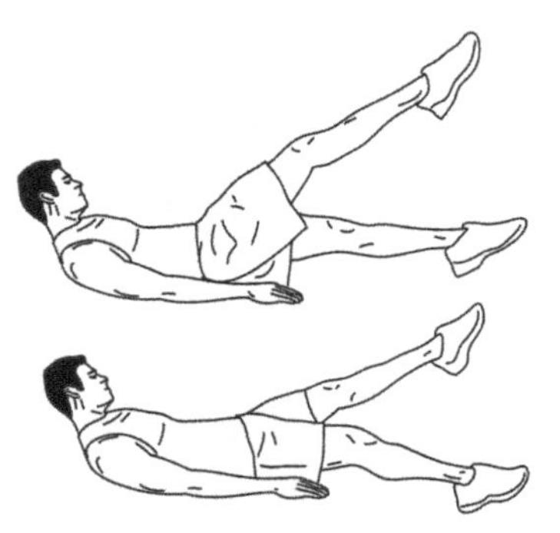

20 flutter kicks

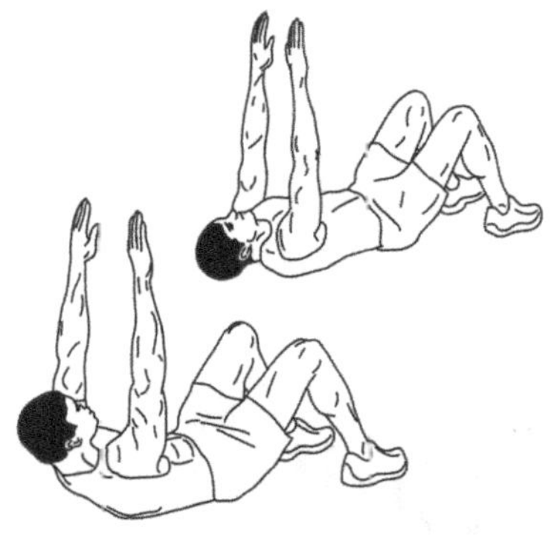

20 high crunches

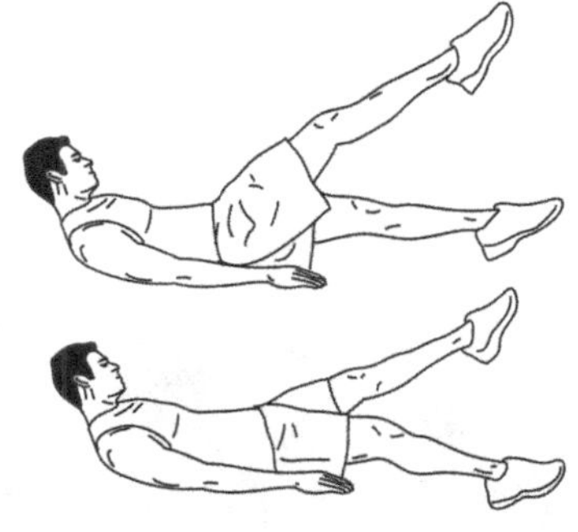

20 flutter kicks

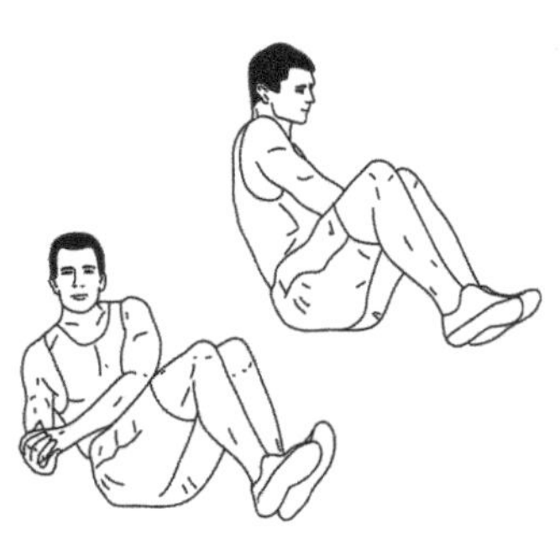

20 sitting twists

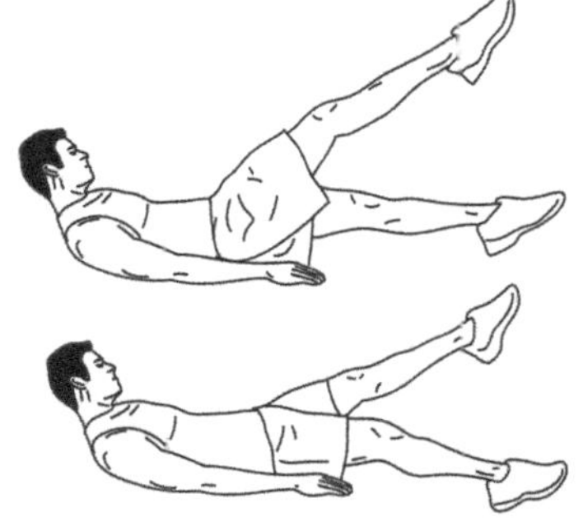

20 flutter kicks

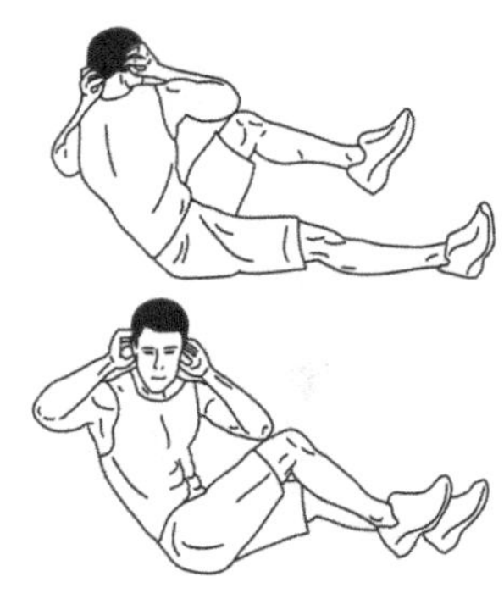

20 knee-to-elbow crunches

4 Ab Builder

Building Abs is about consistent work and precise muscle group targeting and the Ab Builder workout delivers on both of these fronts. This isn't just another workout to 'conquer' and forget. It should be on your regular workouts list and revisiting it will pay off handsomely.

BUILD

ab builder

DARGEBEE WORKOUT © darebee.com

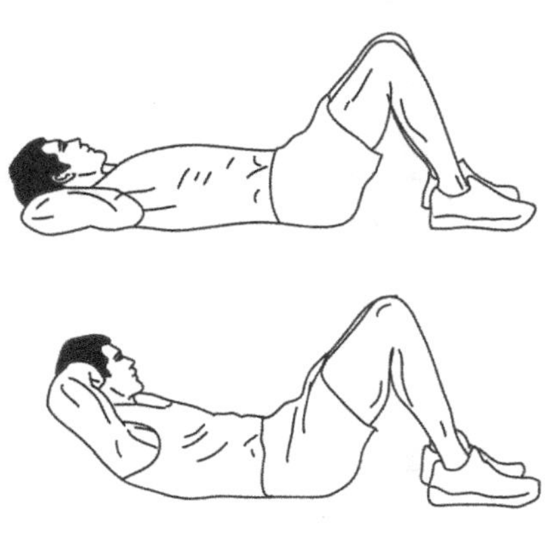

20 crunches **x 3 sets**
20 seconds rest between sets

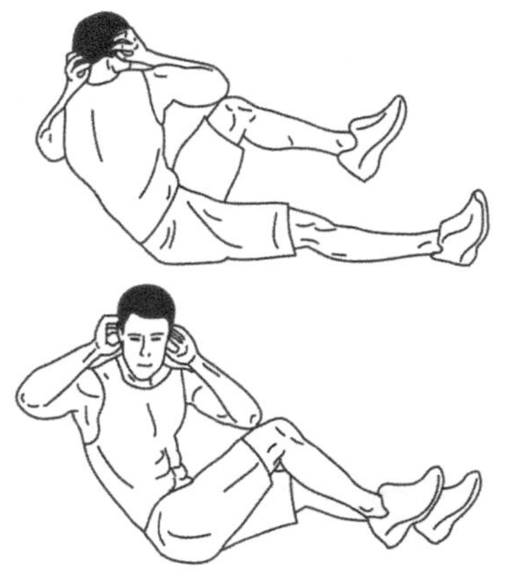

20 knee-to-elbow crunches **x 3 sets**
20 seconds rest between sets

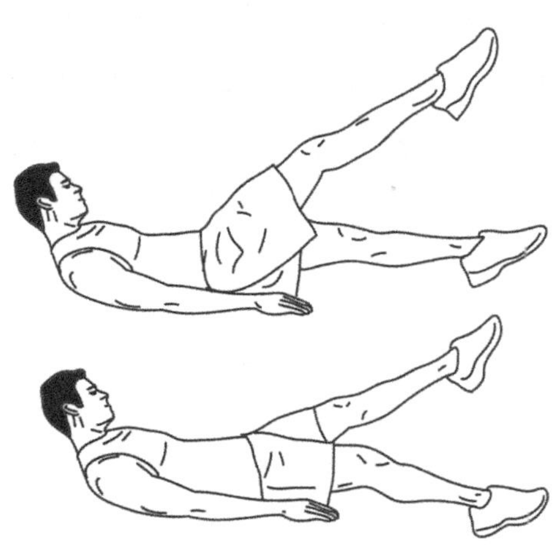

20 flutter kicks **x 3 sets**
20 seconds rest between sets

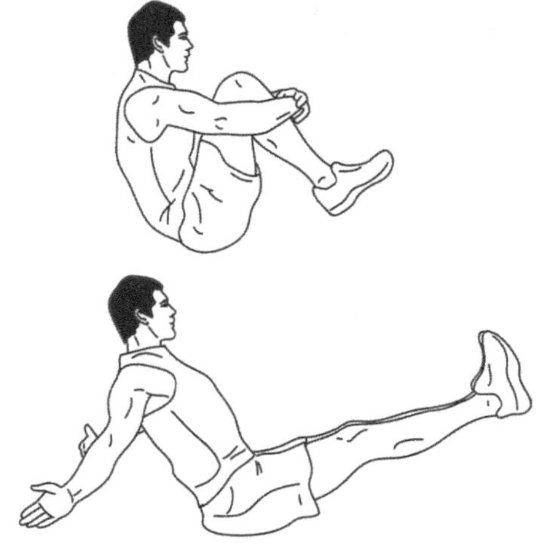

20 knee hug crunches **x 3 sets**
20 seconds rest between sets

5 Ab Crunch

Abdominal muscles are performance engines. No matter what you do, will be done better and easier if you have strong abdominals. This is a set that starts you off on the right path plus you know it feels good to have a rippling torso (go on, admit it).

ab crunch

DAREBEE WORKOUT © darebee.com

LEVEL I 3 sets **LEVEL II** 4 sets **LEVEL III** 5 sets **REST** up to 2 minutes

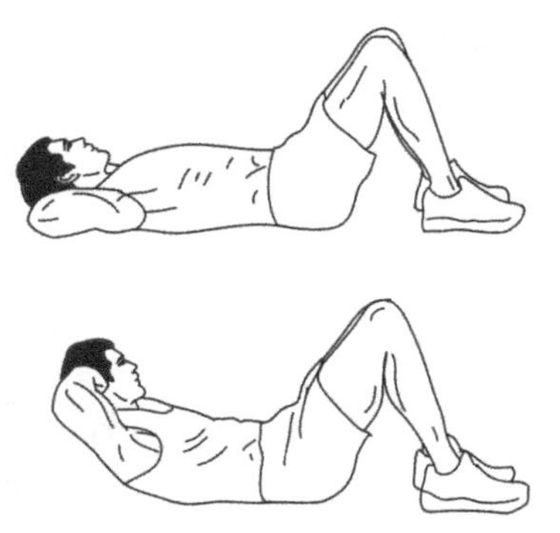

20 crunches

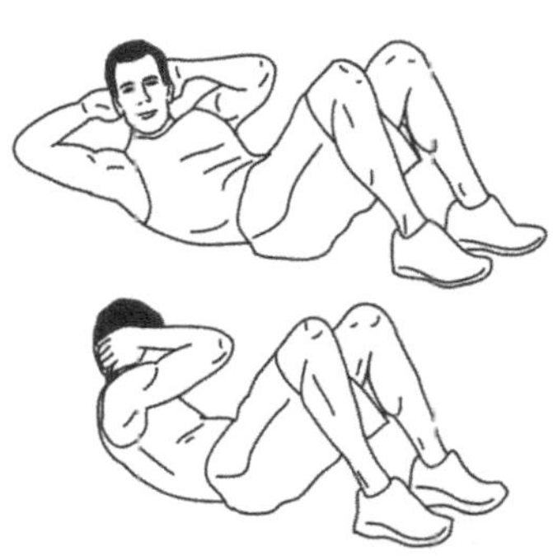

10 cross crunches

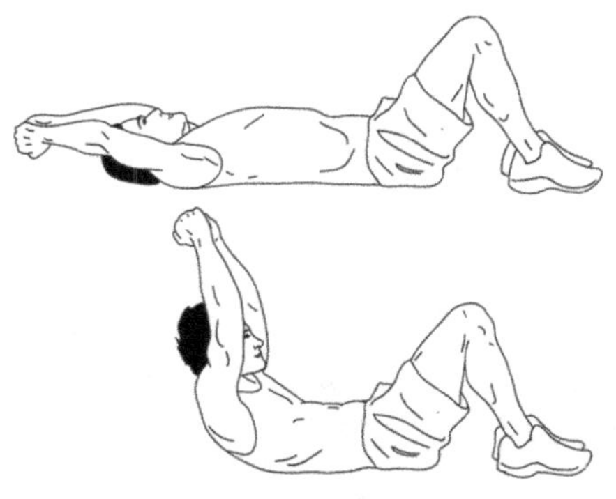

10 long arm crunches

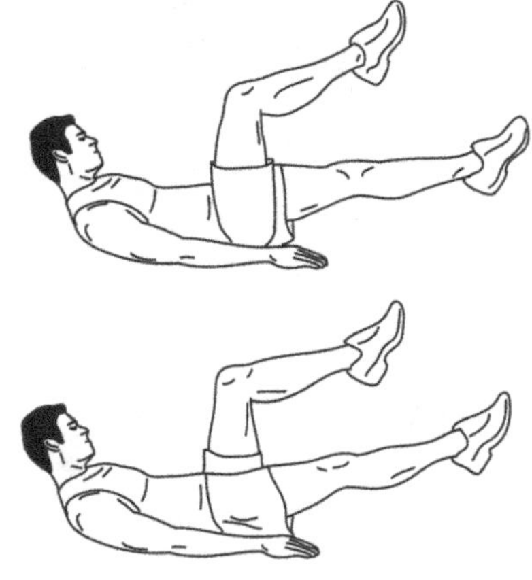

20 air bike crunches

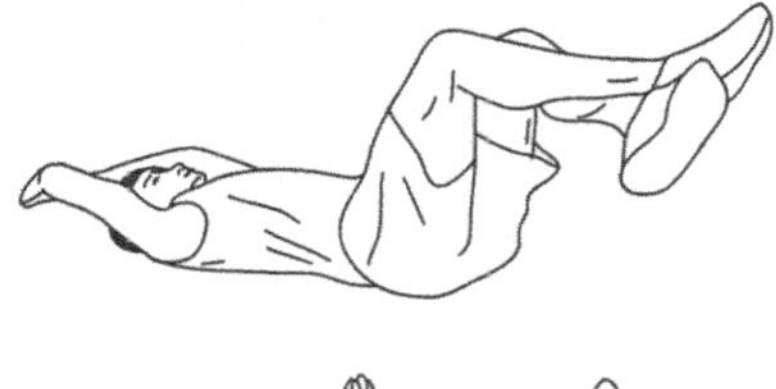

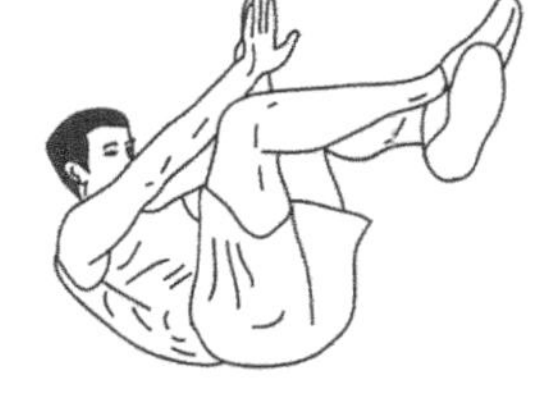

10 knee crunches

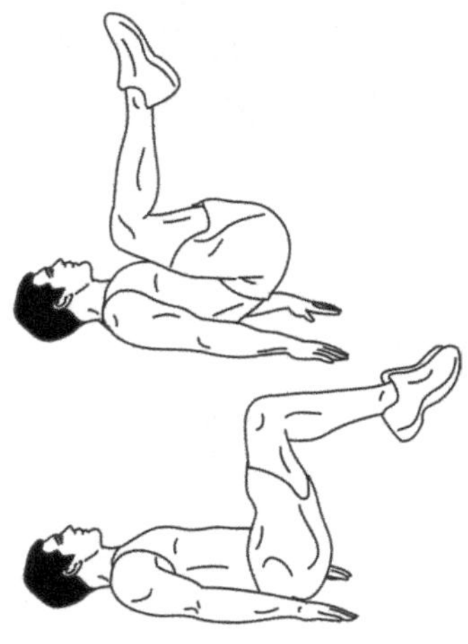

10 reverse crunches

6 Ab Master

One of the biggest challenges your abs can face is the need to keep your lower and upper body together when you are pulled down by gravity. Ab Master uses the Earth's gravity (and a handy pull up bar) to help you develop the abdominal strength you need to fight the entire planet's pull.

ab master

DAREBEE WORKOUT © darebee.com

1 minute rest between exercises

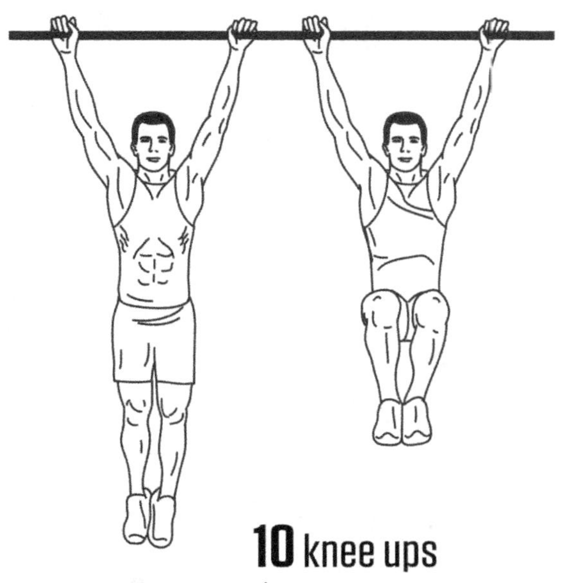

10 knee ups

3 sets | 20 seconds rest

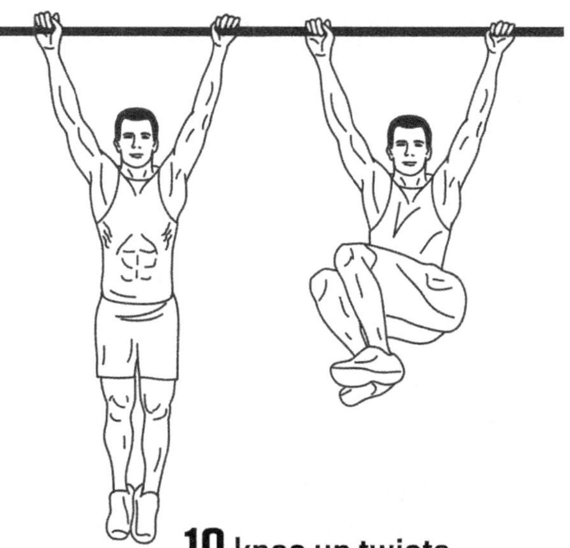

10 knee up twists

3 sets | 20 seconds rest

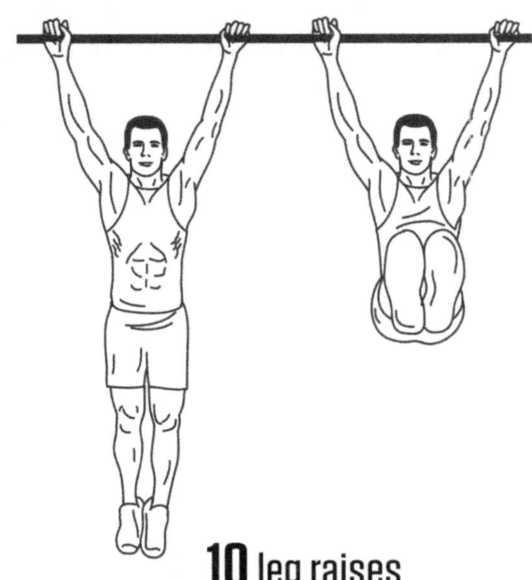

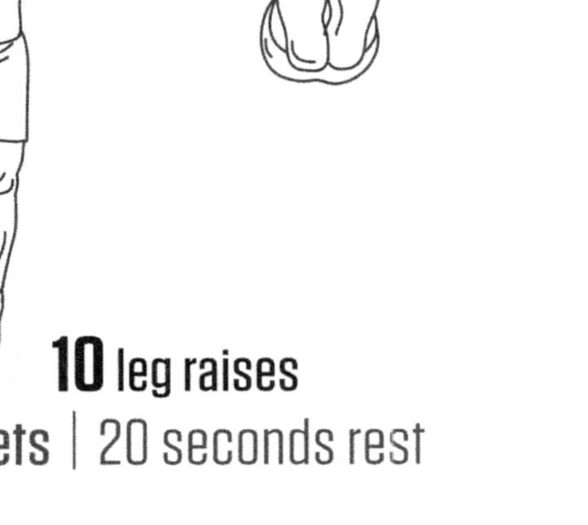

10 leg raises

3 sets | 20 seconds rest

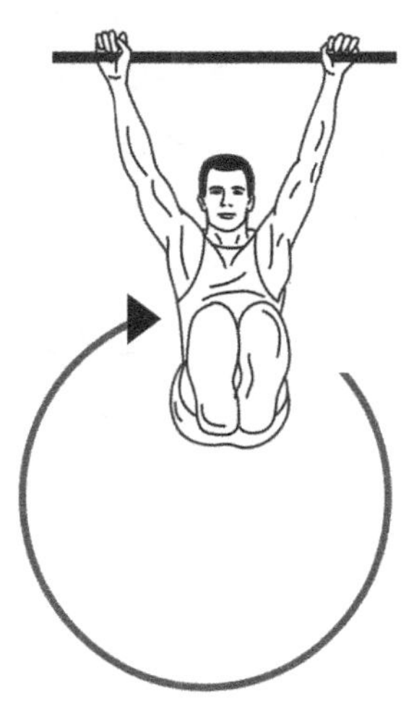

10 raised leg circles

3 sets | 20 seconds rest

7 Ab Mod

Abs are the powerhouse of the body. Strong abs help posture, stability, balance and power transfer between the muscles of the lower body and the upper ones. The Ab Mod workout helps you get your abs to the kind of state where they become a true asset to your overall athletic performance.

ab mod

BUILD

DAREBEE WORKOUT © darebee.com

1 minute rest between exercises

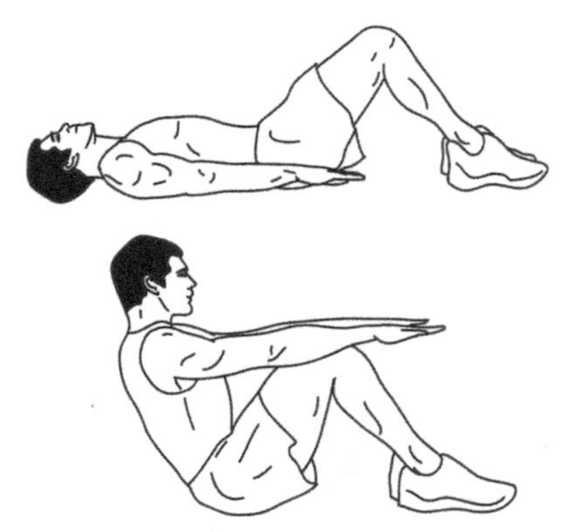

20 sit-ups

3 sets | 20 seconds rest

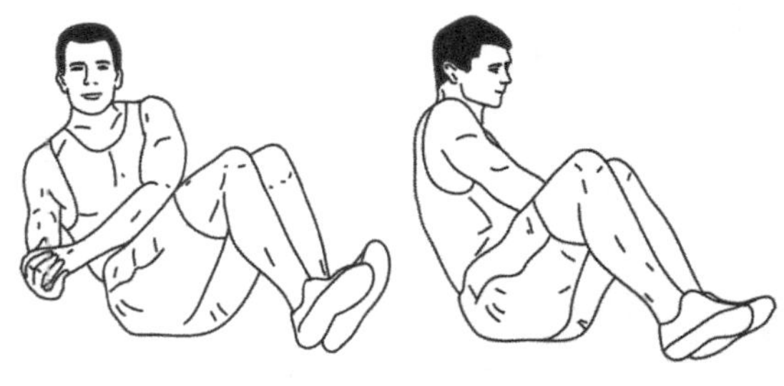

20 sitting twists

3 sets | 20 seconds rest

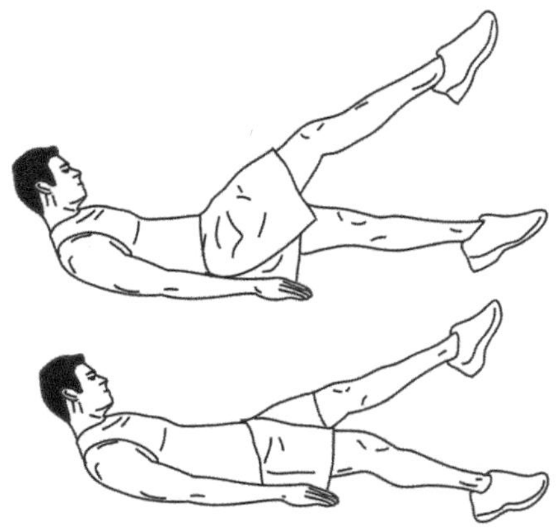

20 flutter kicks

3 sets | 20 seconds rest

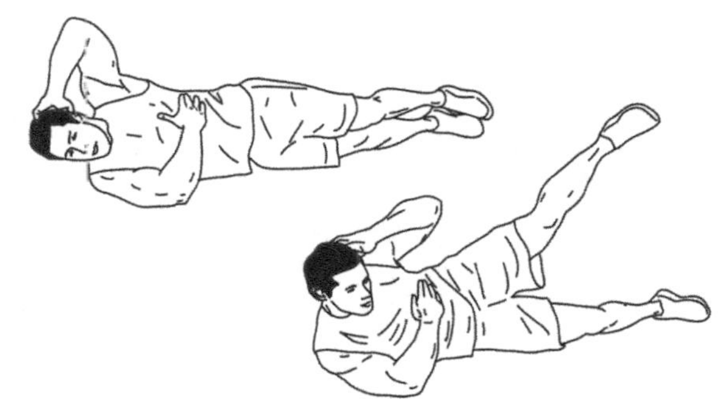

20 side jackknives

3 sets | 20 seconds rest

8 Abs & Core

Desks are not only important pieces of office furniture without which we wouldn't be able to get much work done, they can also be transformed into a handy multi-gym station that allows us to train some of the major muscle groups in our body.

Abs & Core

desk edition

DARBEE WORKOUT © darebee.com

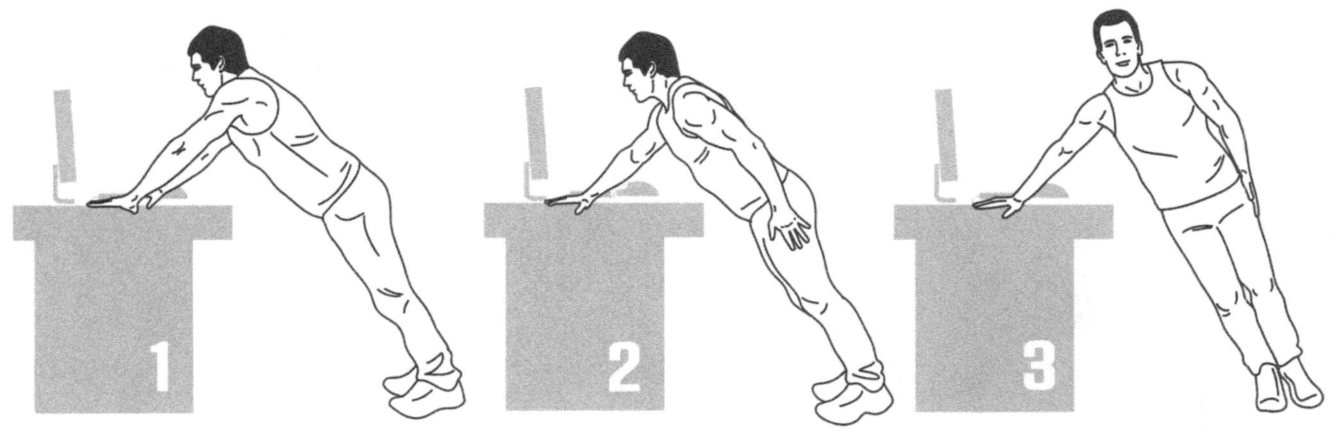

30 seconds
table plank

60 seconds
one arm table plank

60 seconds
side table plank

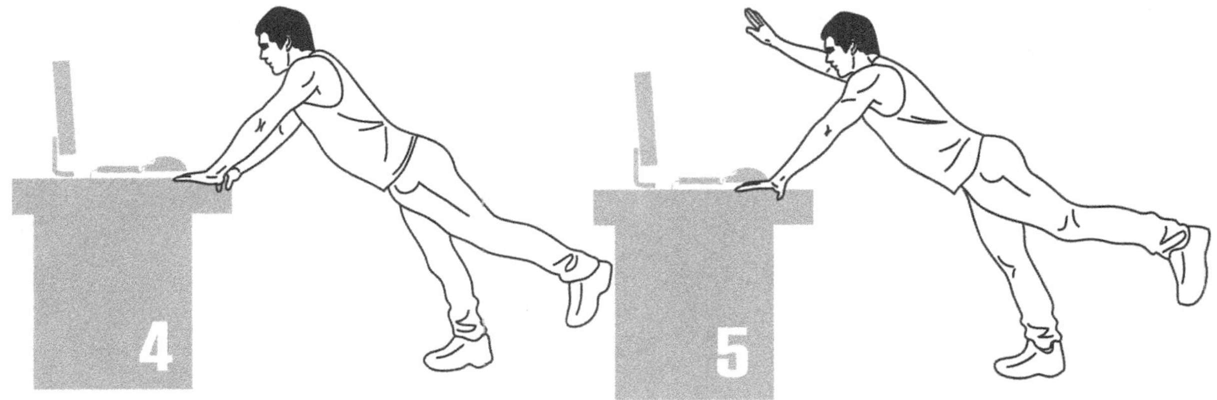

60 seconds
raised leg table plank

60 seconds
alternative arm and leg raise table plank

9 Ab Sculpt

Training the abs and core requires training the back and arms and shoulders and lateral abs. No muscle group works in isolation so in order to have that tight, sculpted abs look you need to work all the supporting muscle groups as well as tendons and upper body. Add EC for that extra load that activates the adaptive response and you have got yourself quite the workout.

ab sculpt

BUILD

DAREBEE WORKOUT © darebee.com

2 minutes rest between exercises

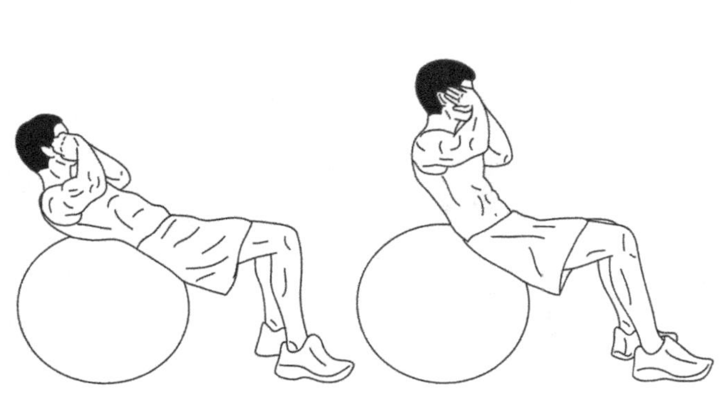

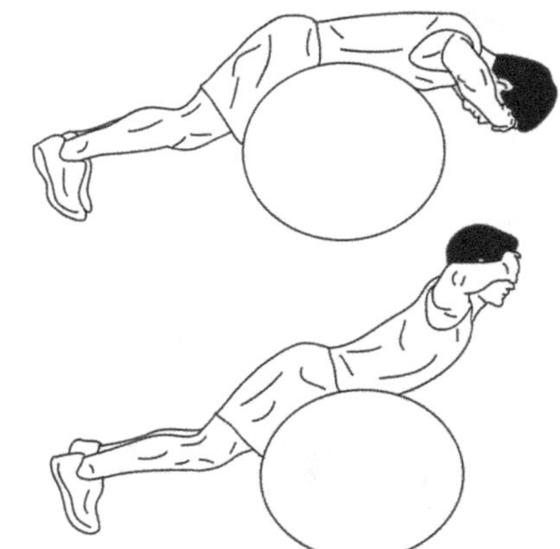

20 sit-ups **x 5 sets** in total
30 seconds rest between sets

10 back extensions **x 5 sets** in total
30 seconds rest between sets

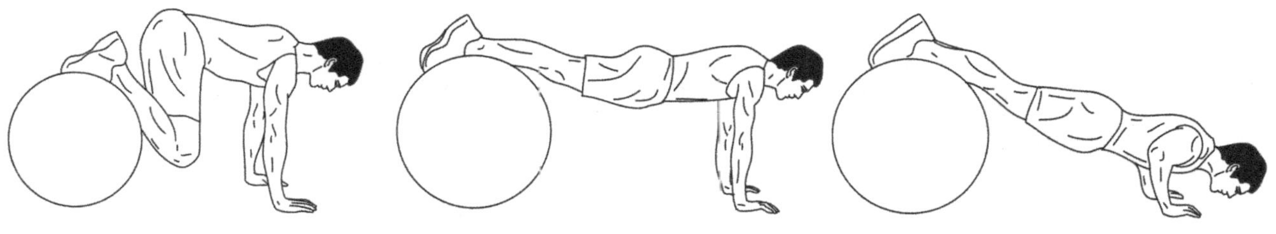

10combos roll out + push-up **x 5 sets** in total
30 seconds rest between sets

10 Abs Defined

Streamline your body, change your posture and add additional power to your every routine with the Abs Defined workout. Not only will you be able to feel the change in the way you walk but you will also see the difference every time you perform any exercise.

BUILD

abs defined

DAREBEE WORKOUT © darebee.com

LEVEL I 3 sets **LEVEL II** 4 sets **LEVEL III** 5 sets **REST** up to 2 minutes

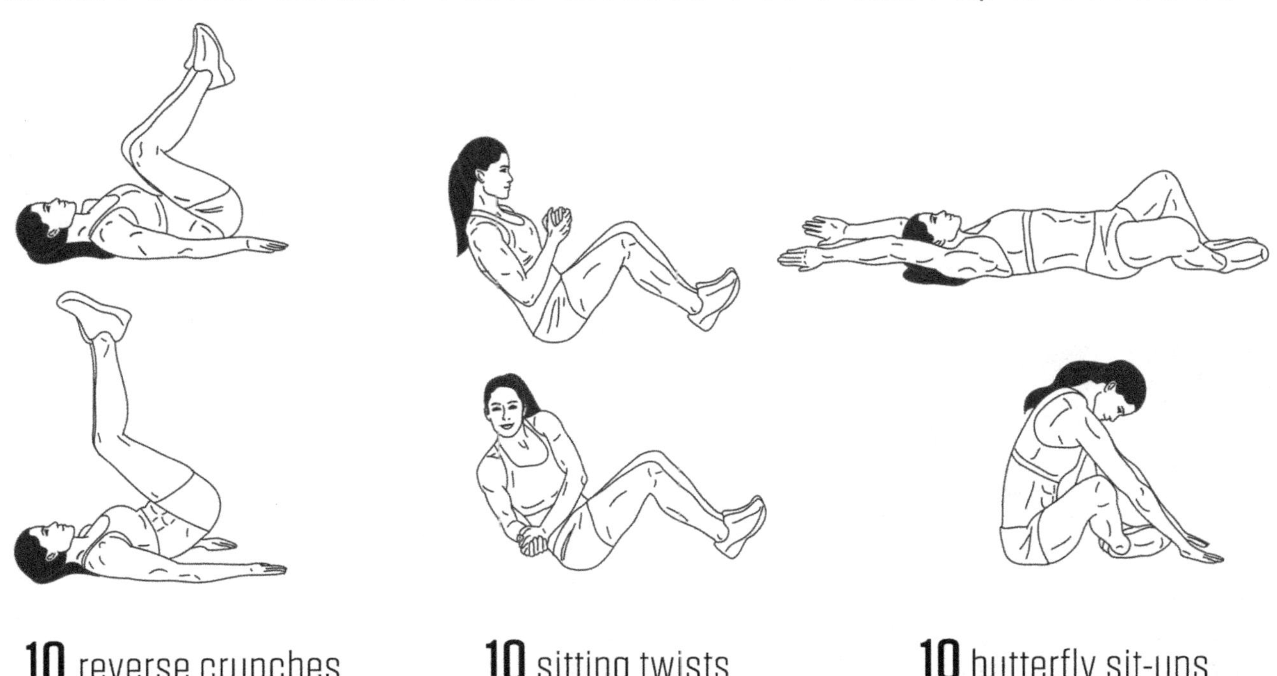

10 reverse crunches

10 sitting twists

10 butterfly sit-ups

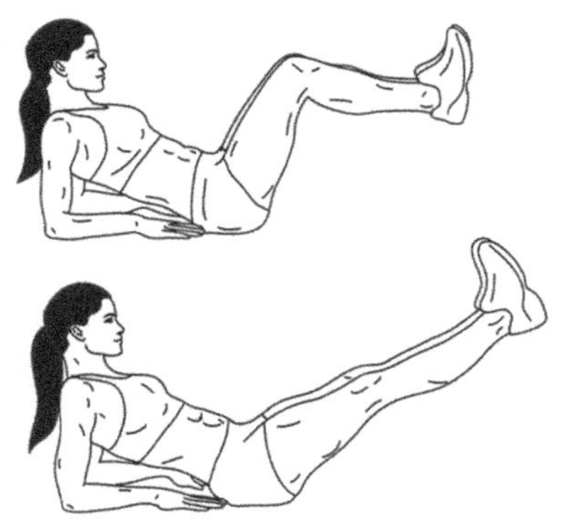

10 crunch kicks

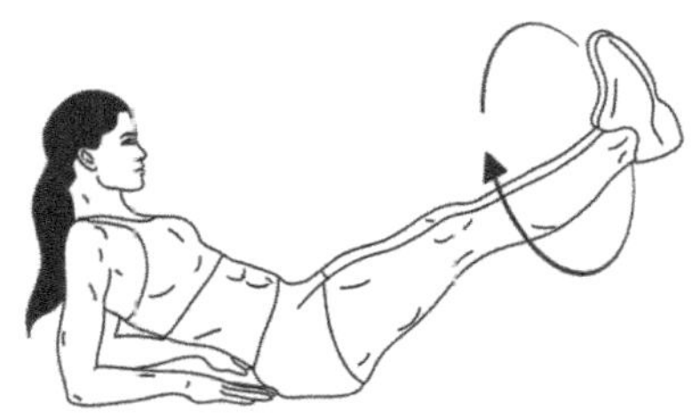

10 raised leg circles

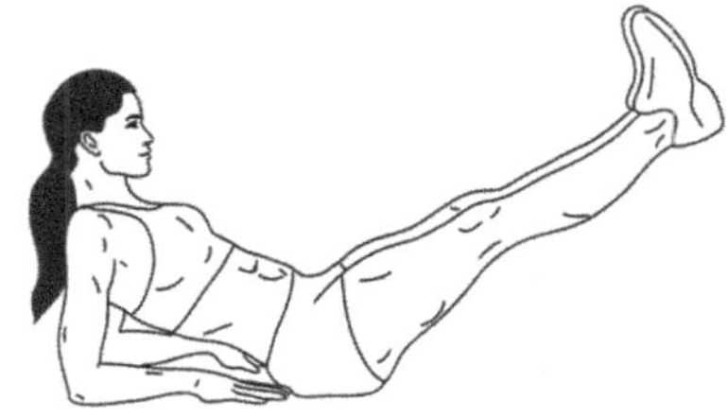

10-count raised leg hold

11 Abs Fold

When it comes to adding some real pressure on the abdominal muscle group to adapt and get stronger Abs Fold is your go-to workout. This is a difficulty level IV workout which means that it's not suitable for beginners, but its challenge is one everyone should aspire to. Abs are key to athletic performance and our ability to train them to a high strength level unlocks the potential of the body in just about any athletic endeavour.

abs fold

DAREBEE WORKOUT © darebee.com

Repeat 3 times | 2 minutes rest between sets

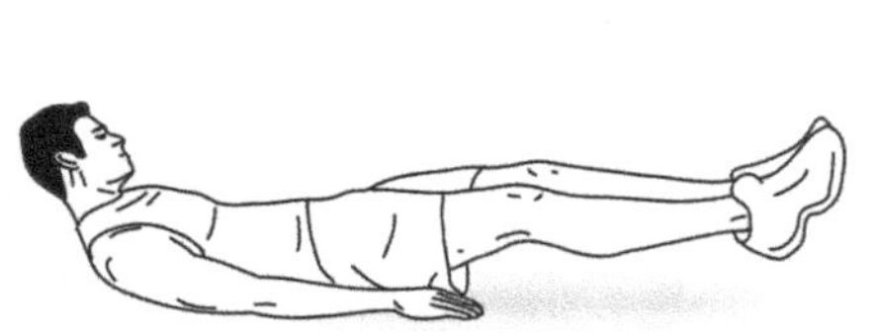

20sec hold
raised leg hold
just off the floor

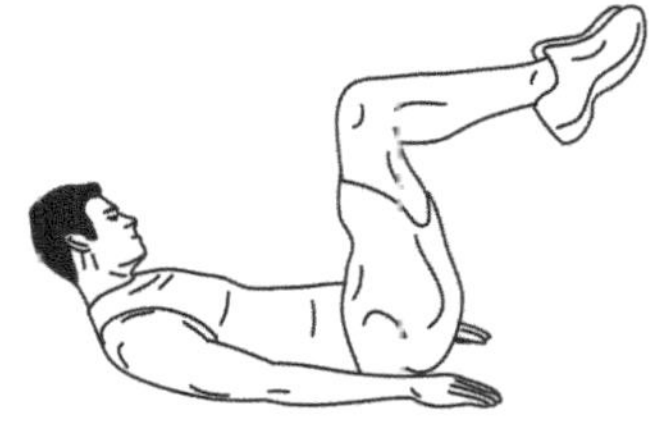

20sec hold
bring your knees in
and hold

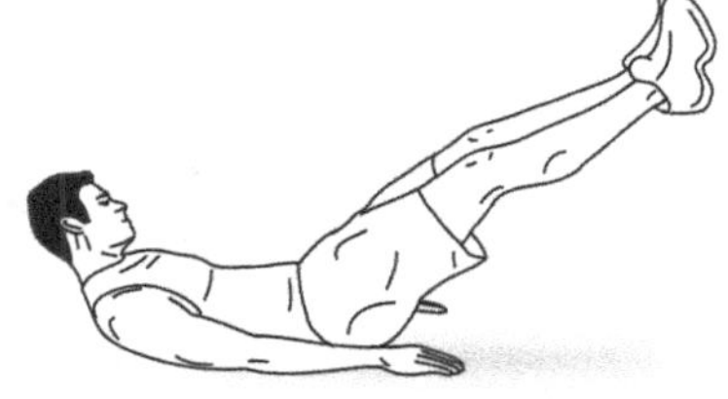

20sec hold
extend your legs
at ~45 degrees and hold

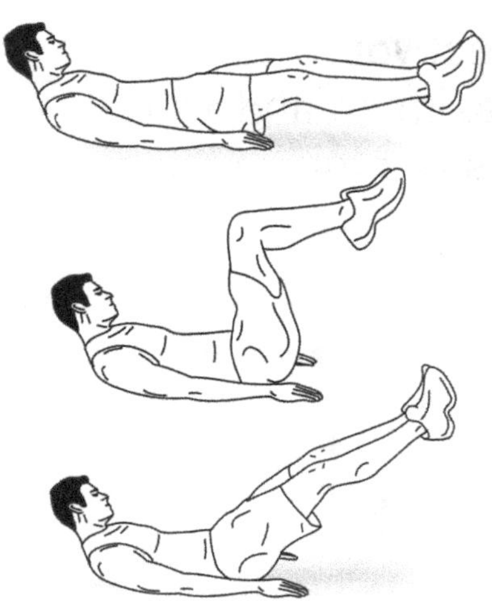

20sec folds
fold in & out
as fast as you can

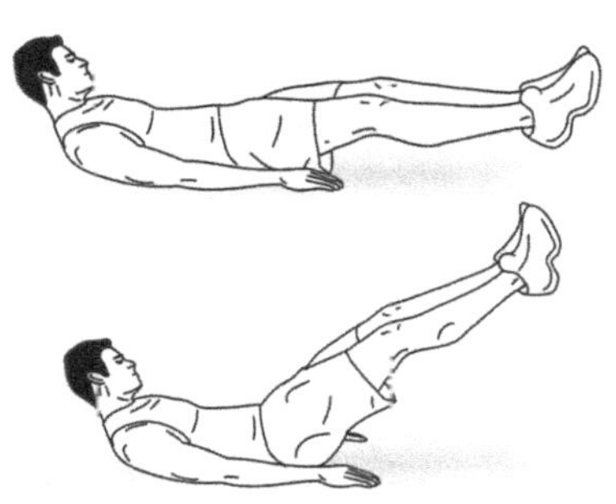

20sec leg raises
do leg raises -
keep legs off the floor

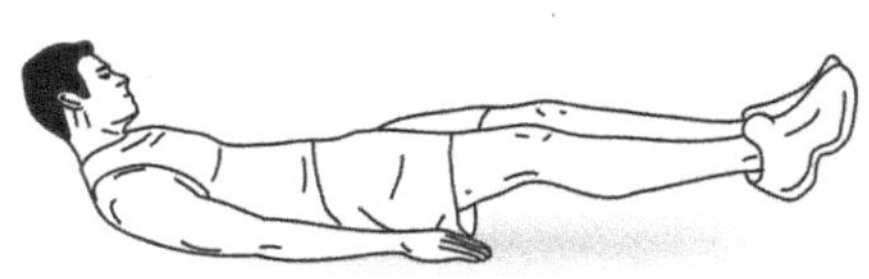

20sec hold
raised leg hold
just off the floor

12 Abs of Steel

Abdominal muscles are body armour. They help protect your vital organs from damage. They keep your body performing at maximum and, when the clothes come off, they make you look terrific. This workout is the anvil where that armour is fashioned.

abs of steel

BUILD

DARBEE WORKOUT © darebee.com

LEVEL I 3 sets **LEVEL II** 4 sets **LEVEL III** 5 sets **REST** up to 2 minutes

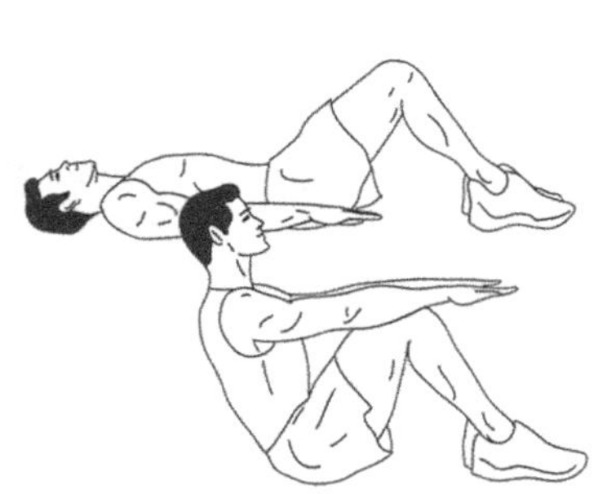

10 sit-ups

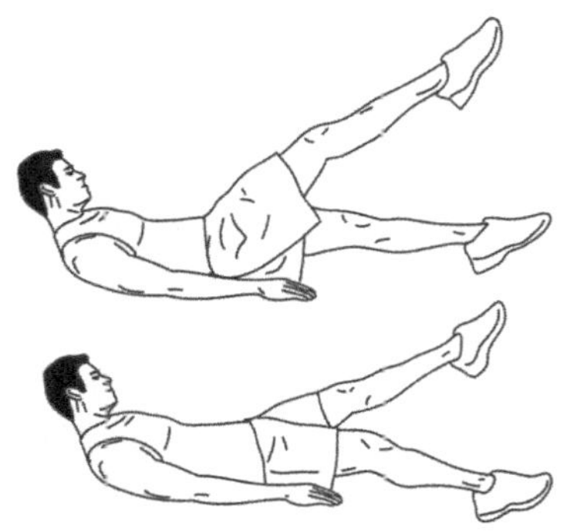

10 flutter kicks

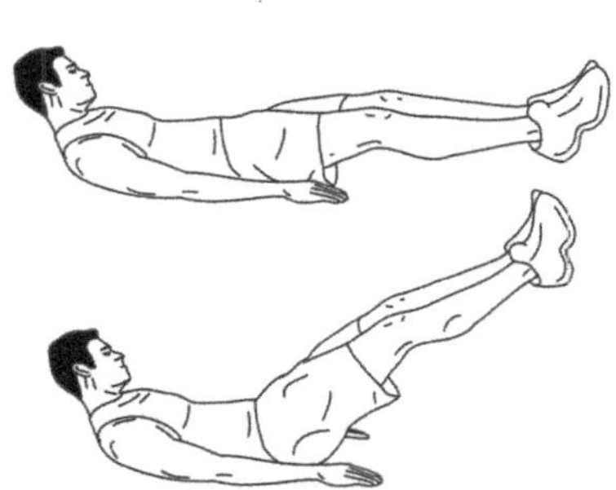

10 leg raises

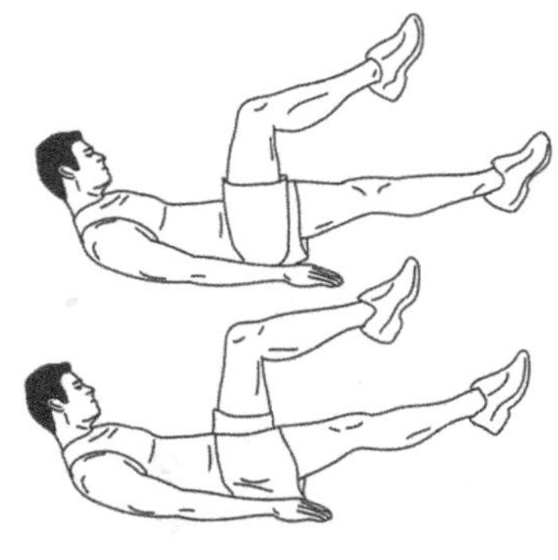

10 air bike crunches

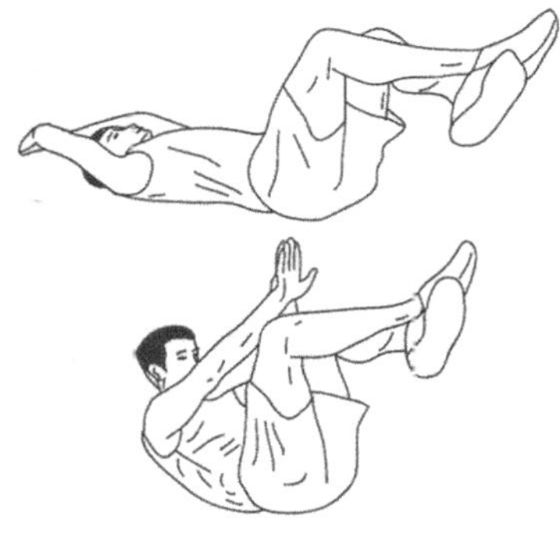

10 knee crunches

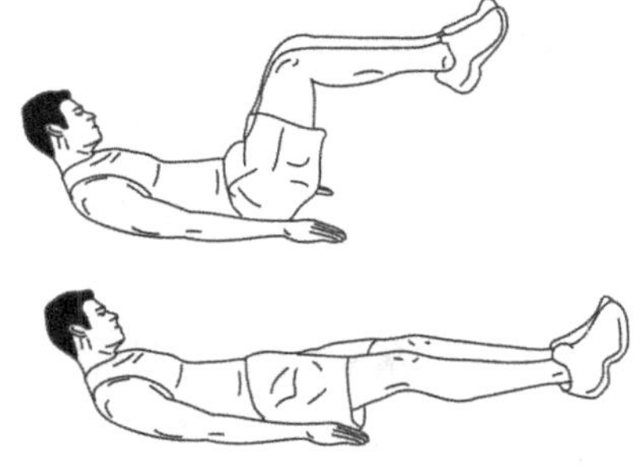

10 crunch kicks

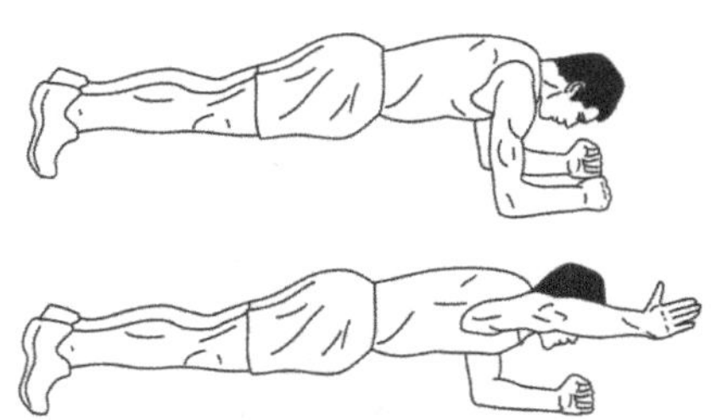

10 plank arm raises

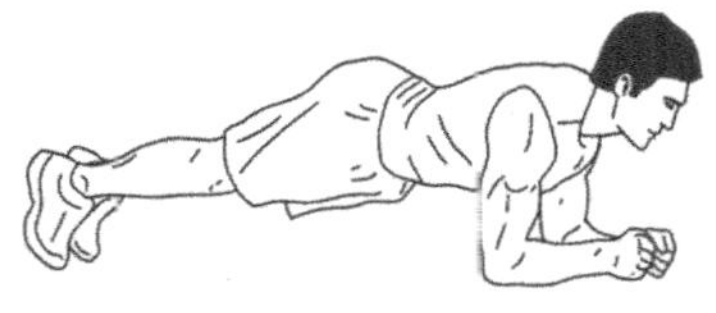

30sec elbow plank

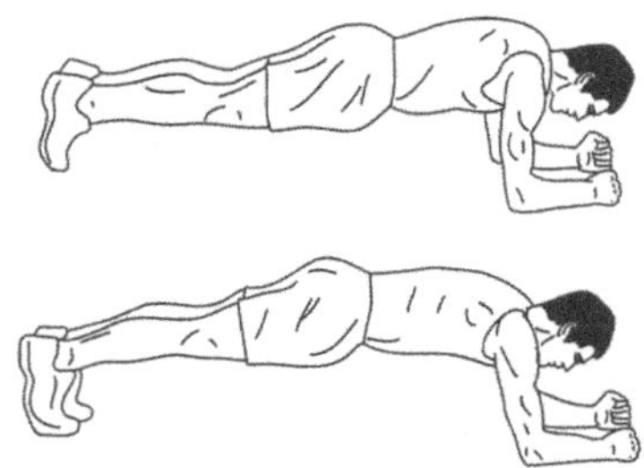

10 body saw

13 Abs on Fire

Set your abs and core on fire with a workout that specifically targets these particular muscle groups. The Abs On Fire workout ought to be part of your regular workout library. Abs are a muscle group that needs regular work to maintain tone and strength. And you know the drill: EC is needed here.

abs on fire

DAREBEE WORKOUT © darebee.com

LEVEL I 3 sets **LEVEL II** 4 sets **LEVEL III** 5 sets **REST** up to 2 minutes

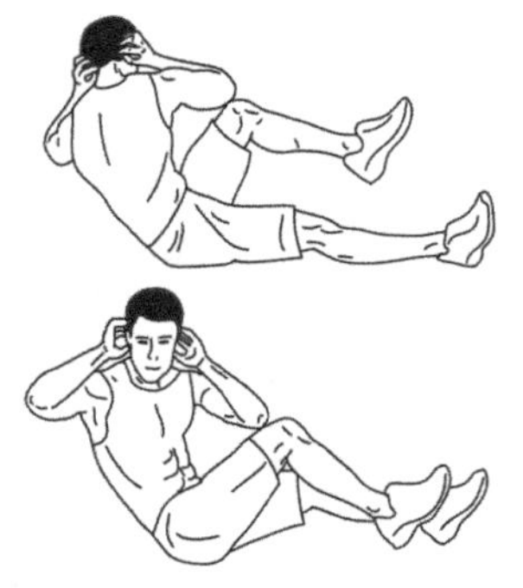

10 knee-to-elbows

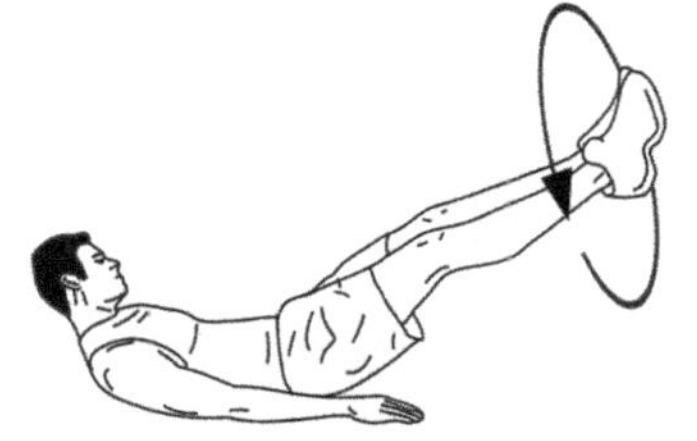

10 raised leg circles

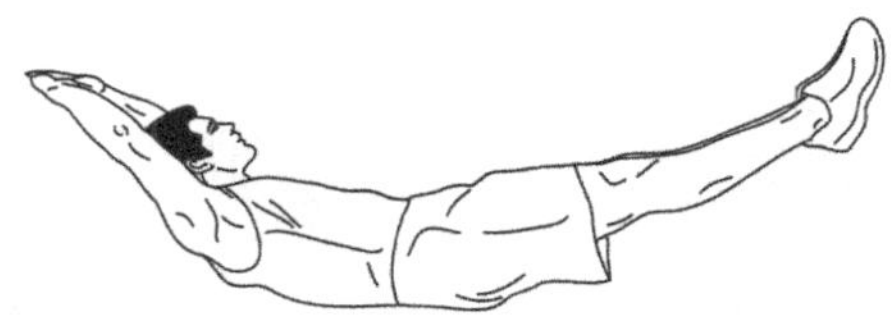

20sec hollow hold

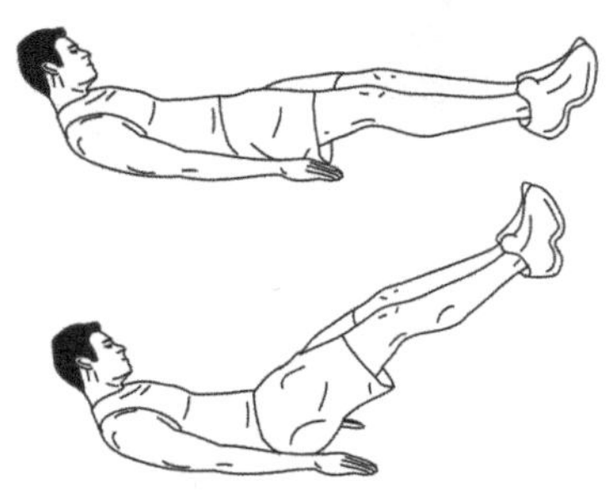

10 leg raises

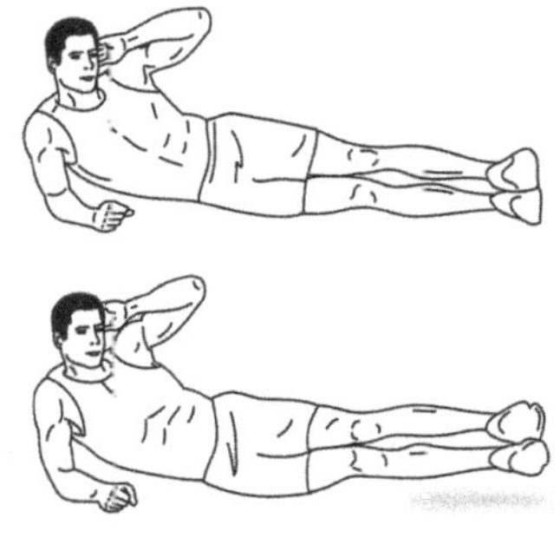

10 side leg raises

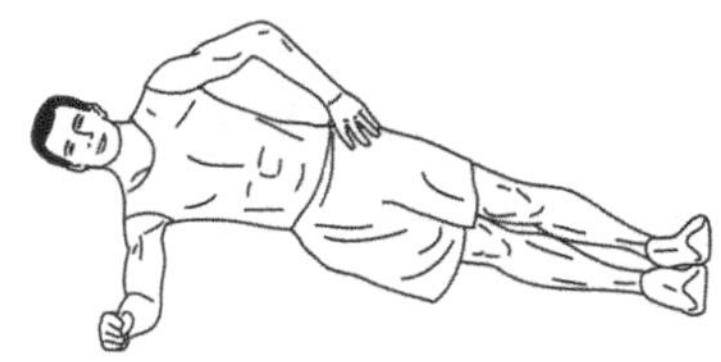

20sec side plank hold

14 Abs Pro

There are four abdominal muscle groups: frontal abs, internal and external obliques and core. Abs Pro targets them all in a workout that is designed to totally test your abs muscle strength and help you develop the kind of abdominals that enhance athletic performance. Add EC and you have a really challenging abs fitness routine.

abs pro

DAREBEE AB WORKOUT © darebee.com

LEVEL I 3 sets **LEVEL II** 4 sets **LEVEL III** 5 sets **REST** up to 2 minutes

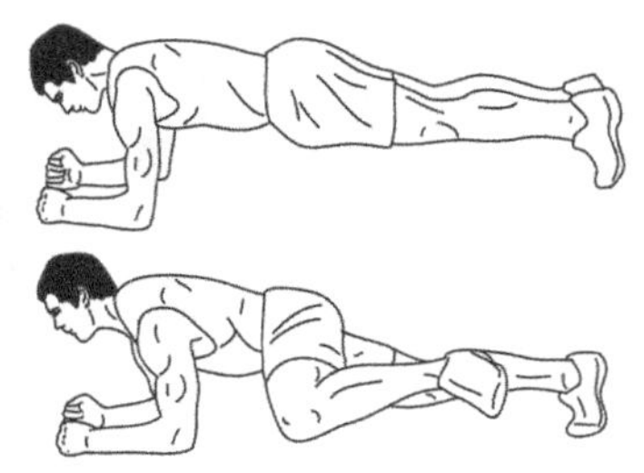

10 plank crunches

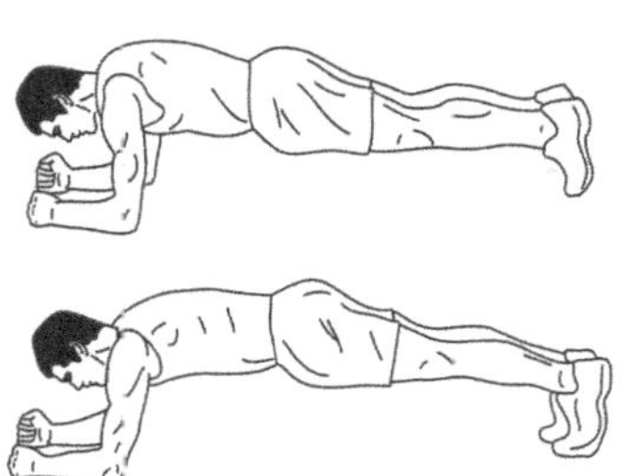

10 body saw

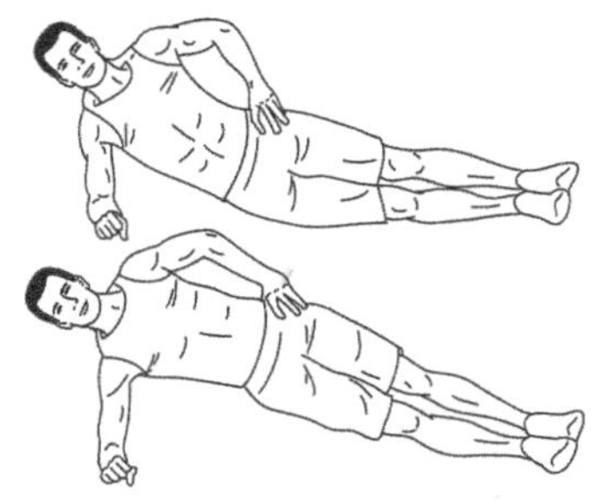

10 side bridges

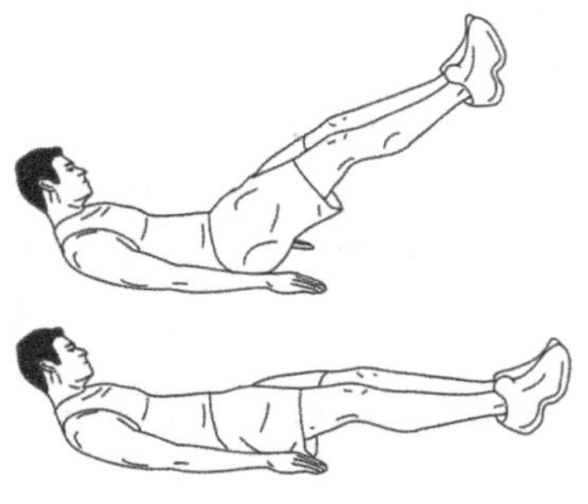

20 leg raises

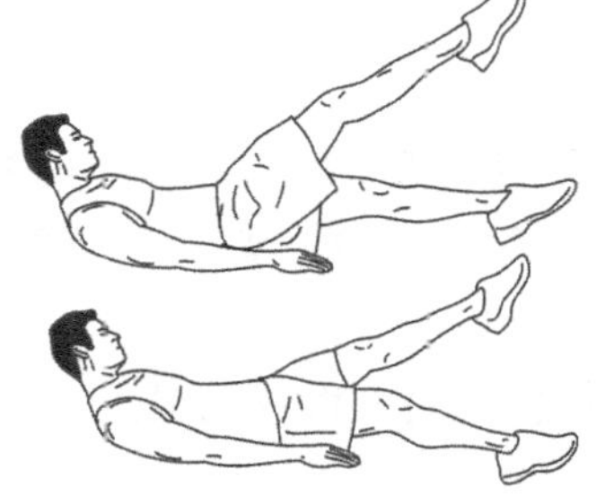

20 flutter kicks

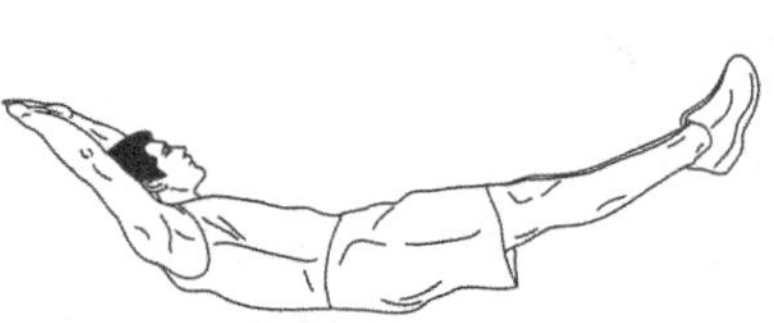

20sec hollow hold

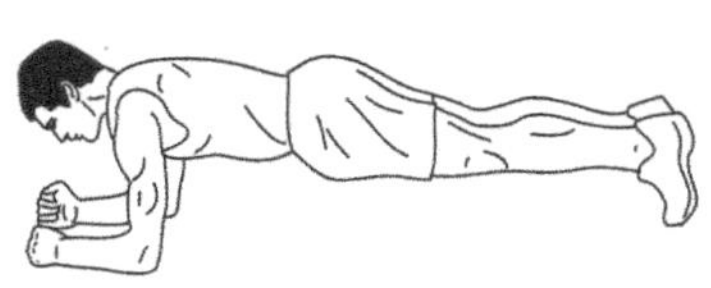

20sec elbow plank

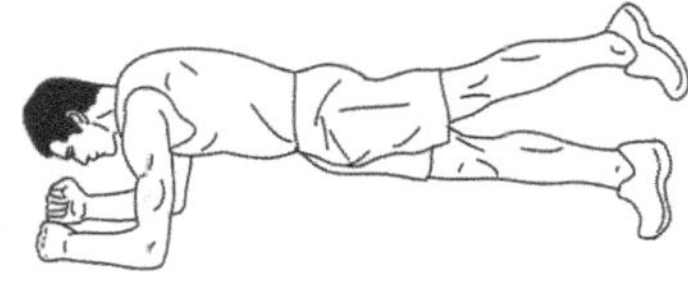

20sec raised leg plank

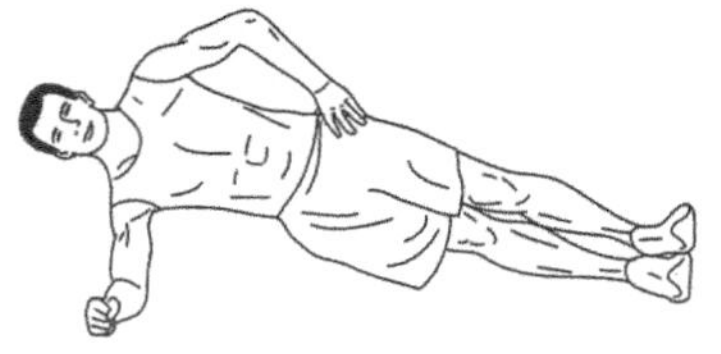

20sec side plank

15 Abs Unlocked

There are four major muscle groups that constitute the abdominal muscle wall and each of them does something very specific. In no particular order they are Rectus Abdominis (the frontal abs which can also be divided into upper and lower abs and make up the six-pack), External Abdominal Obliques, Internal Abdominal Obliques and Transverse Abdominis which we most popularly refer to as core. The Abs Unlocked workout works them all.

abs unlocked

BUILD

DARELBEE WORKOUT © darebee.com

LEVEL I 3 sets **LEVEL II** 5 sets **LEVEL III** 7 sets **REST** up to 2 minutes

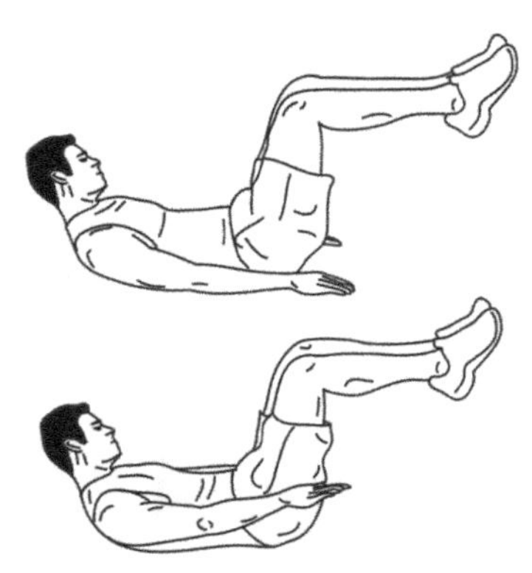

20 hundreds

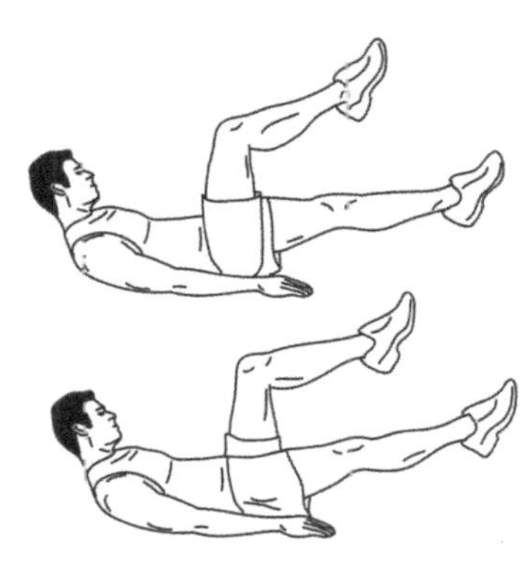

20 air bike crunches

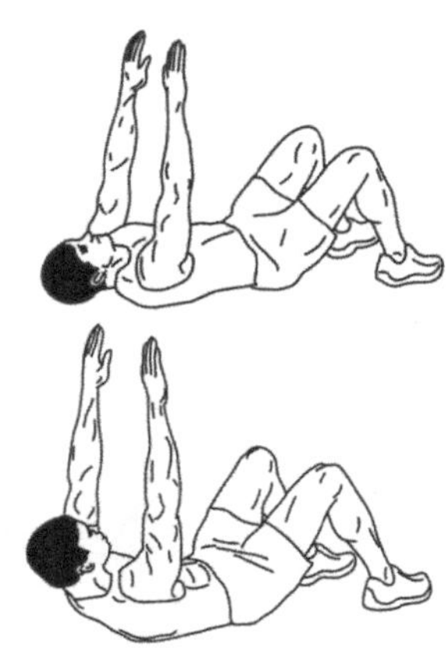

20 high crunches

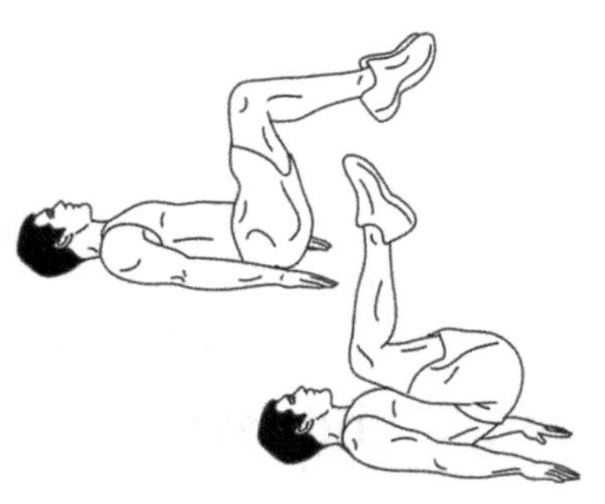

10 reverse crunches

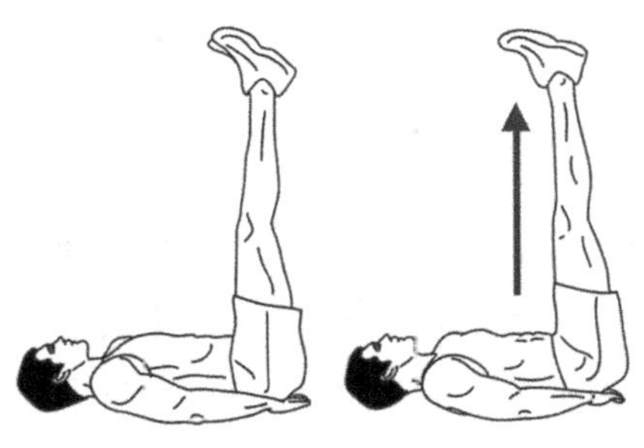

10 pulse-ups

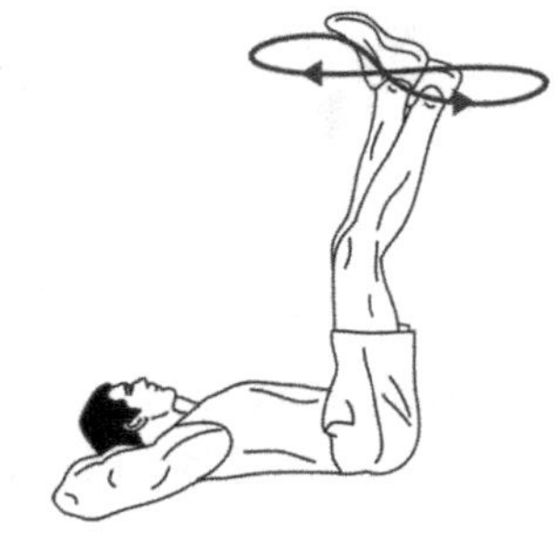

10 infinity circles

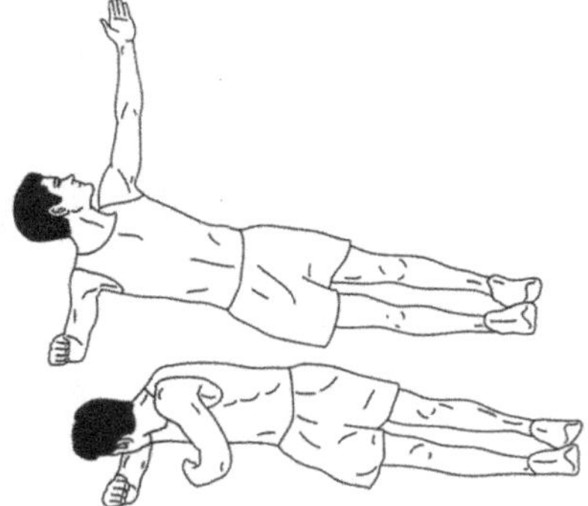

10 side plank rotations

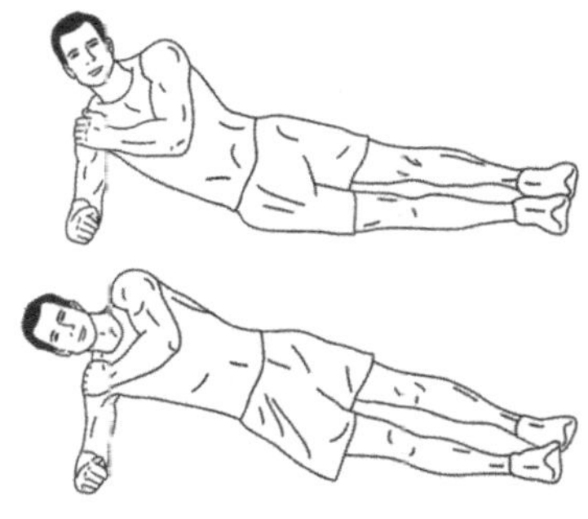

10 side bridges

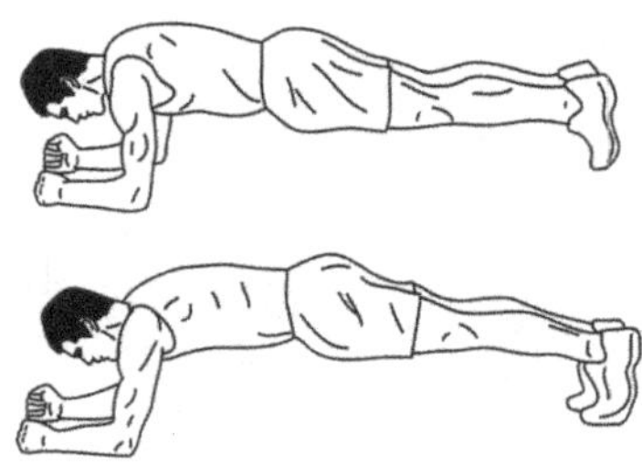

10 body saw

16 Abs Upgrade

Abs are not just the engine that powers some of your most energetic movements, they also play a vital role in protecting a vulnerable part of your body. The Abs Upgrade workout works each of the four major abdominal muscle groups for that all-in feeling.

BUILD

abs upgrade

DAREBEE WORKOUT © darebee.com

LEVEL I 3 sets **LEVEL II** 4 sets **LEVEL III** 5 sets **REST** up to 2 minutes

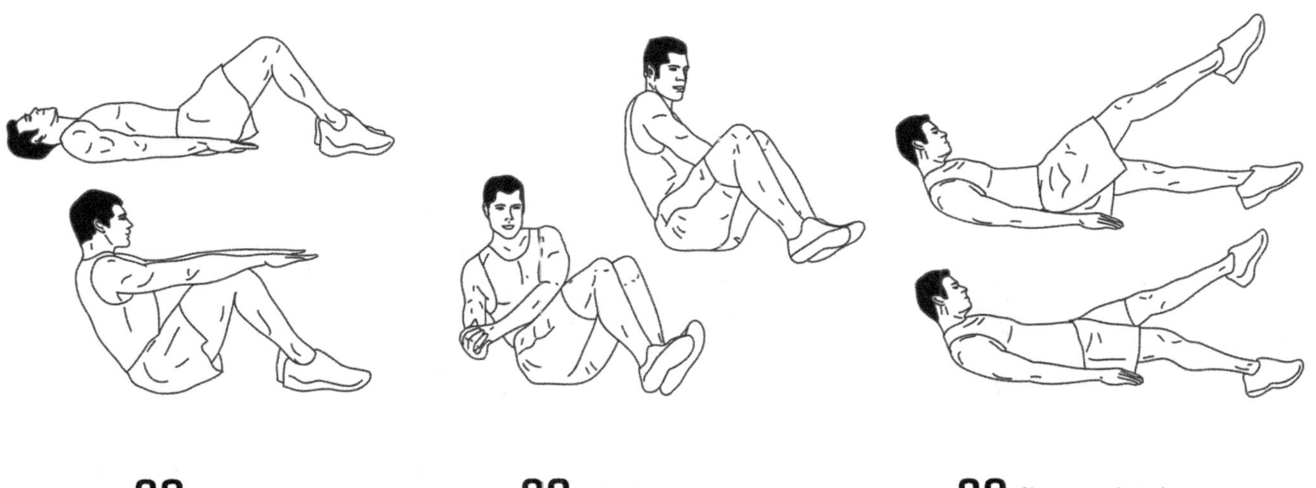

20 sit-ups **20** sitting twists **20** flutter kicks

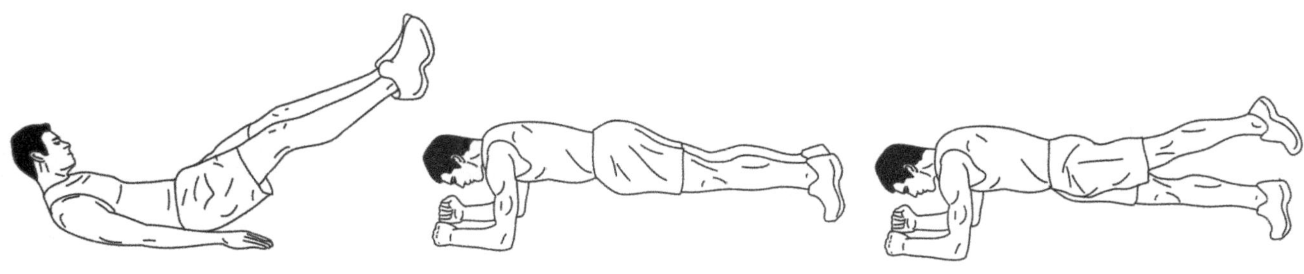

20-count raised leg hold **20-count** plank **20-count** raised leg plank

17 Active Plank

The core is one of the hardest muscle groups of the abdominal group to train. It requires specific exercises, sustained work and an approach that takes into account how this critical muscle group functions when the body is in action. This is why Active Plank uses a series of static and active exercises to load the core and abs for that athletic-performance enhancing workout you've been looking for.

ACTIVE PLANK

DARBEE WORKOUT © darebee.com

Repeat 3 times 2 minutes rest between sets

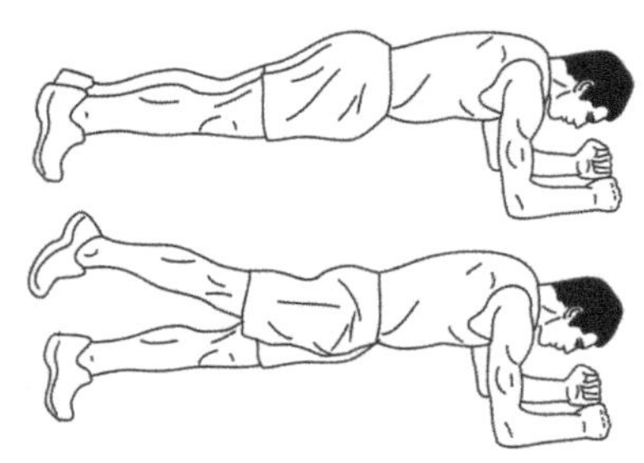

10 plank leg raises

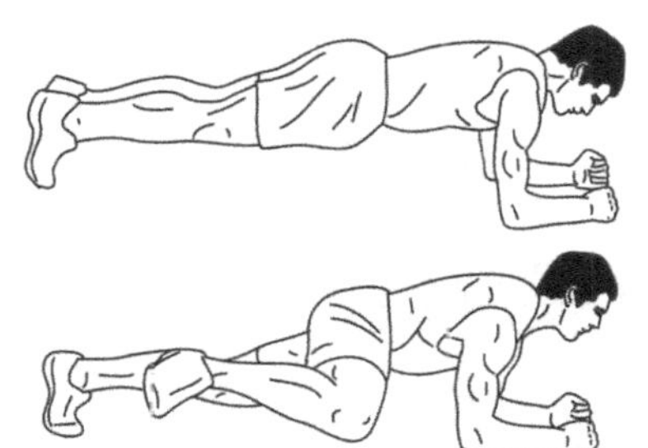

10 plank side crunches

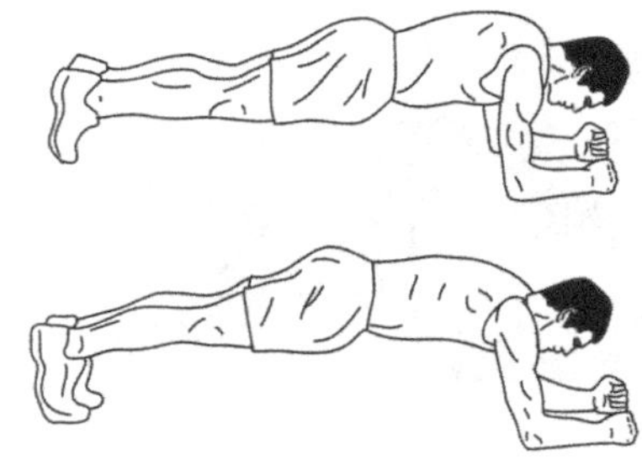

10 body saw

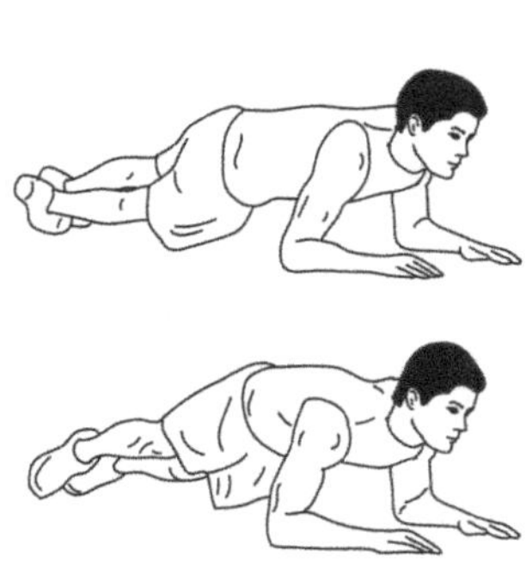

10 plank rolls

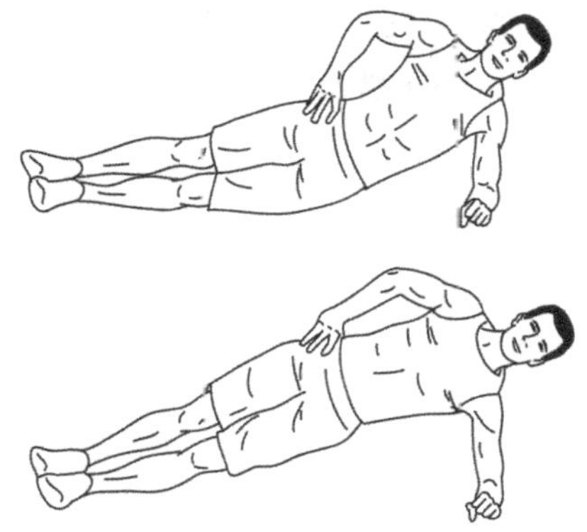

10 side plank dips

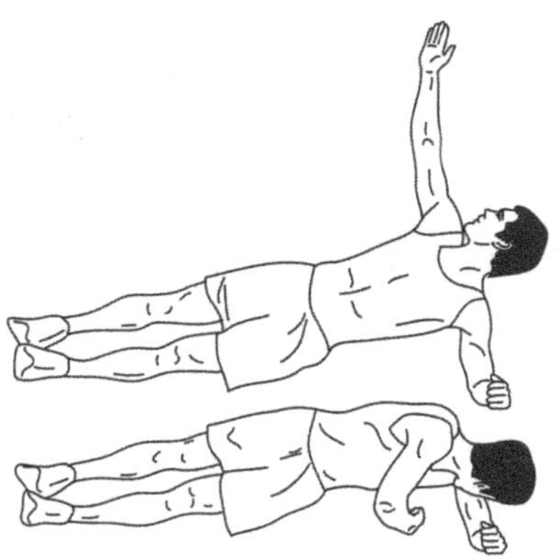

10 side plank rotations

18 Anywhere Abs

If you want abs you need to work for them, but that doesn't just require you to work hard, it needs you to work smart. Anywhere Abs is a workout that helps you get the abs you want by working out even when most people think you can't. These are quick, easy exercises you can do almost any place, in almost any clothing. The result is an activation of your abs that helps you maintain the edge you need in your fitness.

anywhere abs

DAREBEE WORKOUT © darebee.com

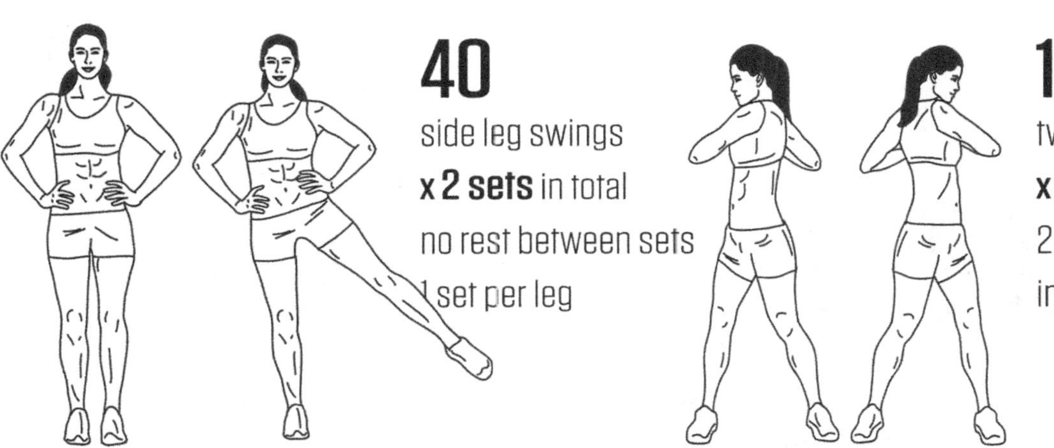

40
side leg swings
x 2 sets in total
no rest between sets
1 set per leg

10
twists
x 4 sets in total
20 seconds rest
in between sets

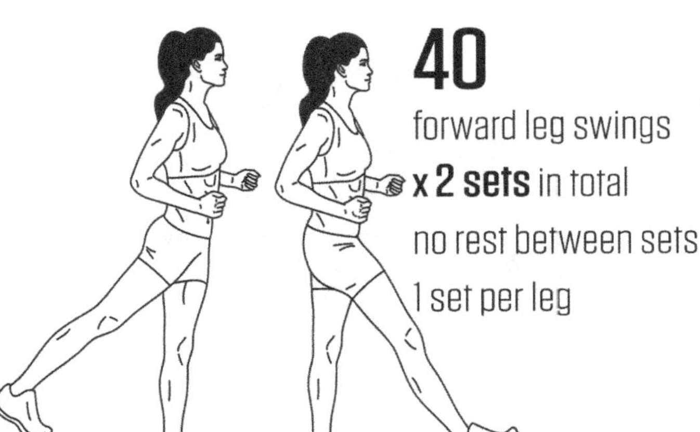

40
forward leg swings
x 2 sets in total
no rest between sets
1 set per leg

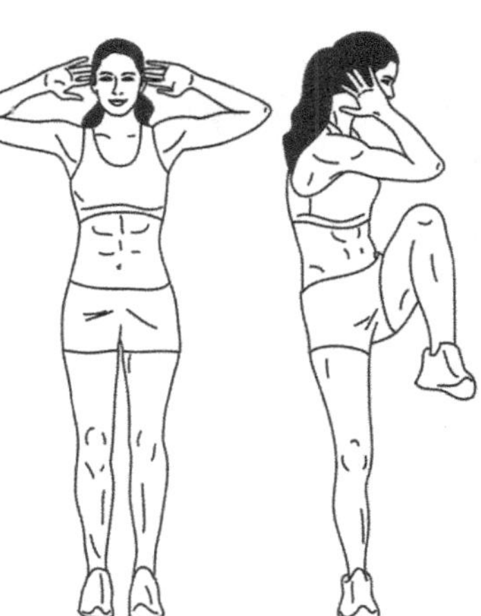

10
knee-to-elbows
x 4 sets in total
20 seconds rest
in between sets

19 Armor Abs

A strong abdominal wall affects everything. The way you sit. How you walk. Your performance in every kind of sport. How quickly you get tired and how smoothly you move. This is a workout that presses all the right buttons, helping you tone up and build your abs, plus come summer you're going to be thankful you did it.

armor abs

BUILD

DARERBEE WORKOUT © darebee.com

LEVEL I 3 sets **LEVEL II** 5 sets **LEVEL III** 7 sets **REST** up to 2 minutes

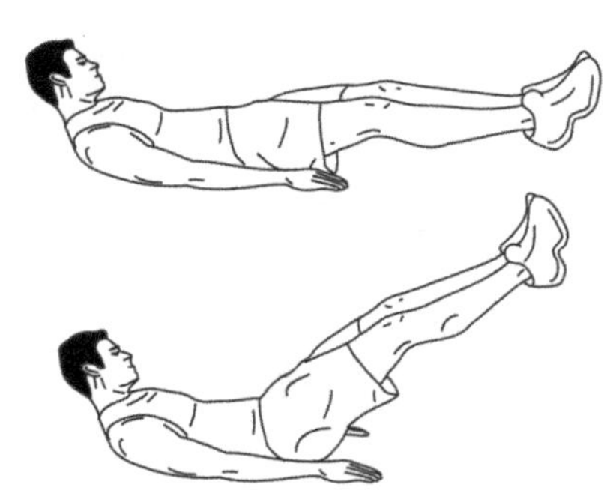

10 leg raises

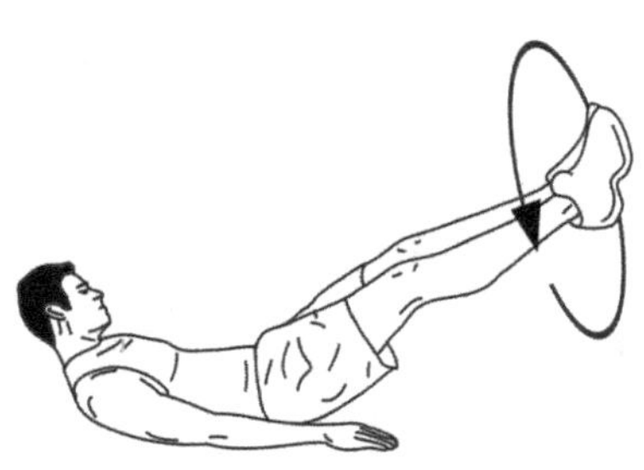

10 raised leg circles

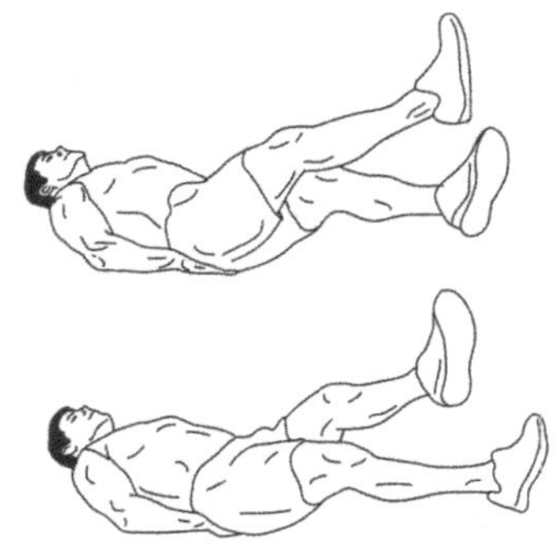

10 scissors

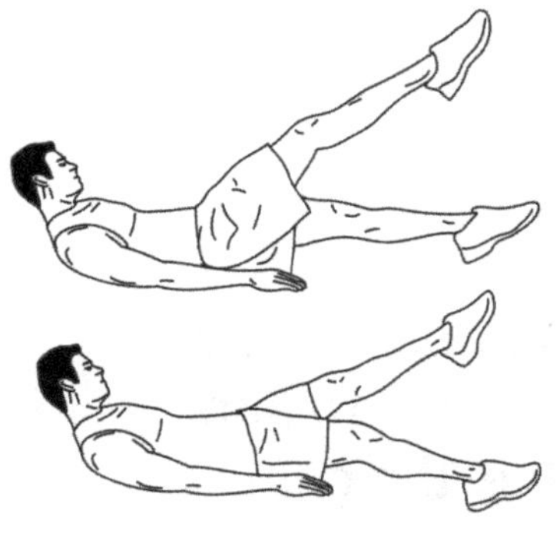

20 flutter kicks

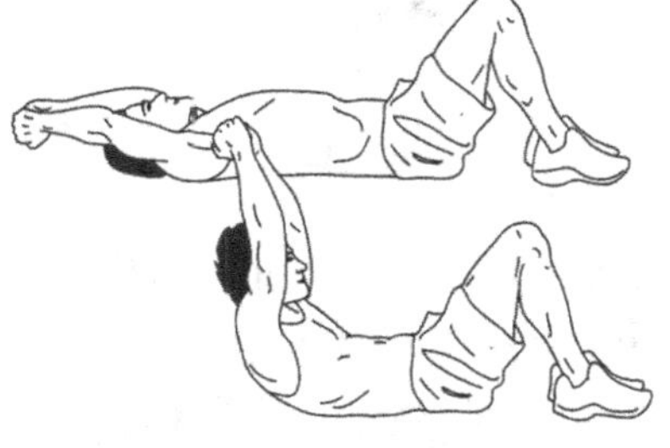

5 long arm crunches

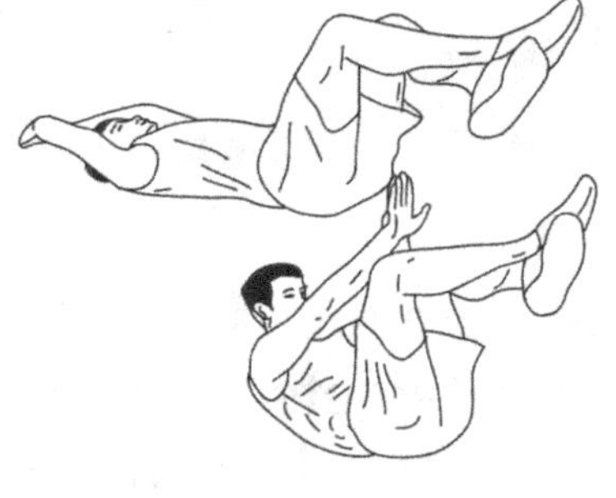

5 knee crunches

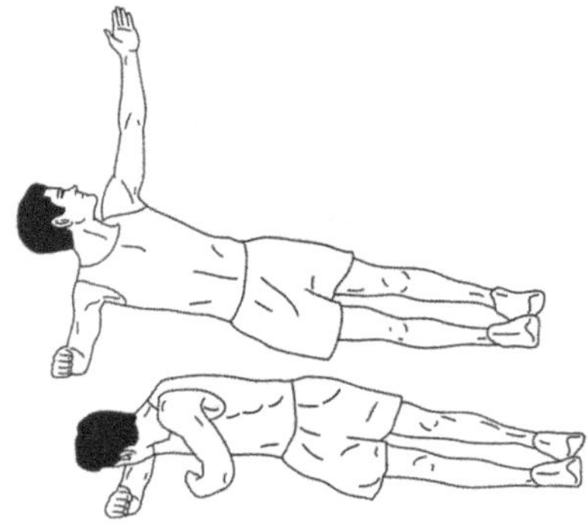

10 side planks rotations

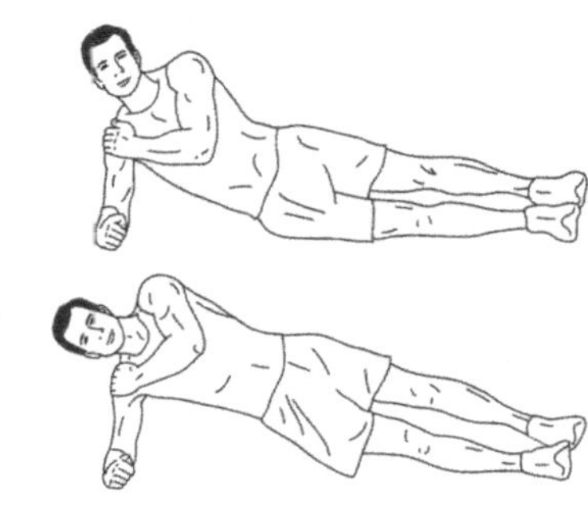

10 side bridges

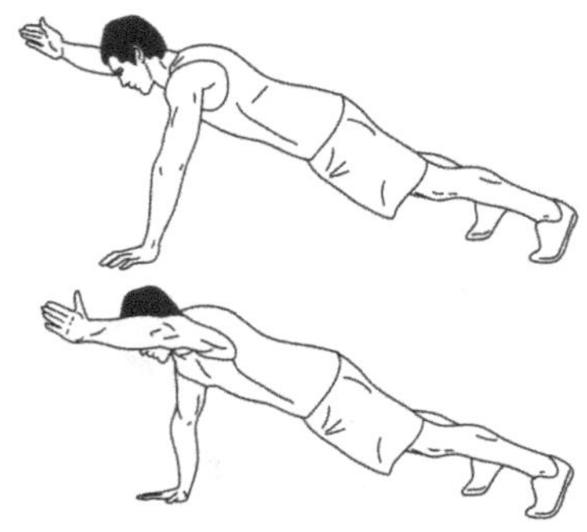

10 plank arm raises

20 Art of Abs

There are four separate muscle groups that make up our abs. The Art of Abs targets them all. This is not a workout where you need to aim for anything less than perfect form. You will definitely feel the gains afterwards.

the art of abs

DAREBEE WORKOUT

2 minutes rest between exercises

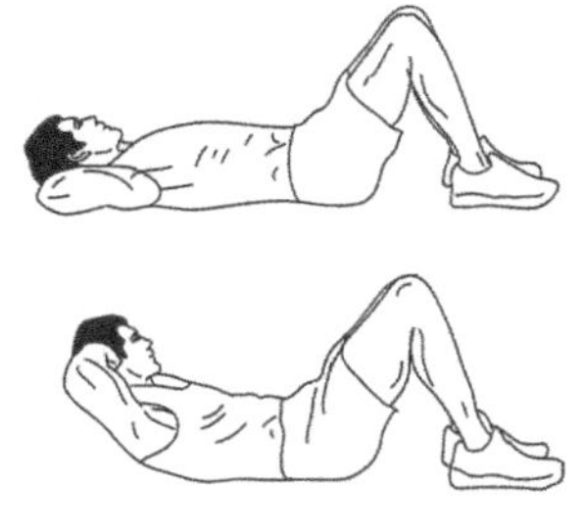

14 crunches
x **5 sets** in total
20 seconds rest between sets

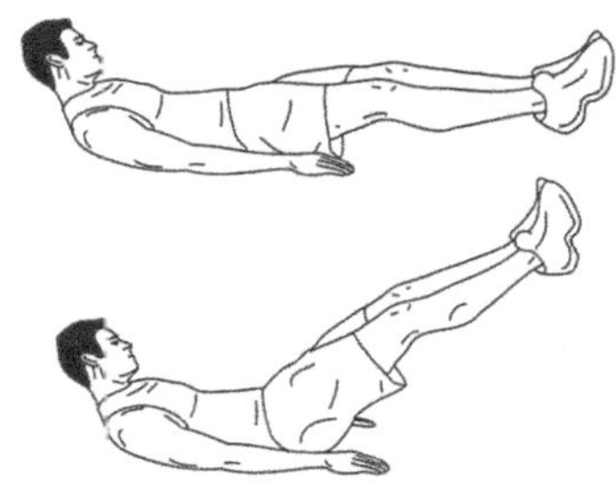

14 leg raises
x **5 sets** in total
20 seconds rest between sets

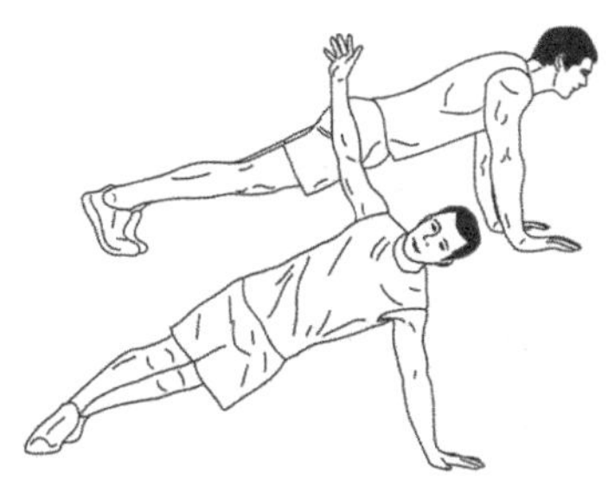

14 plank rotations
x **5 sets** in total
20 seconds rest between sets

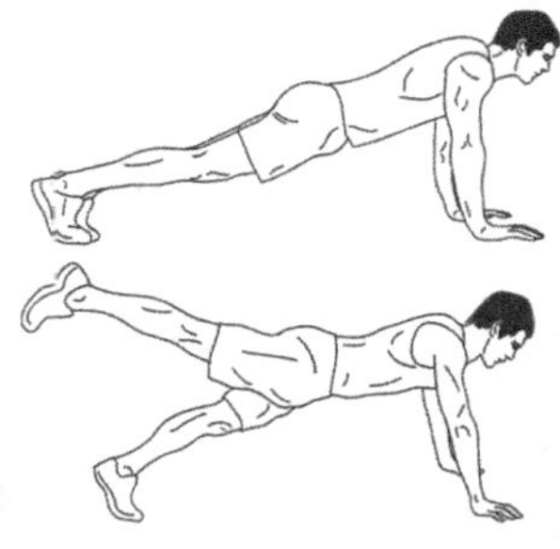

14 plank leg raises
x **5 sets** in total
20 seconds rest between sets

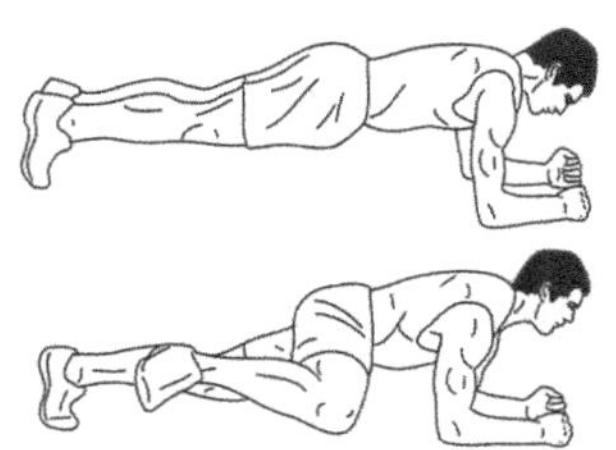

14 plank crunches
x **5 sets** in total
20 seconds rest between sets

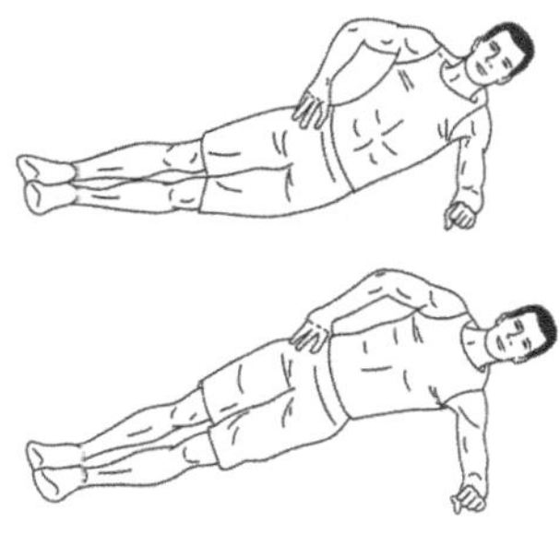

14 side bridges
x **5 sets** in total
20 seconds rest between sets

21 At-Home Abs

Great-looking abs are an on-going project. You're never off the clock on them, which means that whether you're at home, at the office, high up on a telephone tower or practicing trampeze wire walking, you'd better get your abs workout in. In this case, thankfully, the focus is on the home environment so no risky business.

at-home abs

DAREBEE WORKOUT © darebee.com

LEVEL I 3 sets **LEVEL II** 4 sets **LEVEL III** 5 sets

REST up to 2 minutes

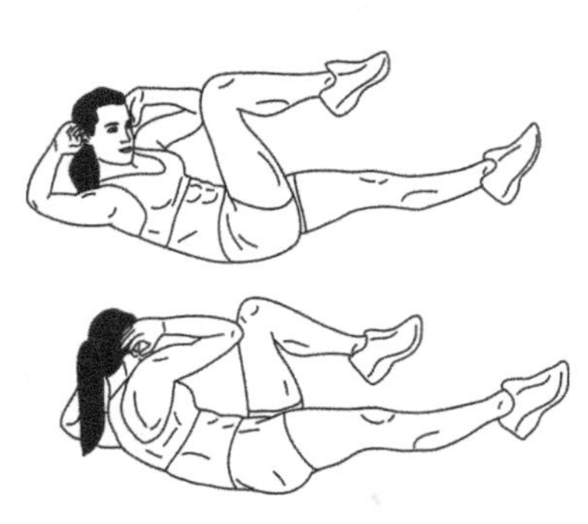

10 knee-to-elbow crunches

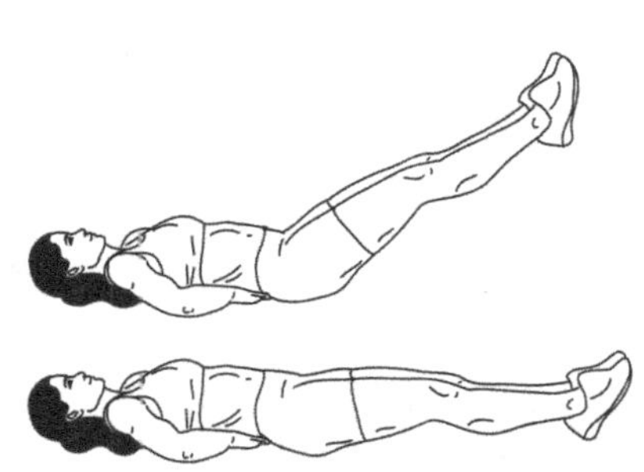

8 leg raises

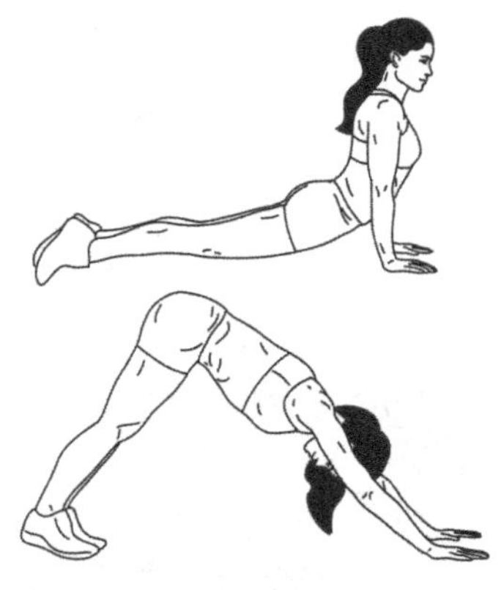

8 upward downward dog

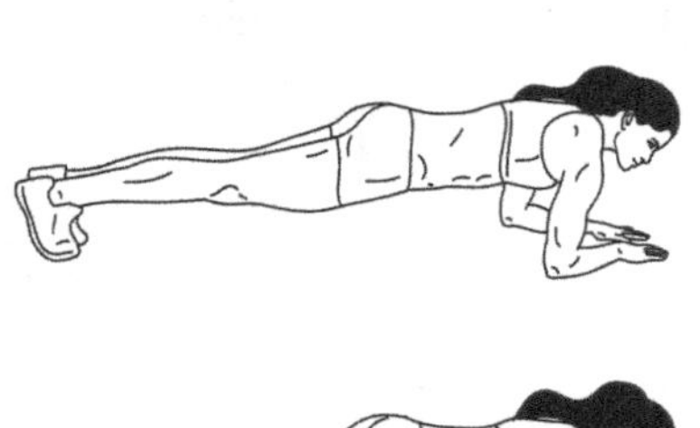

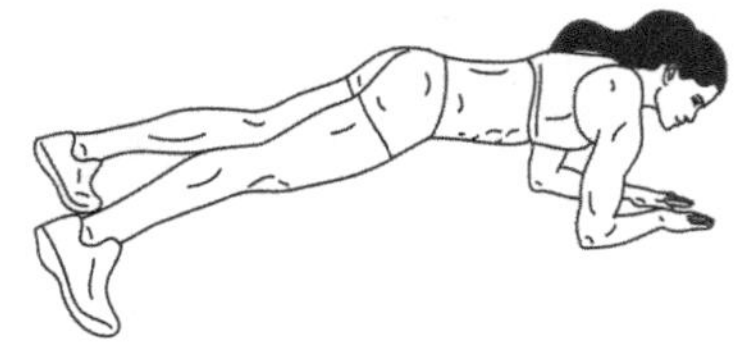

10 elbow plank step-outs

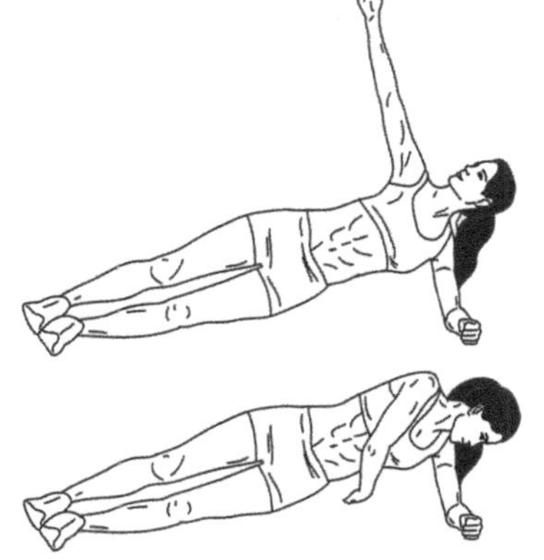

8 side plank rotations

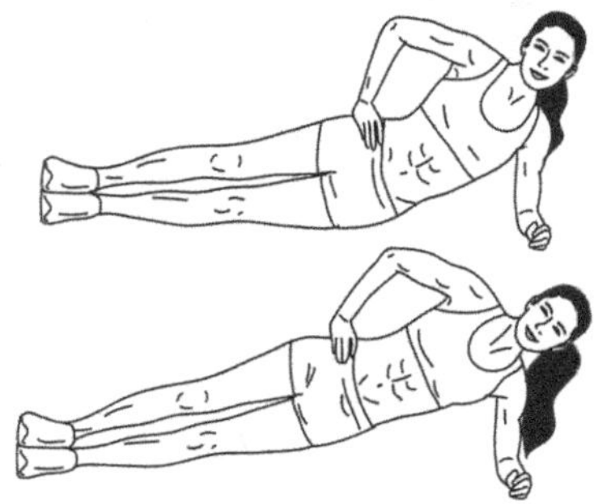

8 side bridges

22 Back Up

Our back is vulnerable not because we stand upright but because we end up not doing so most of the day. The Backup workout addresses that problem with exercises that target the abs and core strengthening spinal support and reducing the opportunity for those niggling aches and pains, to develop.

backup

DAREBEE WORKOUT © darebee.com

LEVEL I 3 sets **LEVEL II** 5 sets **LEVEL III** 7 sets **REST** up to 2 minutes

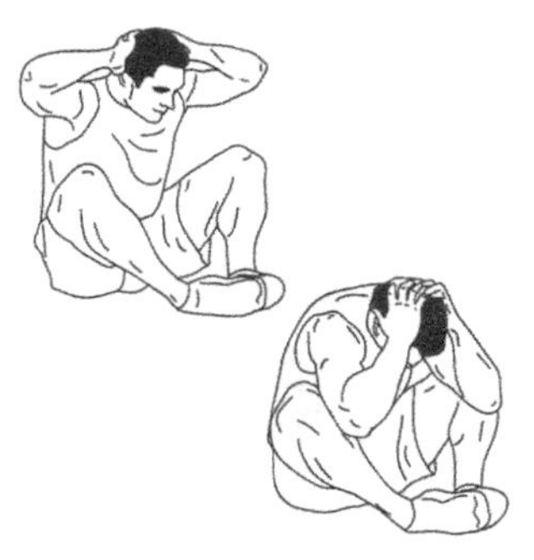

5 groin stretches

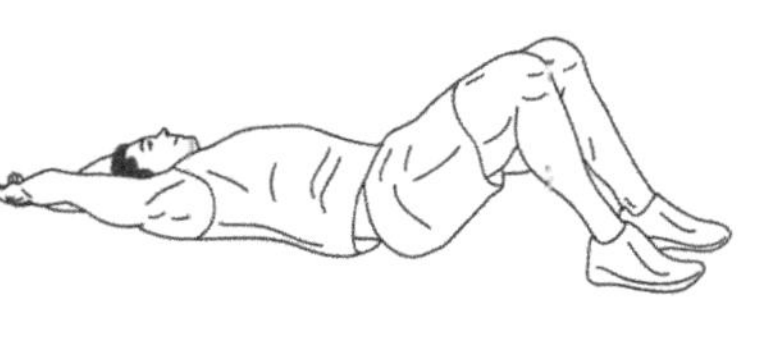

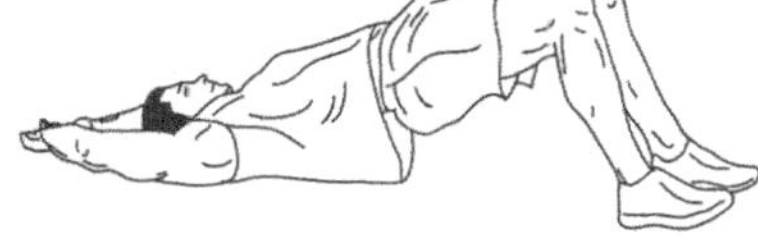

5 bridges

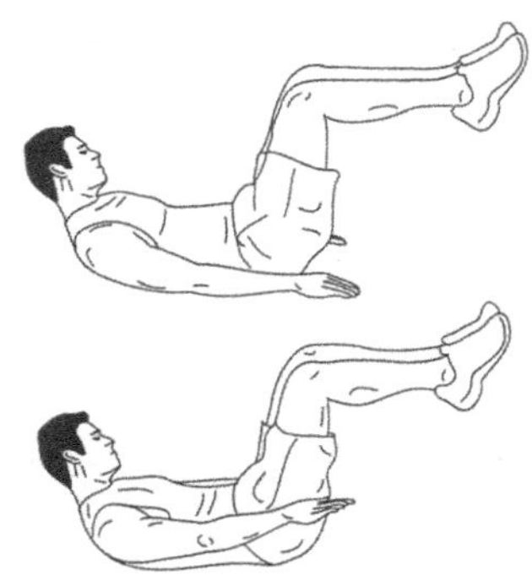

10 hundreds

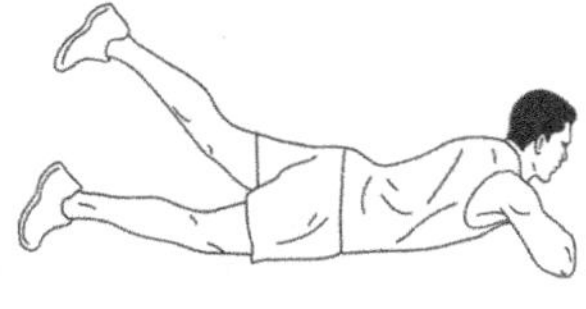

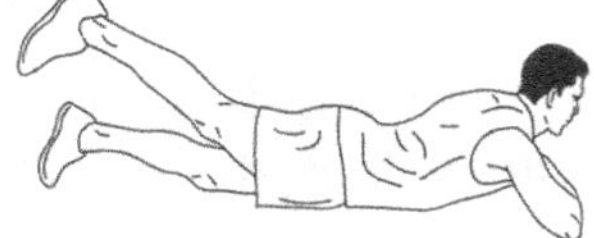

10 reverse flutter kicks

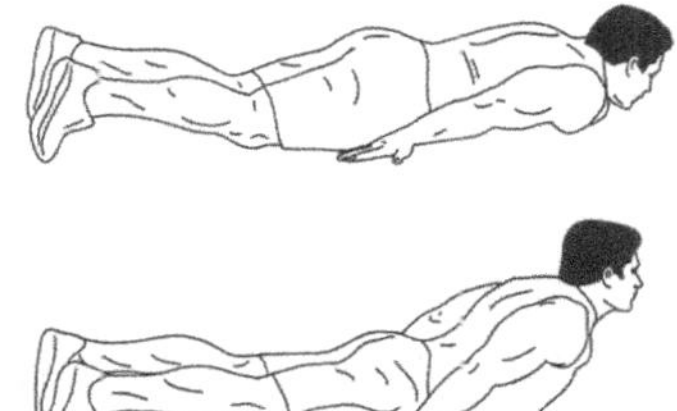

5 lower back curls

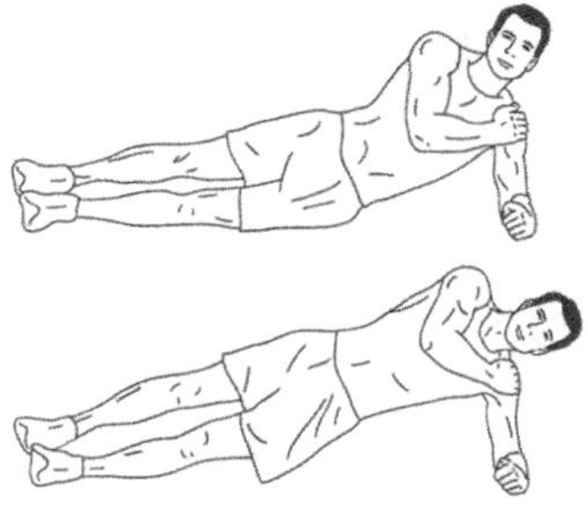

10 side planks

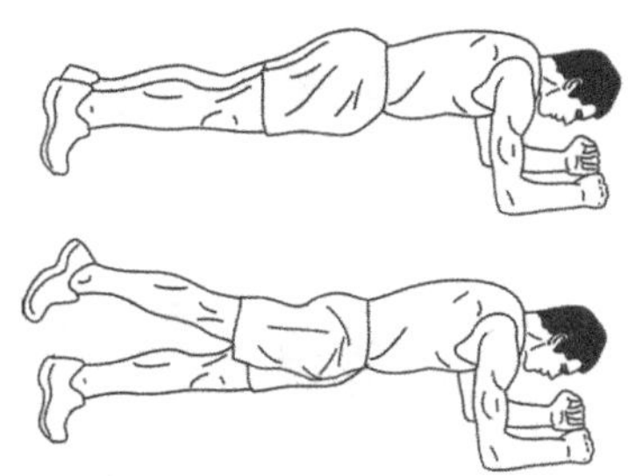

10 plank leg raises

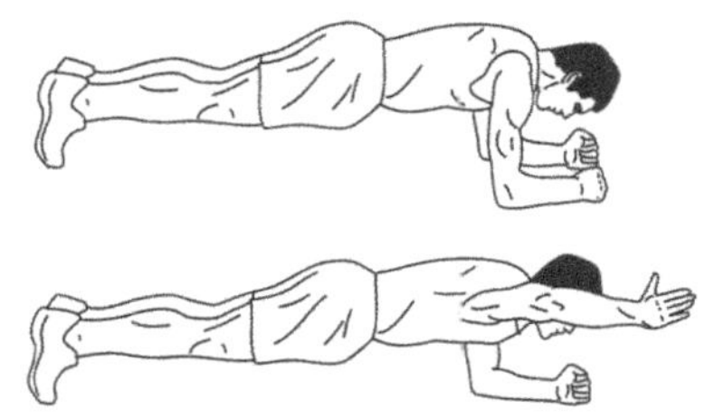

10 plank arm raises

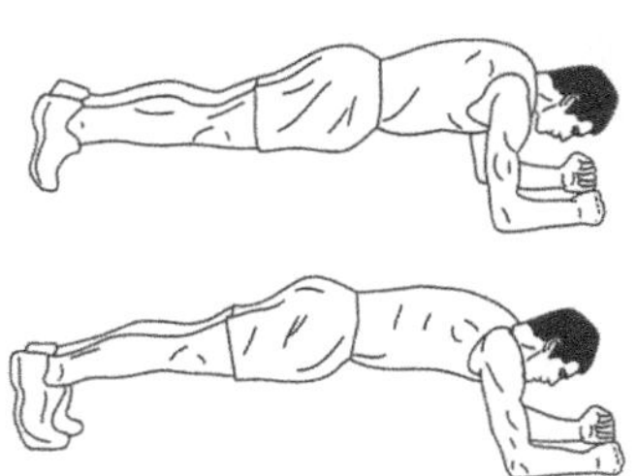

5 body saw

23 Beginner Abs

Rock-hard abs always need to start from somewhere and the Beginner Abs workout is as good a place as any. These are exercises designed to activate your abs (including the core) without putting undue stress in any of the supporting muscle structure. Perfect for beginners but also a great set of abs exercises for those wishing to maintain ab strength.

beginner **abs**

DAREBEE WORKOUT © darebee.com

LEVEL I 3 sets **LEVEL II** 4 sets **LEVEL III** 5 sets **REST** up to 2 minutes

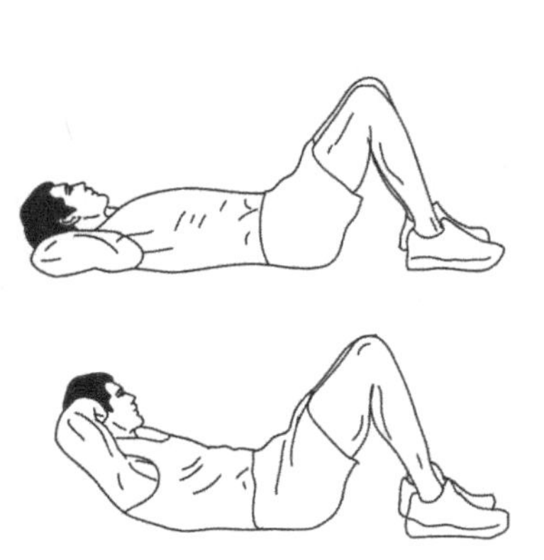

10 crunches

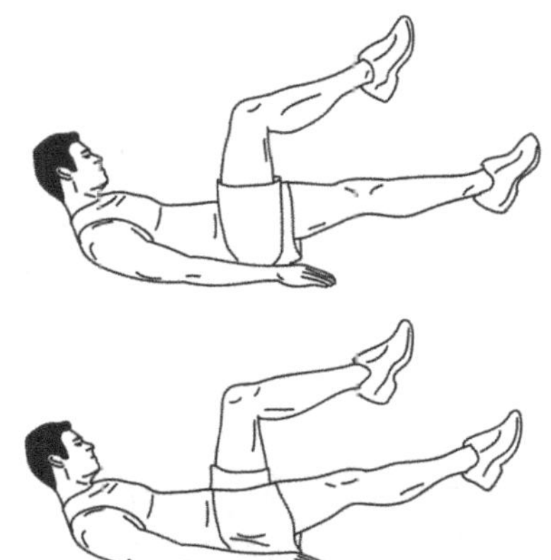

10 air bike crunches

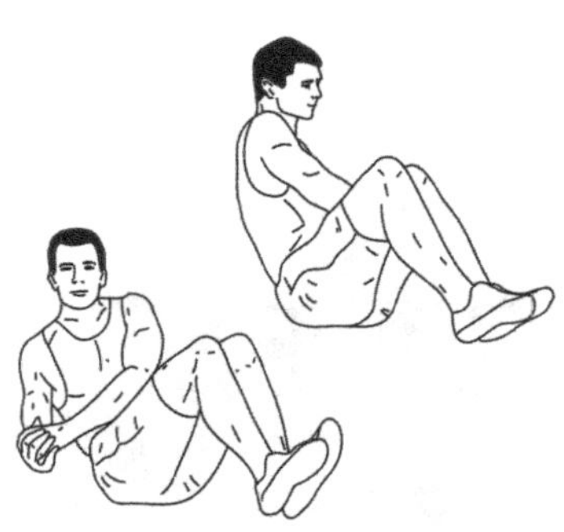

10 sitting twists

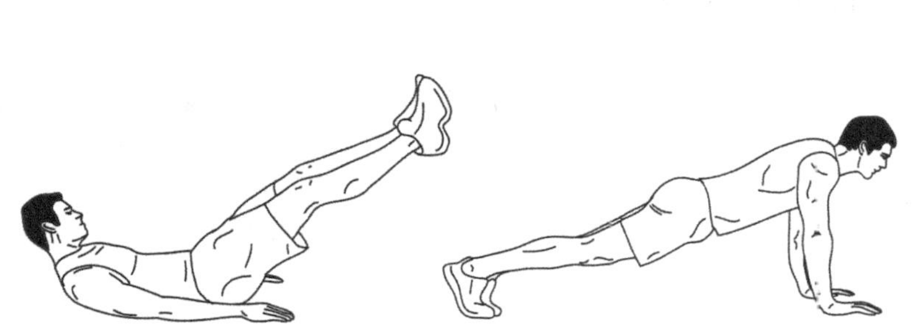

10-count raised leg hold

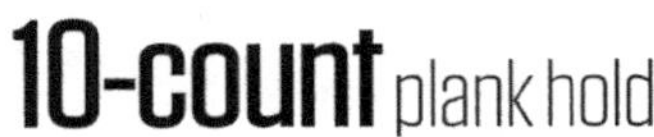

10-count plank hold

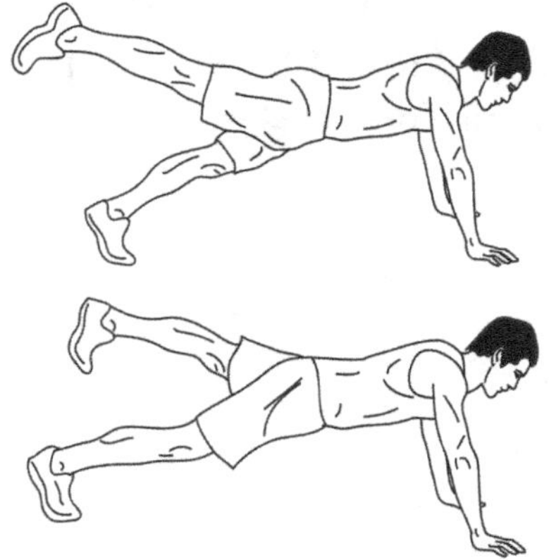

10 plank leg raises

24 Boxer Abs

Boxing without abs work is like trying to row without a paddle. You will simply not get anywhere fast. Boxer Abs addresses this through nine exercises that target the four muscle groups that make us the abdominals. If you really want to train like a boxer here you will forego the rest and simply let your abs scream for a while. Yo will most definitely see and feel the difference in your overall performance.

BOXER | ABS

DAREBEE BOXING WORKOUT © darebee.com

LEVEL I 3 sets **LEVEL II** 4 sets **LEVEL III** 5 sets **REST** 2 minutes

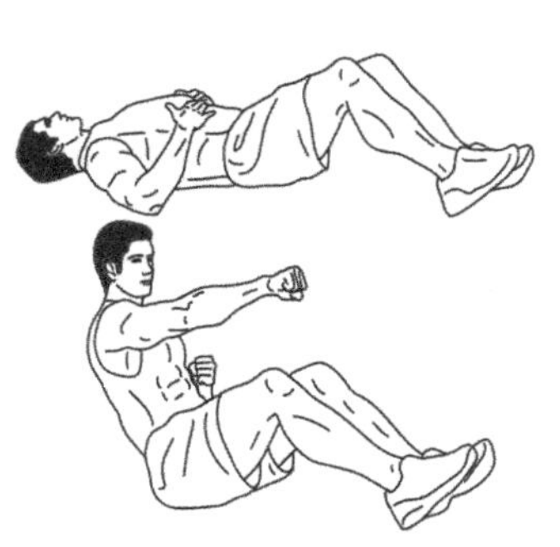

30 sit-up punches

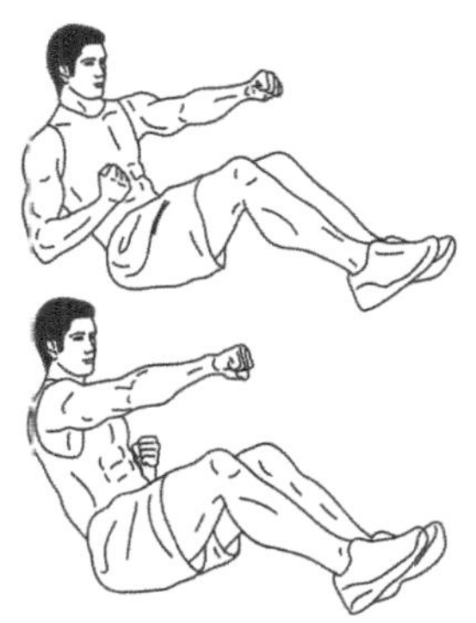

30 siting punches

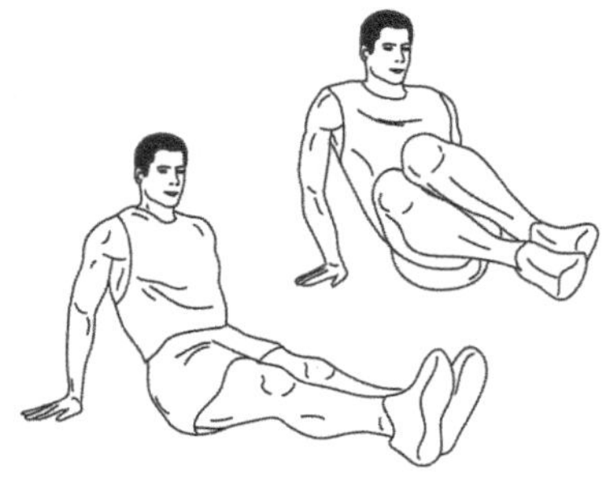

30 knee-ins & twists

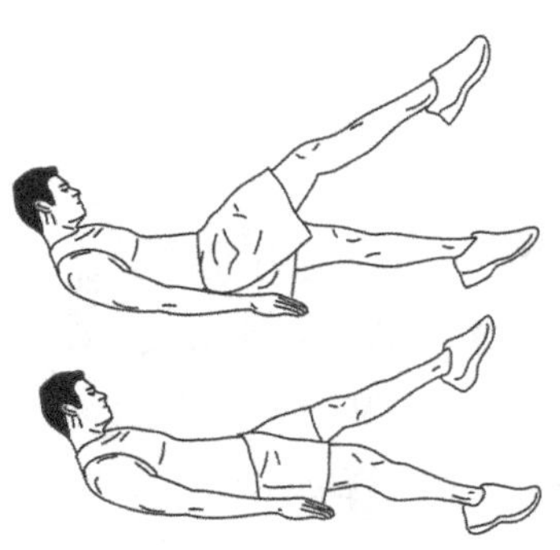

30 flutter kicks

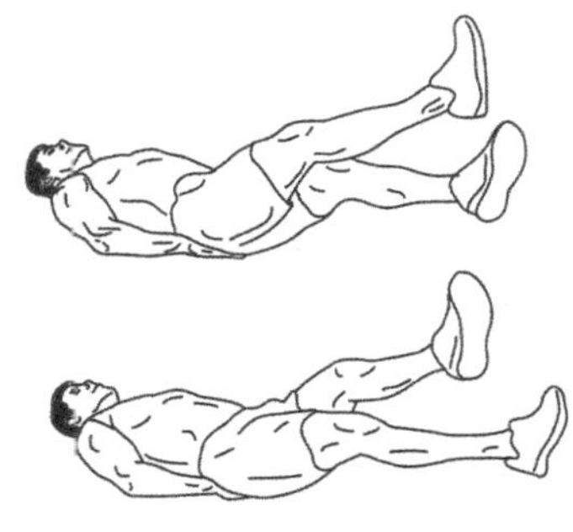

30 scissors

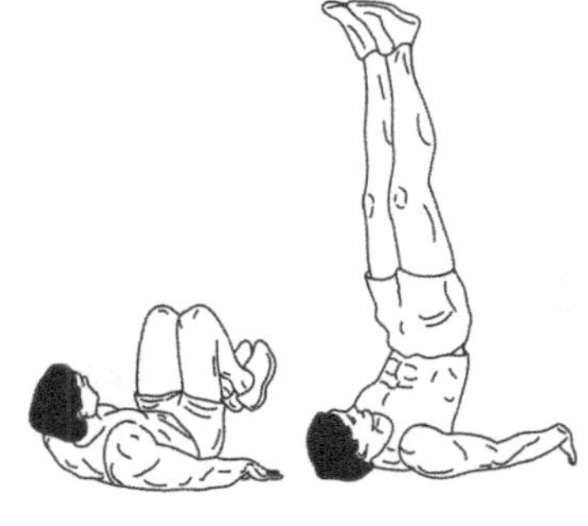

30 butt-ups

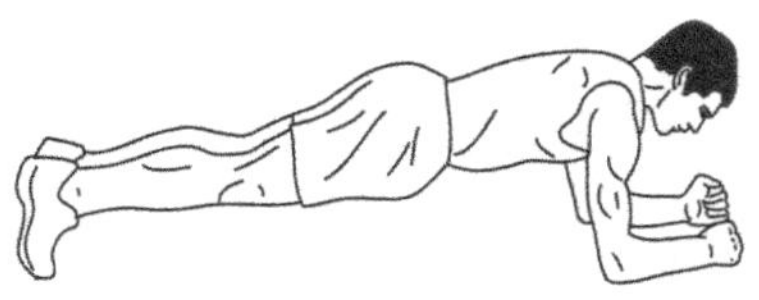

30-count plank

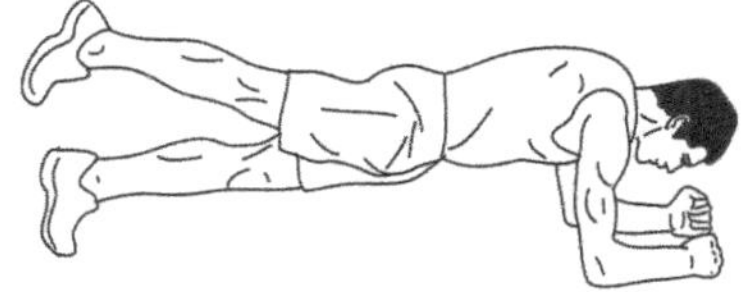

30-count raised leg plank

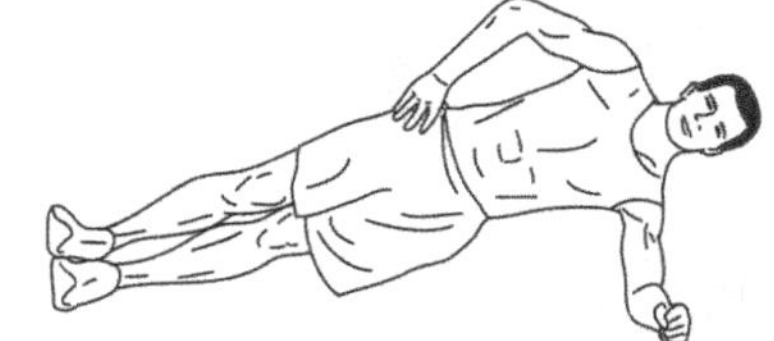

30-count side plank

25 Brute Abs

Because the abdominal muscle group is already pretty strong, eliciting an adaptation response from it requires a lot of extra effort. Enter Brute Abs. This is a workout designed to do just that. If you have a handy dumbbell you can load your abs to elicit the adaptation response, increase their strength and maybe, even, their size. Be slow, methodical and controlled in your execution here and the workout will reward you.

BRUTE

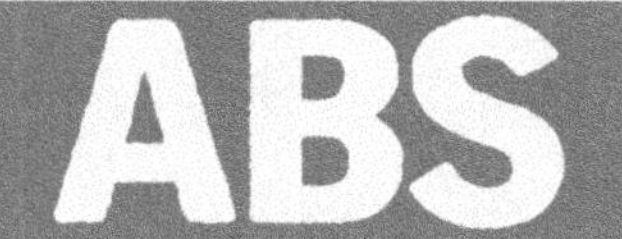

DAREBEE WORKOUT © darebee.com

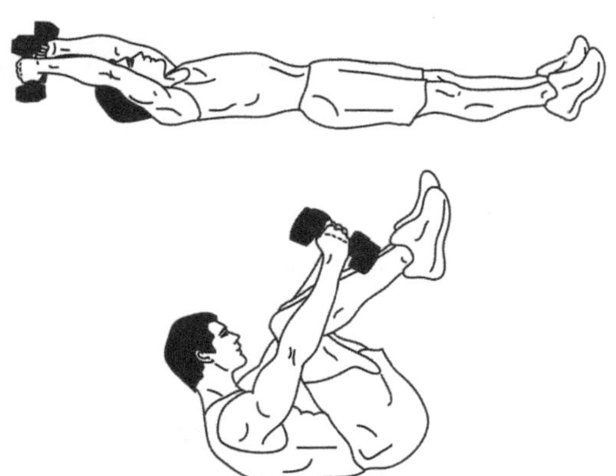

10 sit-up folds
x 4 sets in total
20 seconds rest between sets

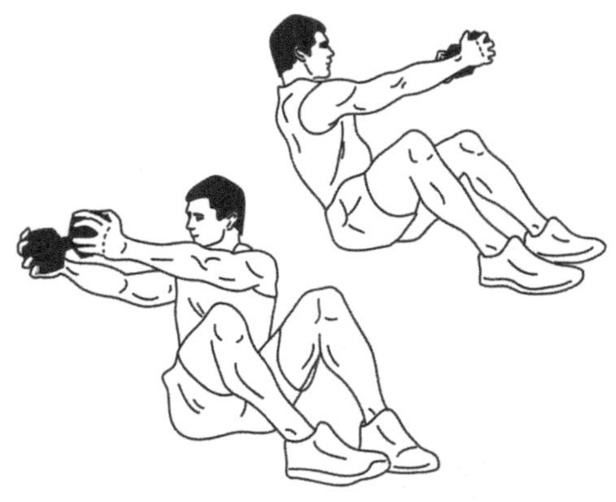

10 sitting twists
x 4 sets in total
20 seconds rest between sets

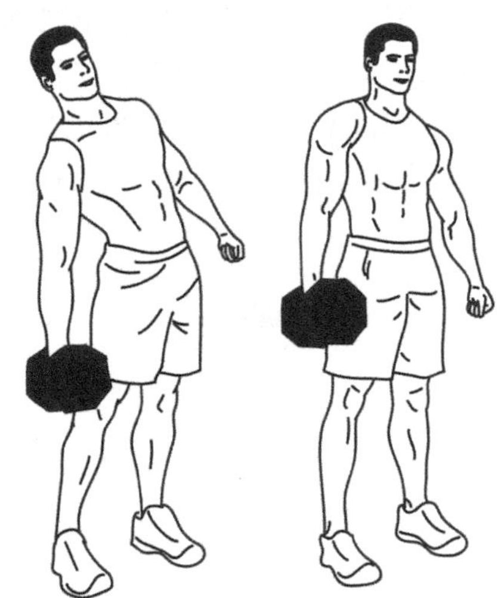

10 side tilts
x 4 sets in total
20 seconds rest between sets

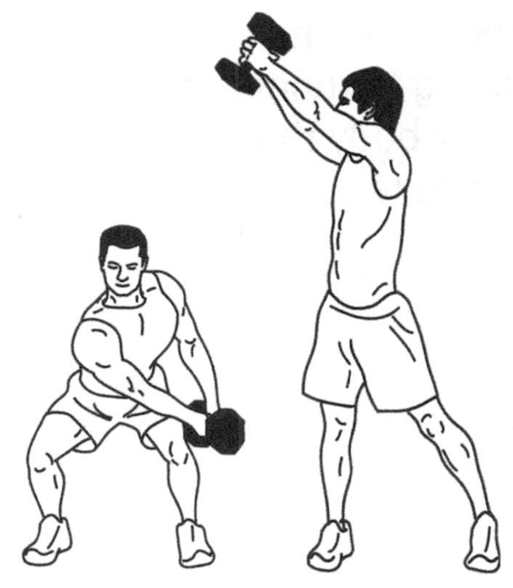

10 cross chops
x 4 sets in total
20 seconds rest between sets

26 Carver

Lower body strength is the powerhouse that moves not just our bodies but also lends strength to everything we do as fitness athletes, from punching and kicking to running and jumping. Carver helps you get there by taking your lower body through a series of exercises targeting specific muscle groups and tendons. The results will make themselves felt the very next day.

BUILD

CARVER

DAREBEE BACK WORKOUT © darebee.com

LEVEL I 3 sets **LEVEL II** 4 sets **LEVEL III** 5 sets **REST** up to 2 minutes

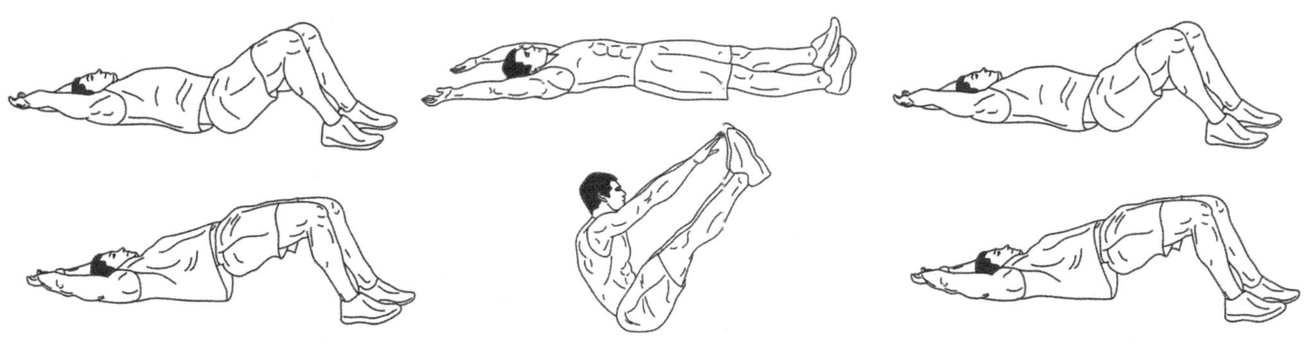

20 bridges

10 V-ups

20 bridges

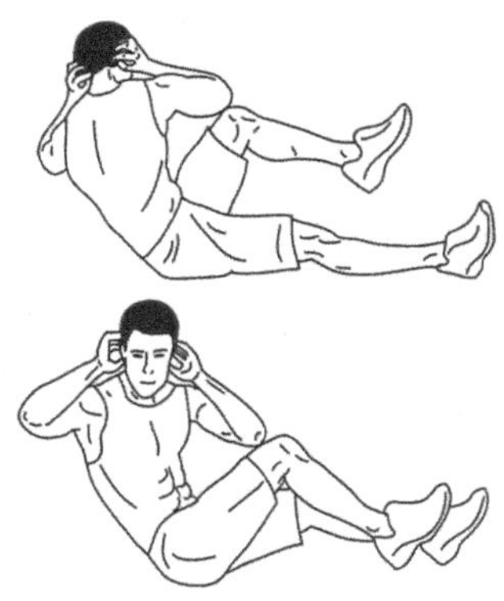

10 knee-to-elbows

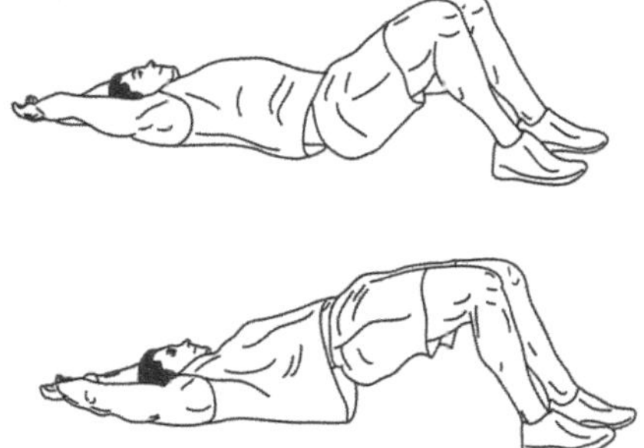

20 bridges

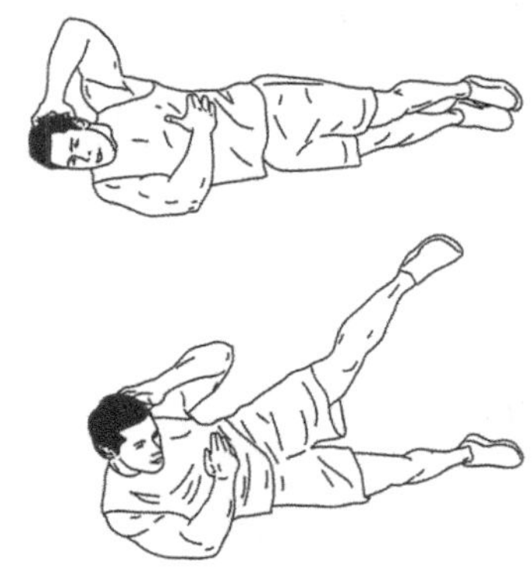

10 side jackknives

27 Chair Abs

Strong abs and core affect posture, relieve back pain and change your mood by helping release dopamine, the feel-good hormone, in your bloodstream when you exercise. The Chair abs workout is proof that you can hold down an office job and still sport rock-hard abs.

chair abs

DAREBEE WORKOUT © darebee.com

BUILD

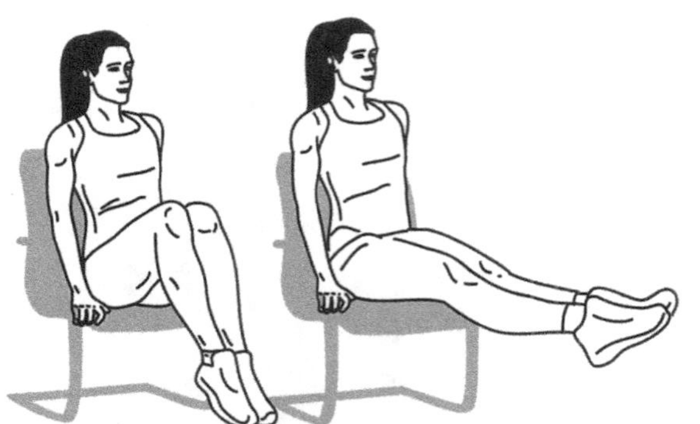

10 crunch kicks

10 side-to-side knee sweeps

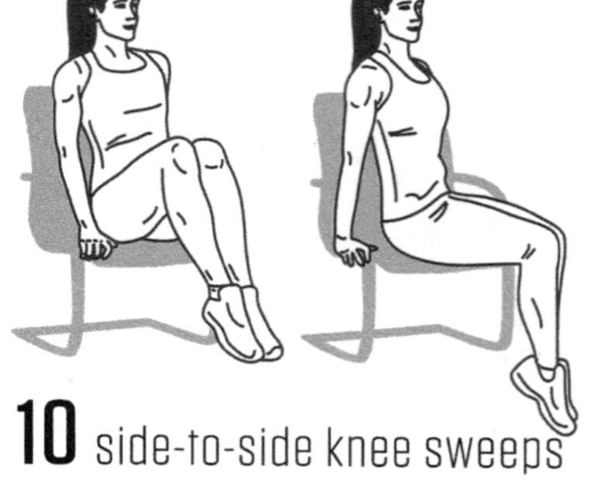

10 knee-to-elbows

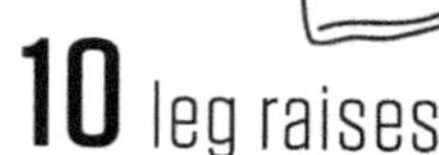

10 leg raises

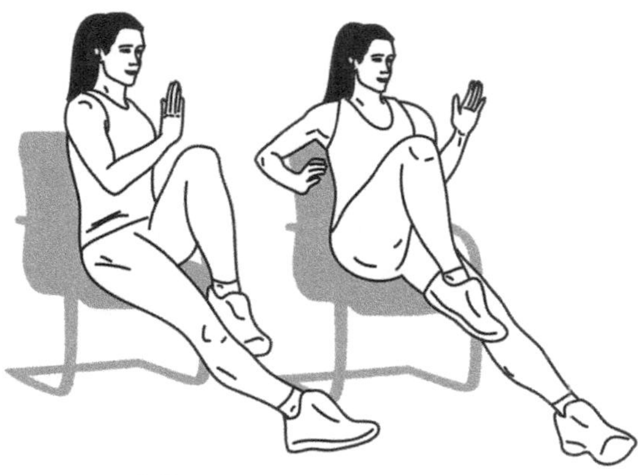

10 cycling crunches

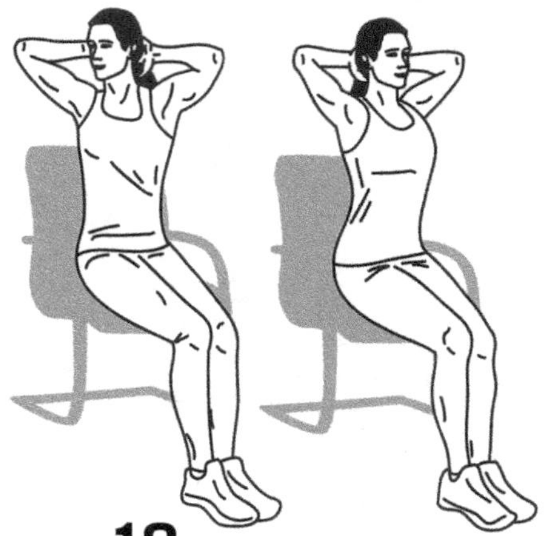

10 sitting twists

28 Code of Abs

e code, the source code. Strong abs are not just the engine that powers ur every move nor are they just the armour that protects some of your al organs. They're also the scaffolding that supports your spine. In short y're really important. That's why you need them. Plus they make you k cool when you take your shirt off.

code of **abs**

BUILD

DAREBEE WORKOUT © **darebee.com**

LEVEL I 3 sets **LEVEL II** 4 sets **LEVEL III** 5 sets **REST** up to 2 minutes

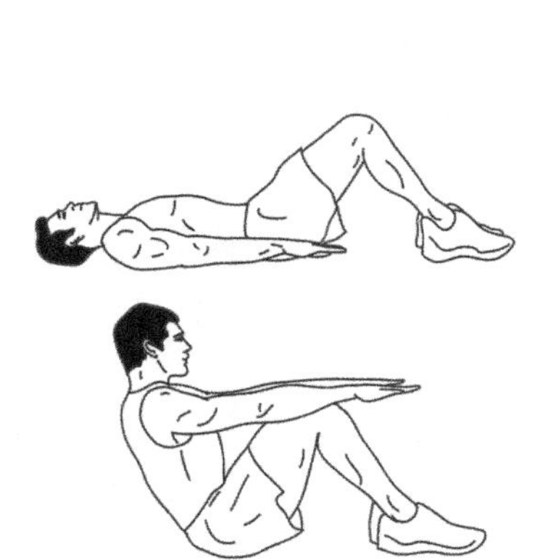

10 sit-ups

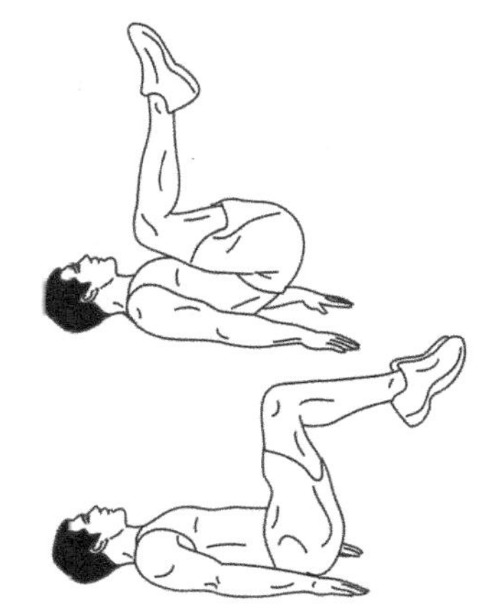

10 reverse crunches

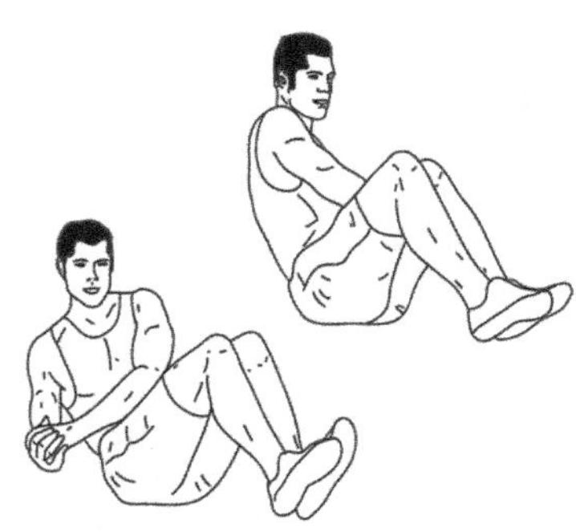

10 sitting twists

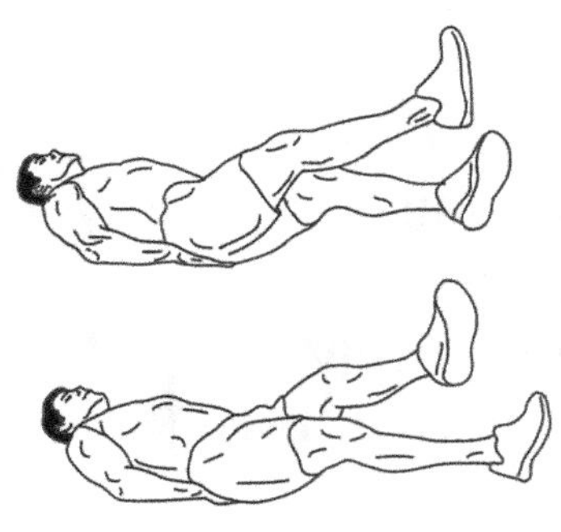

8 scissors

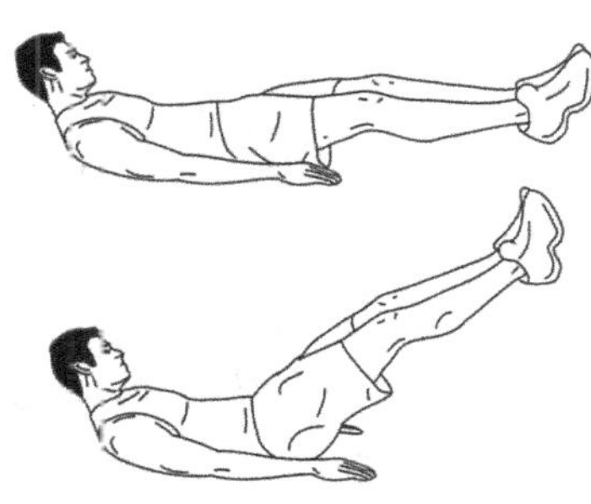

8 leg raises

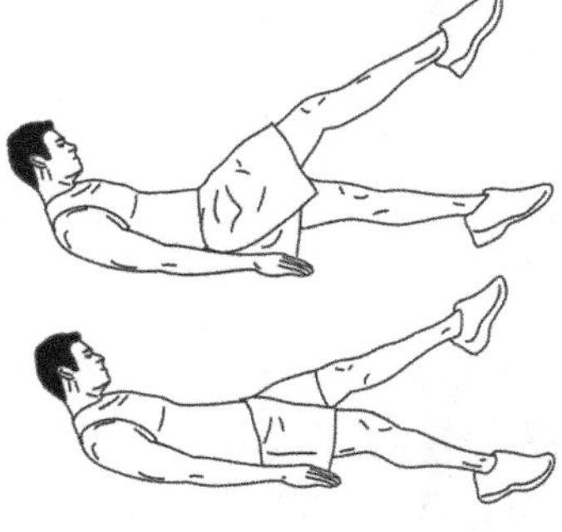

20 flutter kicks

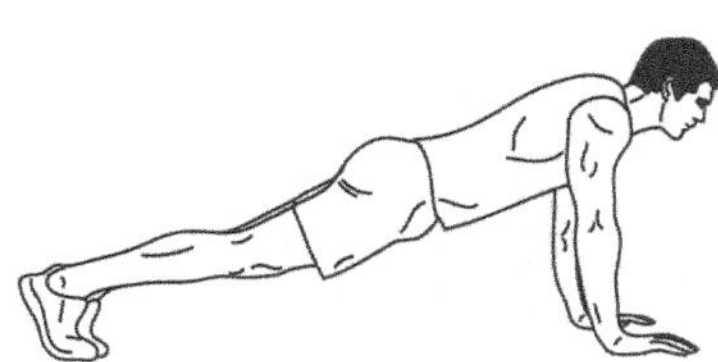

30sec plank

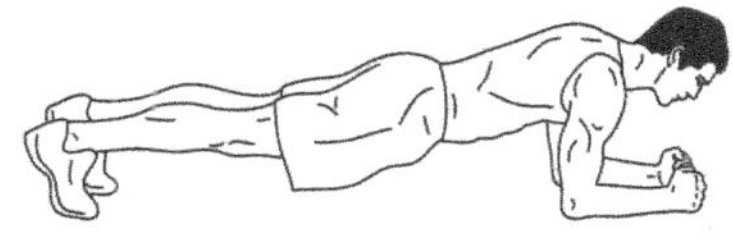

30sec elbow plank

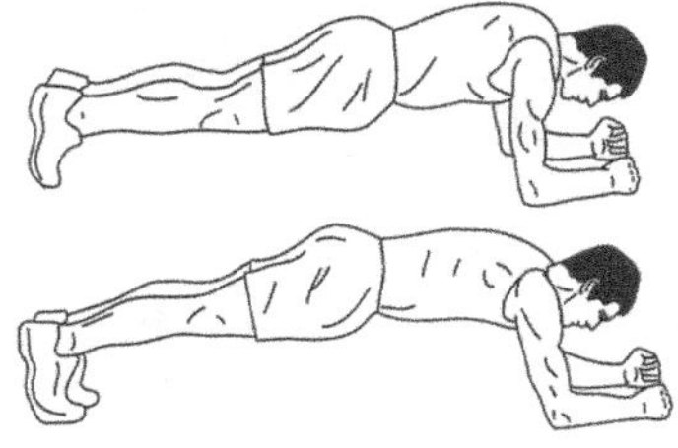

8 body saw

29 Concrete Core

The Concrete Core workout targets your abs and core, works lower body tendons (like the front hip flexors) and the lower back. This is a difficulty Level V workout and as such it will feel way harder than it really is. Key here is to get through each set, recover and then go at it. Do not let the difficulty rating intimidate you. You're better than that!

concrete **core**

DARAREBEE WORKOUT © **darebee.com**

LEVEL I 3 sets **LEVEL II** 4 sets **LEVEL III** 5 sets

REST up to 2 minutes

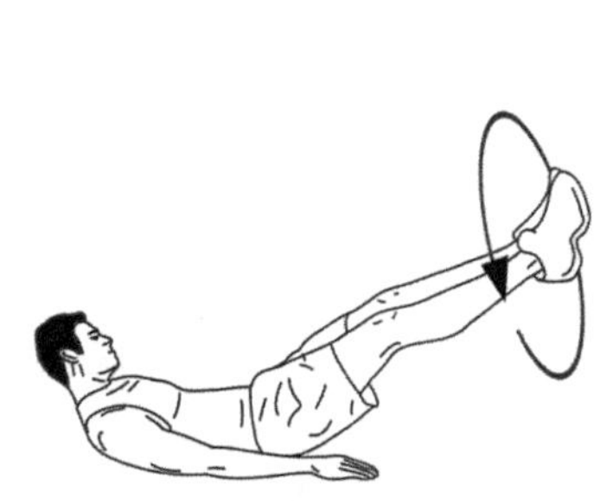

20 raised leg circles

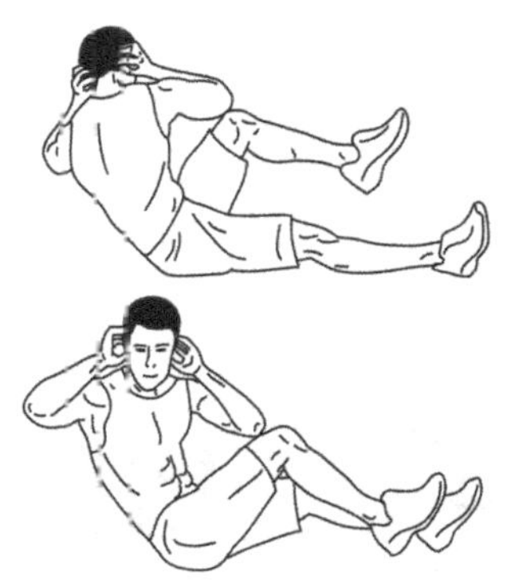

20 knee-to-elbows

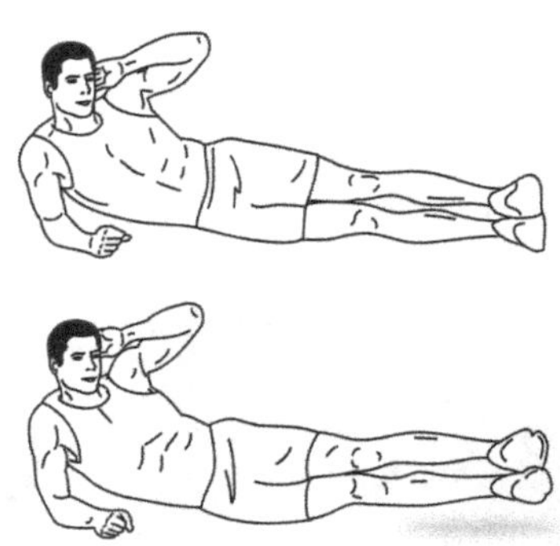

20 side leg lifts

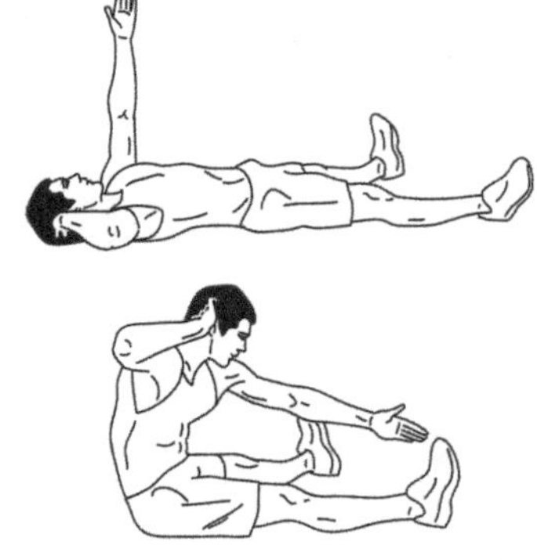

10 sit-up w/reach

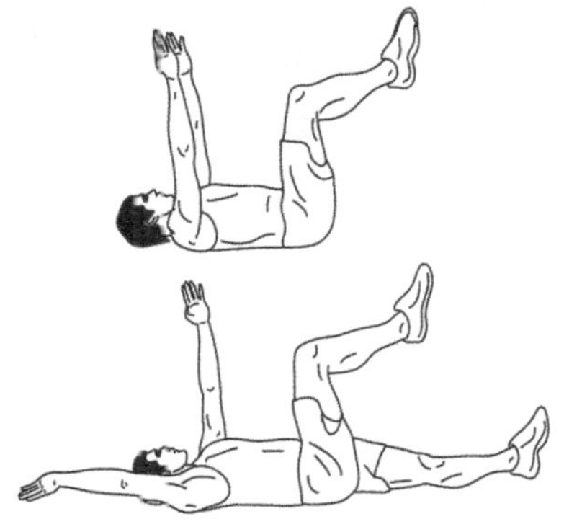

10 dead bug

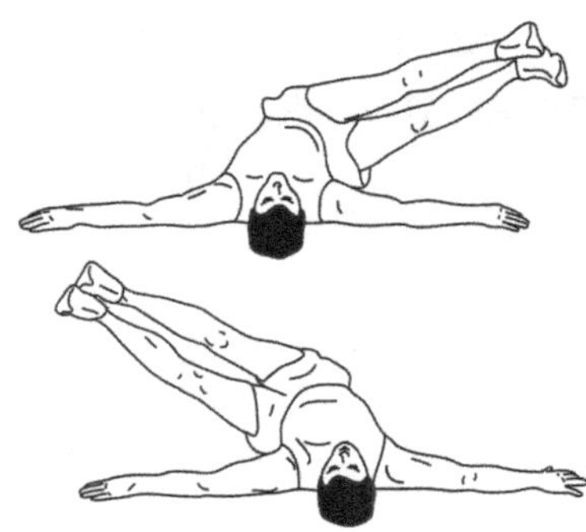

10 windshield wipers

30 Core Builder

No sets - just one killer circuit. Core Builder uses the body's own inertia to target each of the four muscle groups that make up the abdominals. The result is a workout that never feels easy but which gives you what is arguably the perfect exercise when it comes to building stronger abs and core. Perform after a workout or whenever you feel you could do with a good abs workout.

core builder

DAREBEE WORKOUT © darebee.com

Switch sides on the fly, halfway through the exercise.

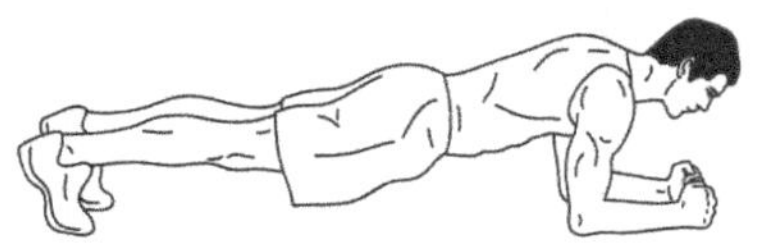

20sec elbow plank

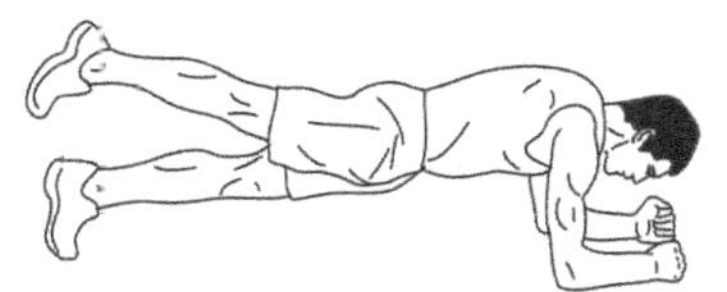

40sec raised leg plank

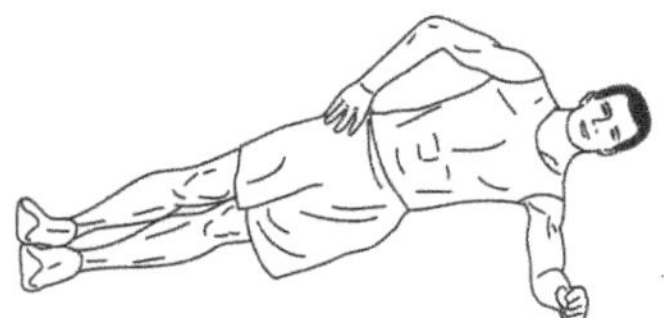

40sec side plank

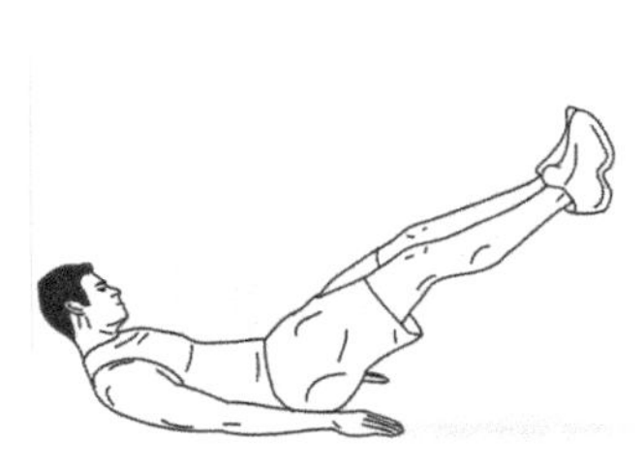

20sec raised leg hold

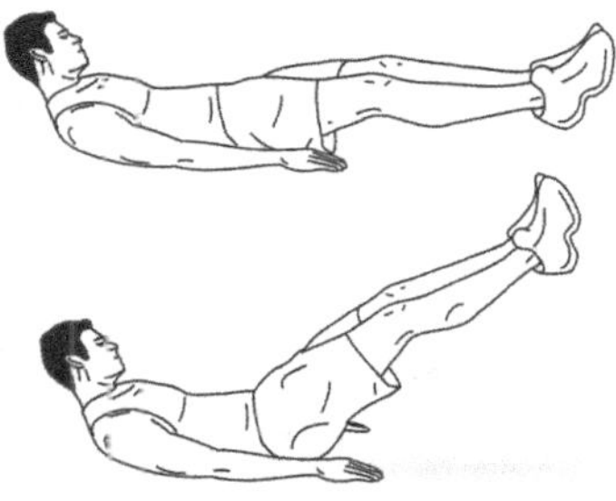

20sec leg raises

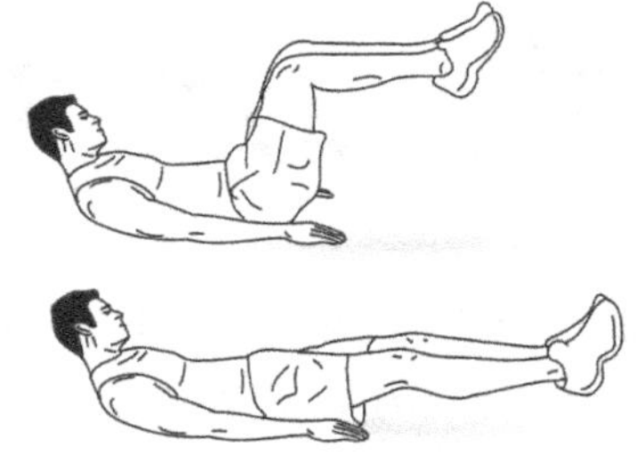

20sec slow kicks

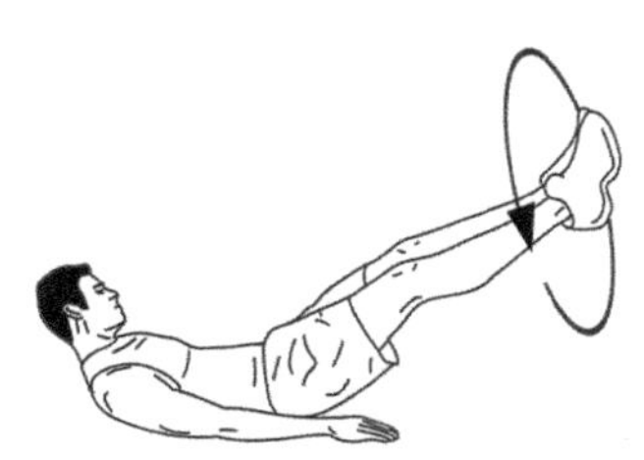

20sec raised leg circles

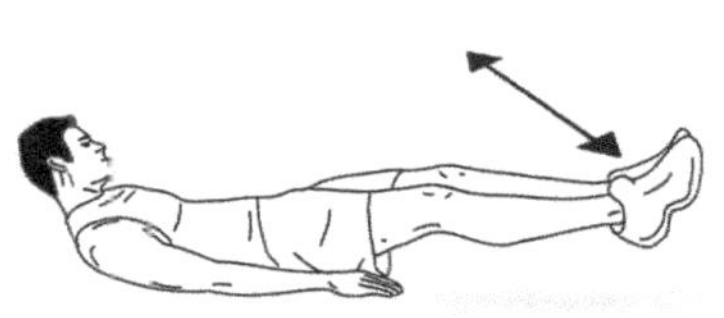

20sec side-to-side tilts

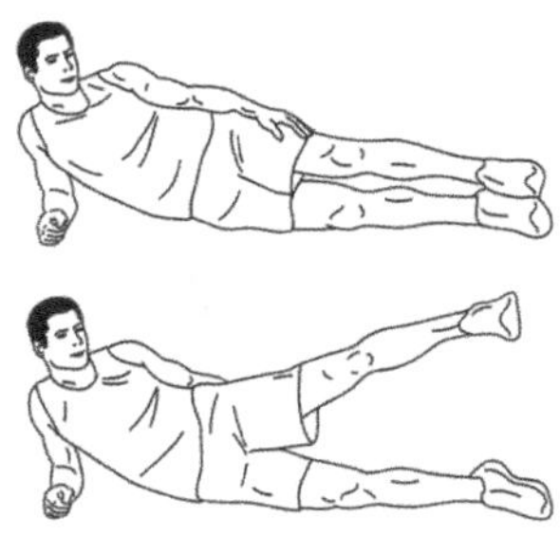

40sec side leg raises

31 Core Connect

A strong core is not easy to come by. The muscles associated with it (transversus abdominis) help develop better functional movements and prevent injury. The core is active in both static and dynamic movements as it brings the skeletal structure into play and allows it to align itself so that it can better absorb and direct specific forces. The Core Connect workout helps strengthen your core and change the way you do, everything.

core connect

DAREBEE WORKOUT © darebee.com

LEVEL I 3 sets **LEVEL II** 5 sets **LEVEL III** 7 sets **REST** up to 2 minutes

10 reps each exercise

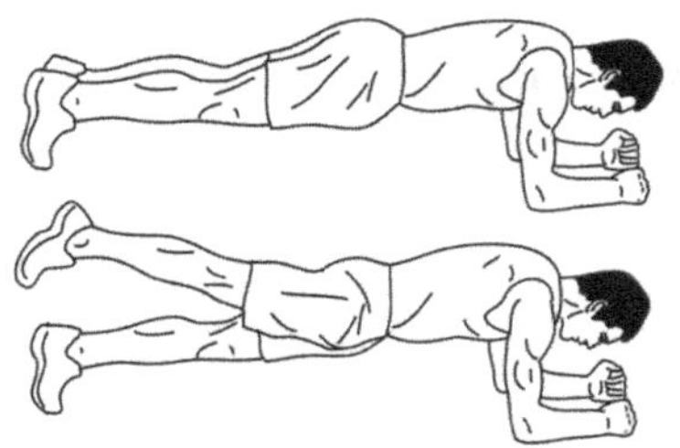

plank leg raises

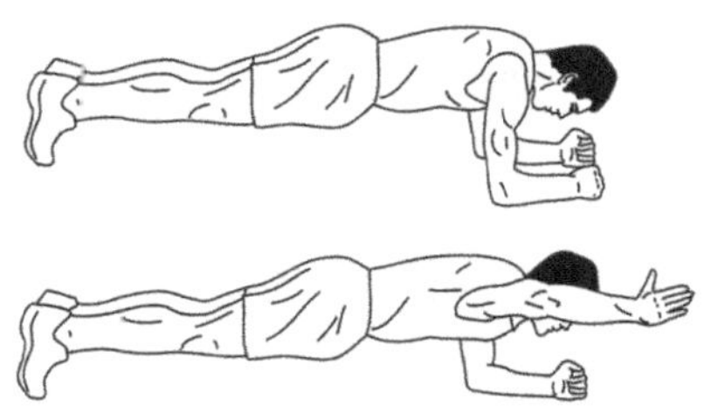

plank arm raises

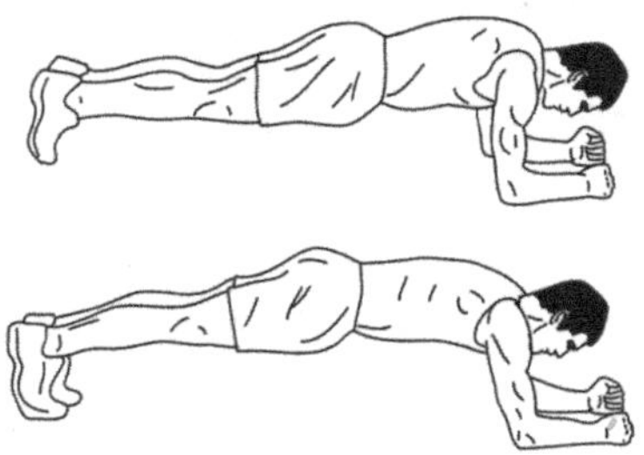

body saw

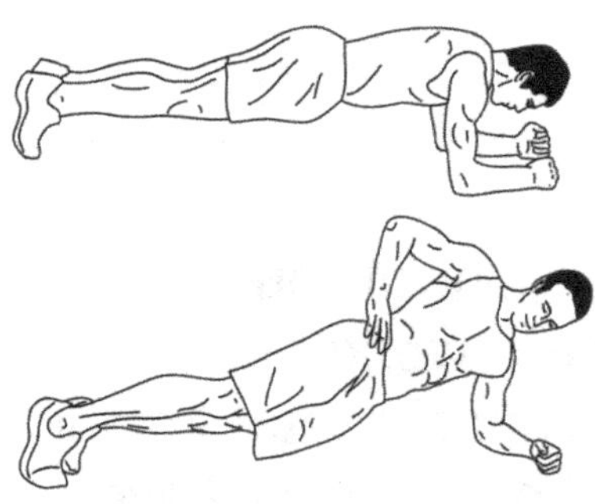

plank rotations

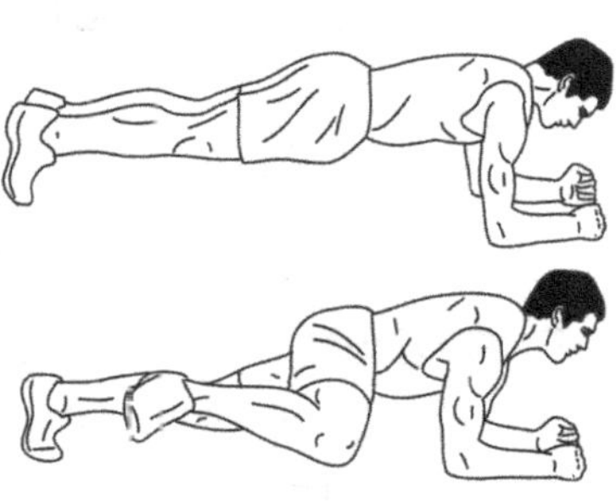

spiderman planks

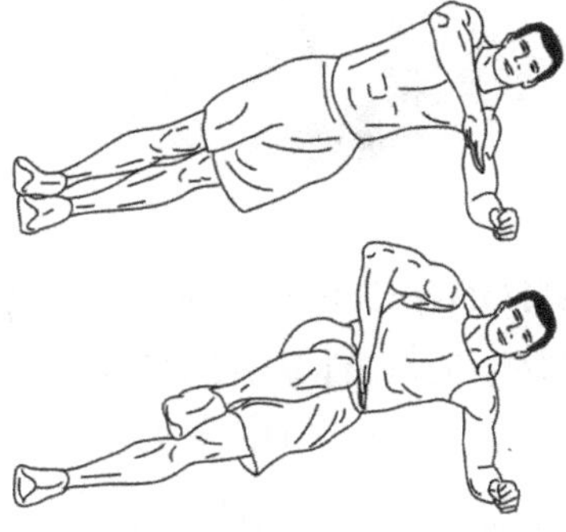

side plank knee taps

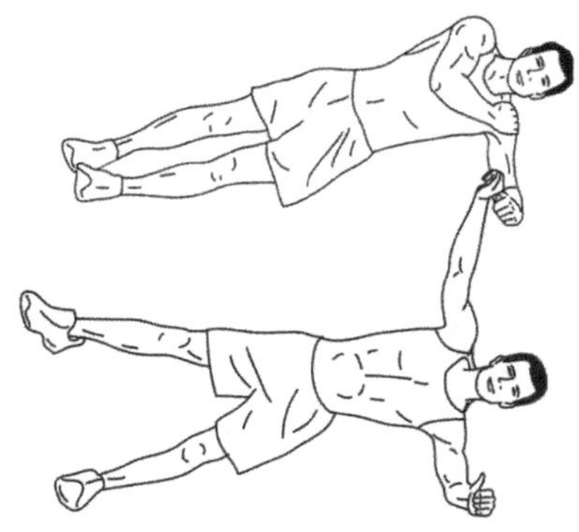

side star plank

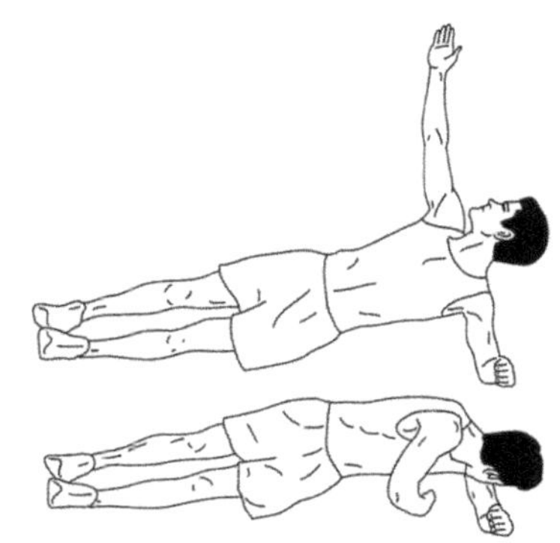

side plank rotations

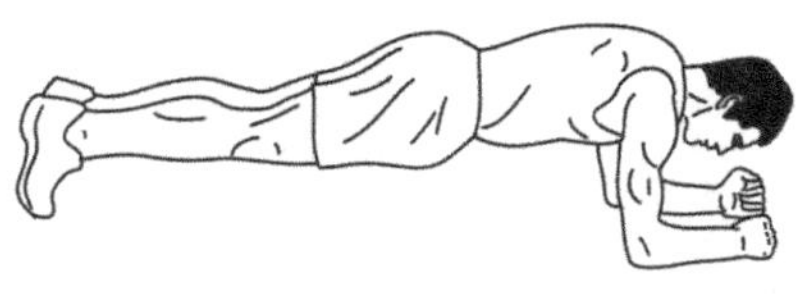

to failure elbow plank

32 Core Control

A strong core changes your posture and allows you to control your body better when you do just about anything. Core Control is a workout aimed to help you build a stronger core. Each exercise works specific abdominal muscles without neglecting other parts of your body. This is only a Level III workout so really go the full length of five sets and add EC and you'll be golden plus you will really feel the difference from the very first session.

CORE
CONTROL

DARBEE WORKOUT © darebee.com

LEVEL I 3 sets **LEVEL II** 4 sets **LEVEL III** 5 sets **REST** up to 2 minutes

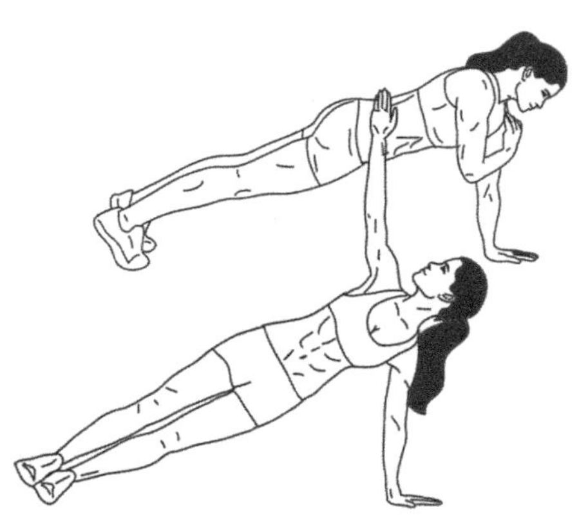

10 shoulder tap + rotation

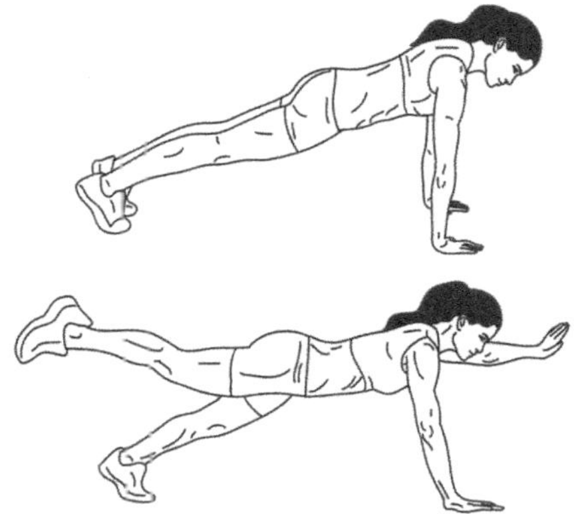

10 alt arm/leg raises

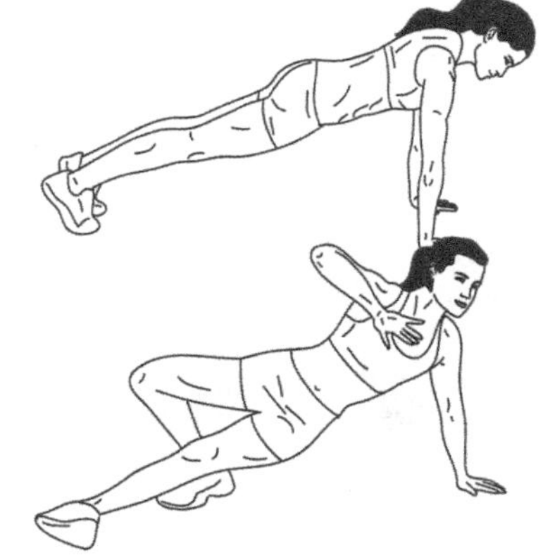

10 sit-outs

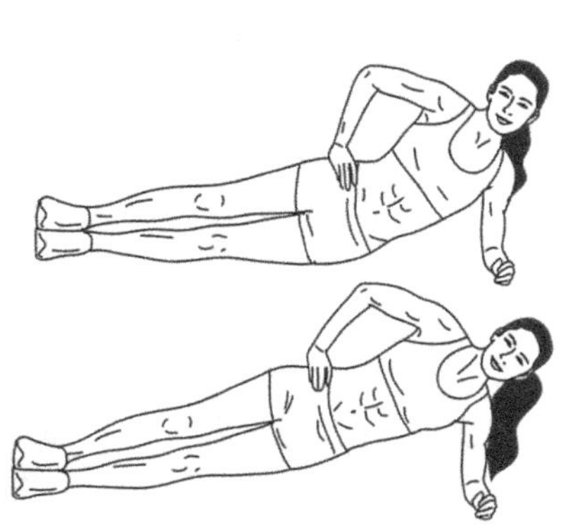

10 side plank raises

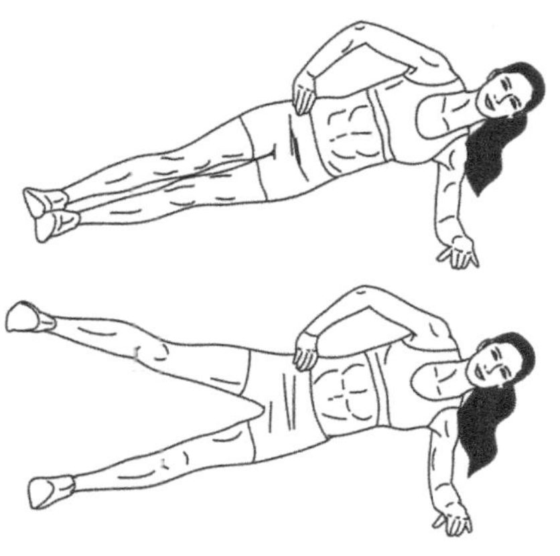

10 side plank leg raises

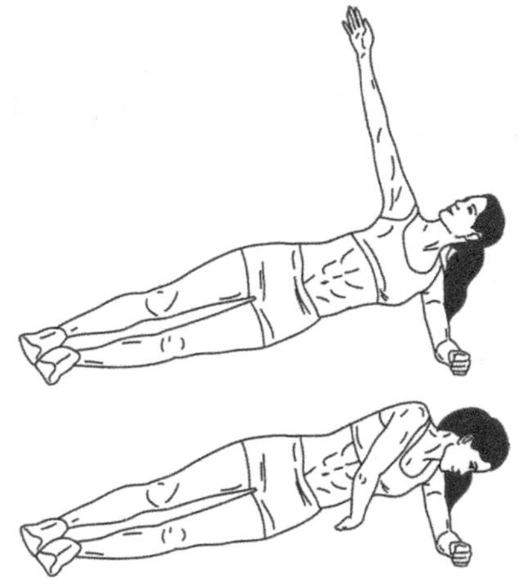

10 side plank rotations

33 Core Crusher

A strong core affects the way strength is transferred from the lower body to the upper body and vice versa which means that a strong core changes almost every aspect of athletic performance. Core Crusher targets the core and the three abdominal muscle groups. As a Level III workout it's not an easy one to do but the benefits from doing it often will be quite tangible.

CORE CRUSHER

DARESEE WORKOUT © darebee.com

LEVEL I 3 sets **LEVEL II** 4 sets **LEVEL III** 5 sets

REST up to 2 minutes

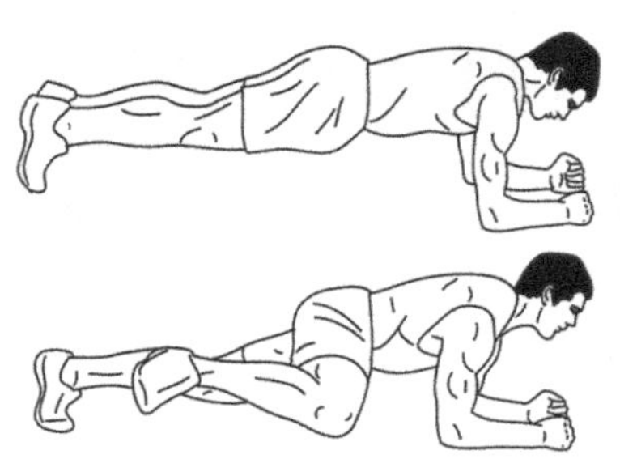

20 plank side crunches

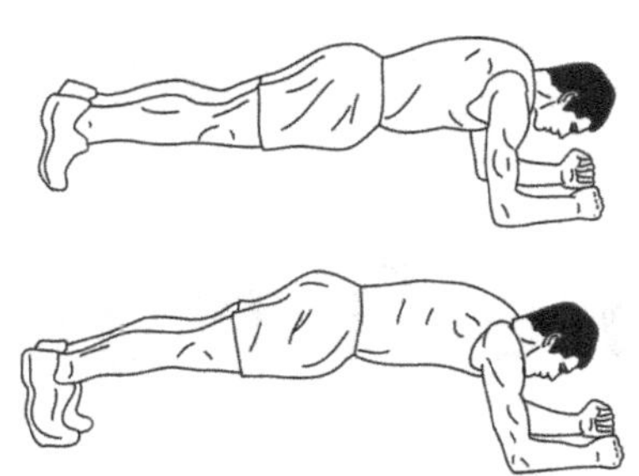

20 body saw

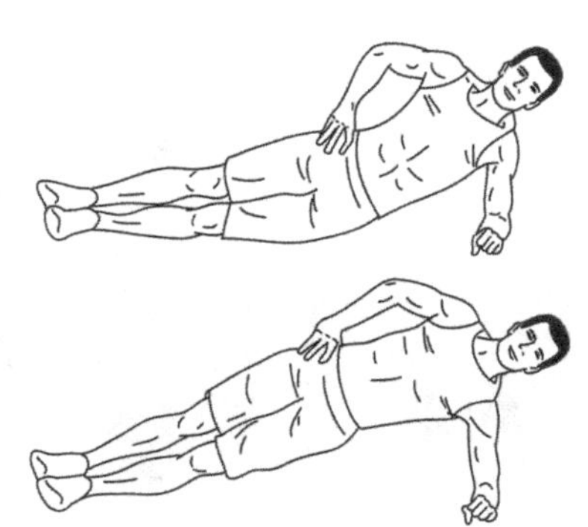

20 side bridges

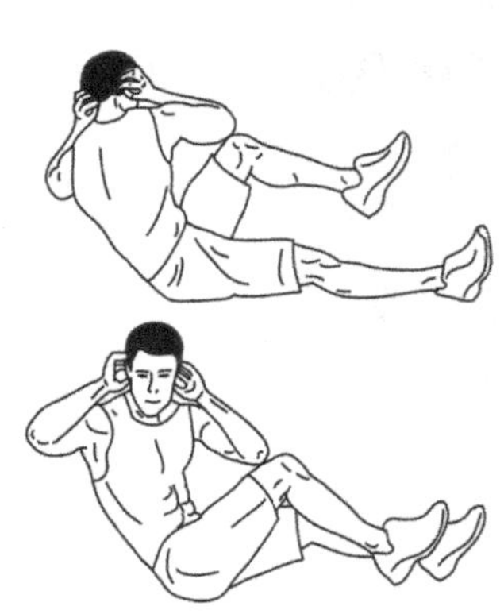

20 knee-to-elbow crunches

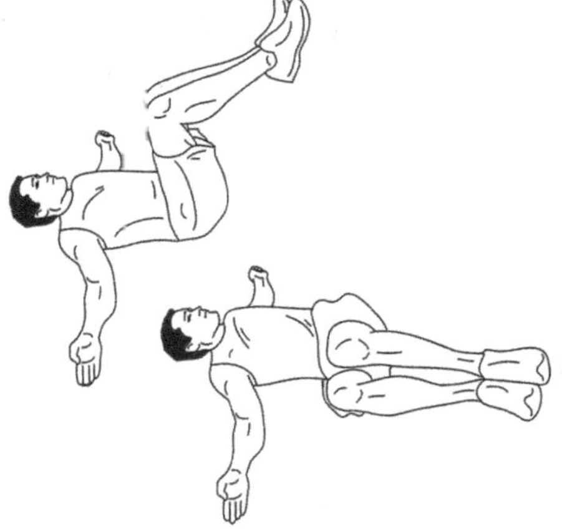

20 half wipers

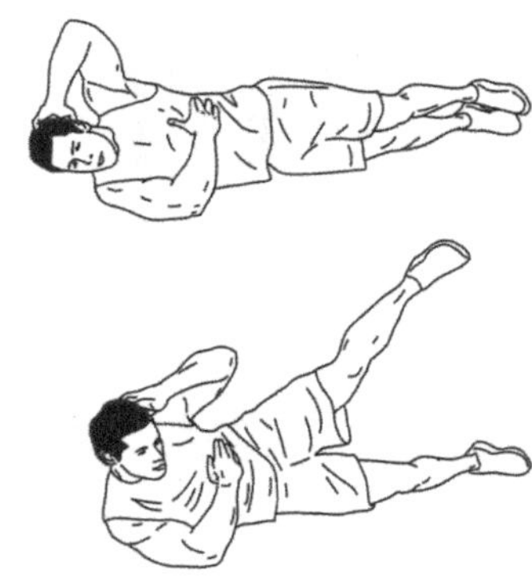

20 side jackknives

34 Core Twister

Abs need work. They require different exercises that place a different load on each of the four abdominal muscle groups. Core Twister lives up to its name. It works the core. It will push your abs. It will make you functionally more powerful by allowing the power transfer from the lower body tot he upper one and vice versa to happen with as little loss of energy as possible. To do all that, you need to do the Core Twister workout.

CORE TWISTER

DAREBEE WORKOUT © darebee.com

Switch sides and repeat the sequence again.

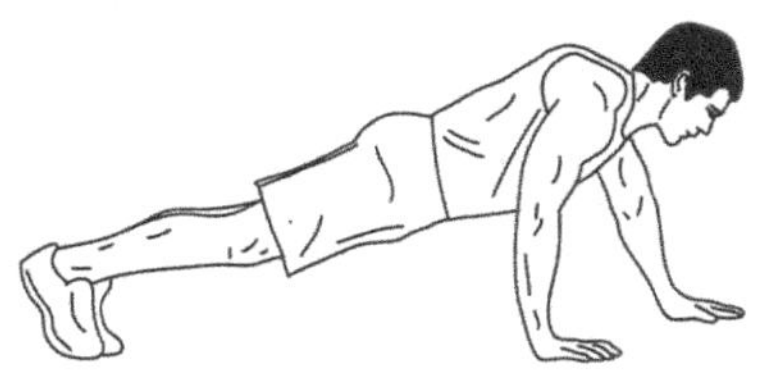

20 seconds
staggered plank hold

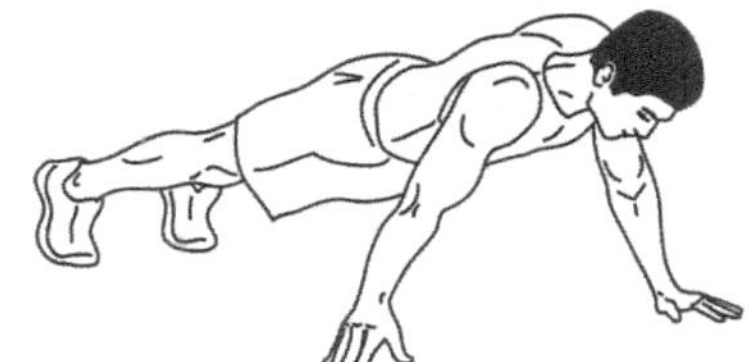

20 seconds
archer plank hold

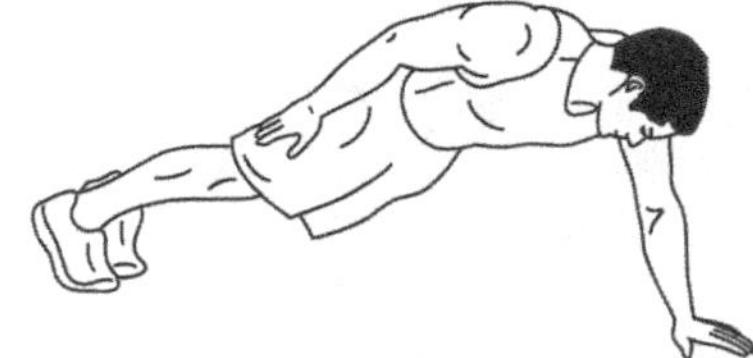

20 seconds
one-arm plank hold

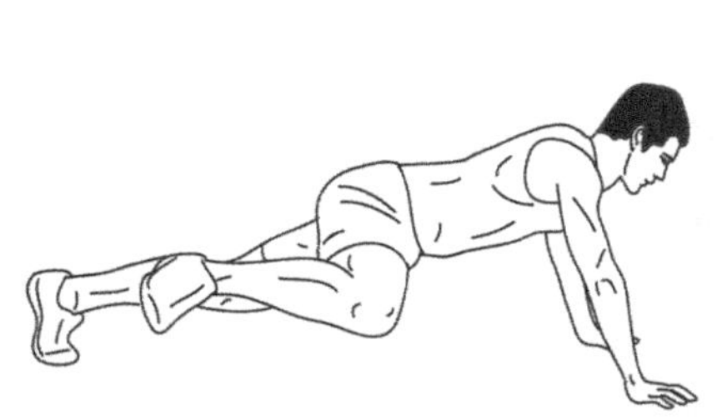

20 seconds
knee-to-the-side plank hold

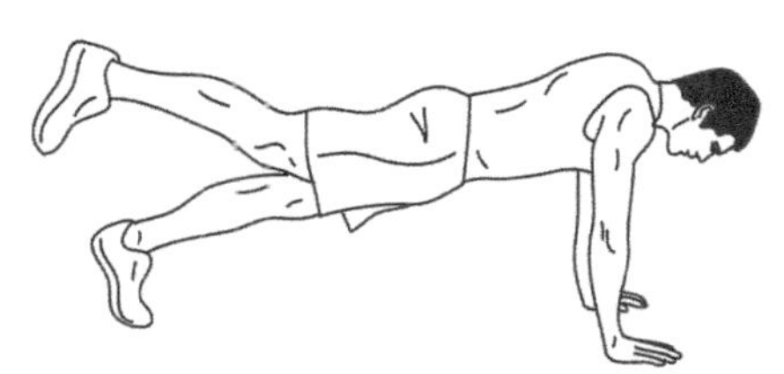

20 seconds
raised leg plank hold

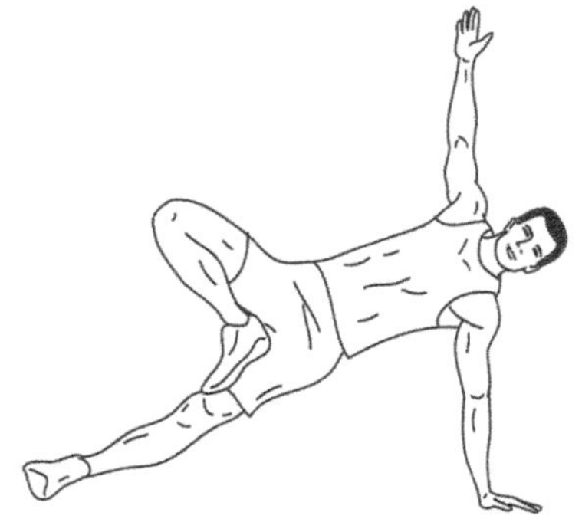

20 seconds
tucked-in side plank hold

35 Crop Top

Strong abs change posture, athletic performance and the power coefficient of a trained body. Plus, let's face it, they also look good in a crop top. The Crop Top workout delivers on its premise (and promise).

CROP TOP WORKOUT

by DAREBEE © darebee.com

5 sets | 2 minutes rest

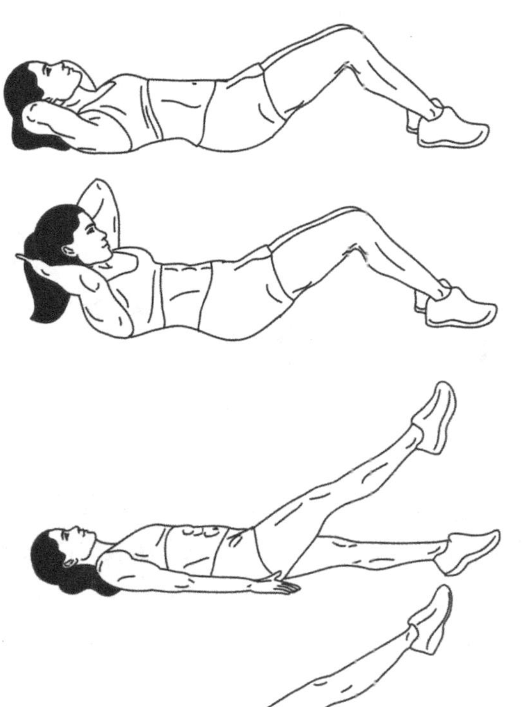

10 crunches

10 flutter kicks

4 sitting twists

10 crunches

10 flutter kicks

4 sitting twists

10 crunches

10 flutter kicks

4 sitting twists

done

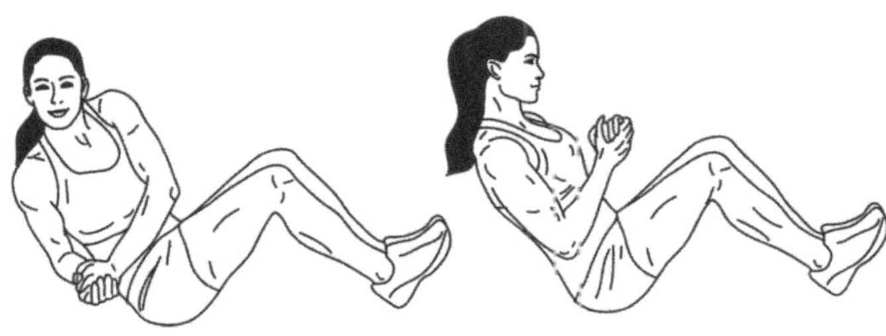

36 Crunch Time

The abdominals are comprised of four separate muscle groups: the external abs (better known as the six-pack), the external and internal obliques and the core. Crunch Time is an abdominal training workout that targets all those muscle groups for an athletic performance-enhancing ab strengthening result.

crunch time

DAREBEE WORKOUT © darebee.com

LEVEL I 3 sets **LEVEL II** 4 sets **LEVEL III** 5 sets **REST** up to 2 minutes

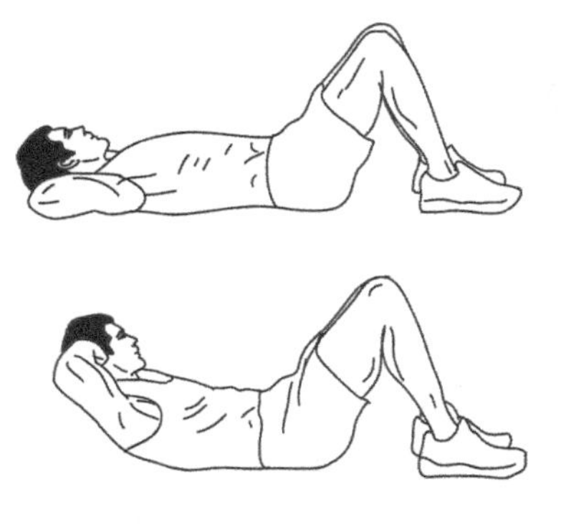

10 crunches

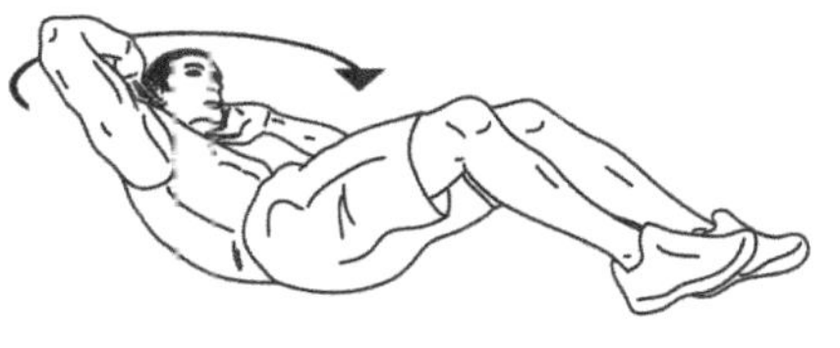

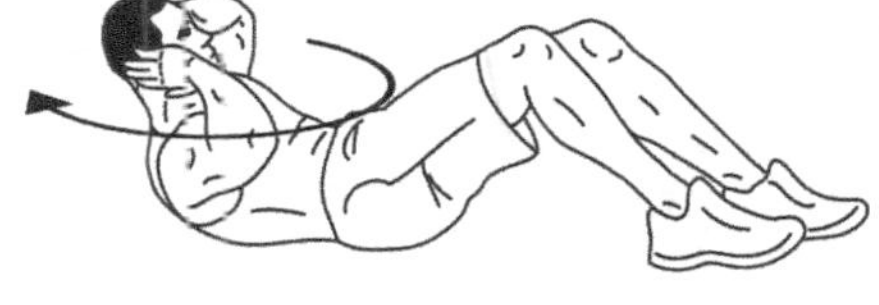

6 circle crunches

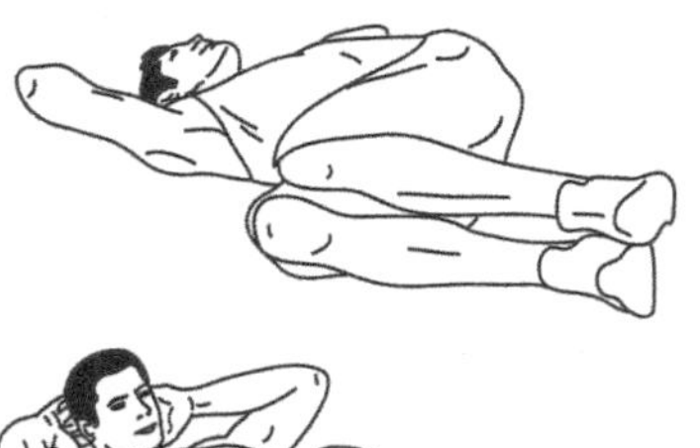

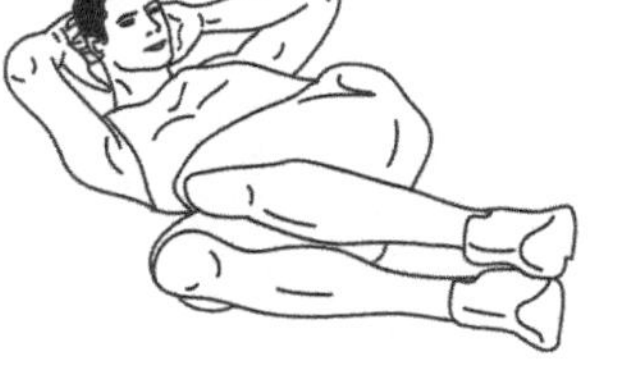

6 folded crunches

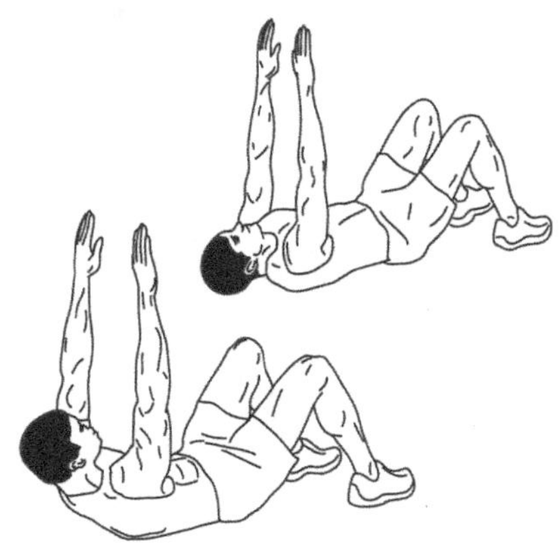

10 high crunches

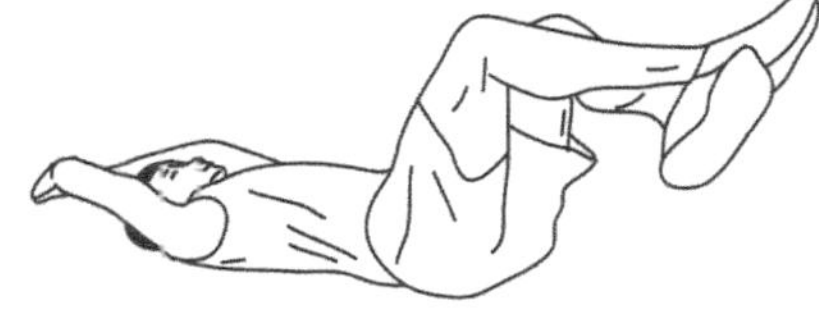

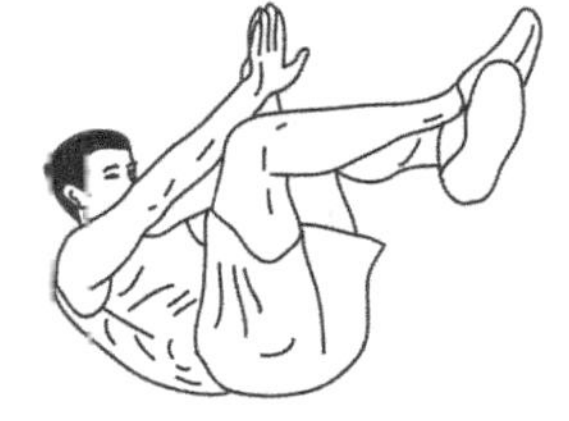

6 knee crunches

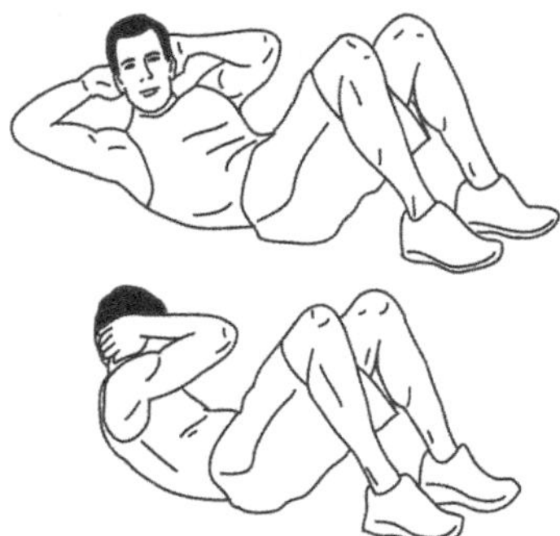

6 cross crunches

37 Daily Abs

You can never have abs that are too strong. But the abdominal muscle groups are hard to train effectively or train well. The Daily Abs workout provides four exercises you can use to address this deficiency. Introduced in your weekly exercise routines this is a workout that will soon begin to deliver a real difference.

daily **abs**

DARKBEE WORKOUT © darebee.com

2 minutes rest between exercises

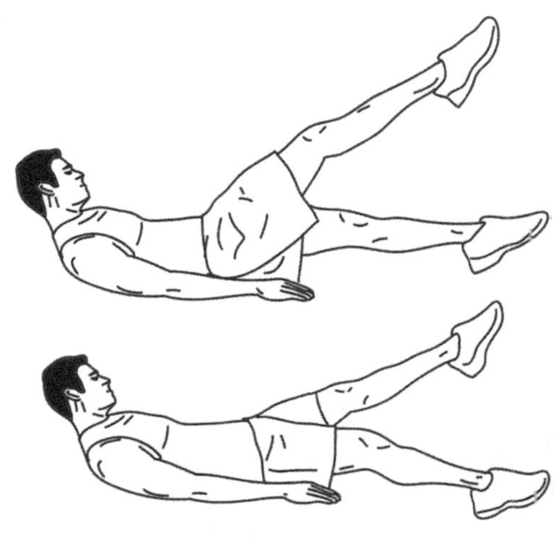

20 flutter kicks
x 3 sets in total
20 seconds rest between sets

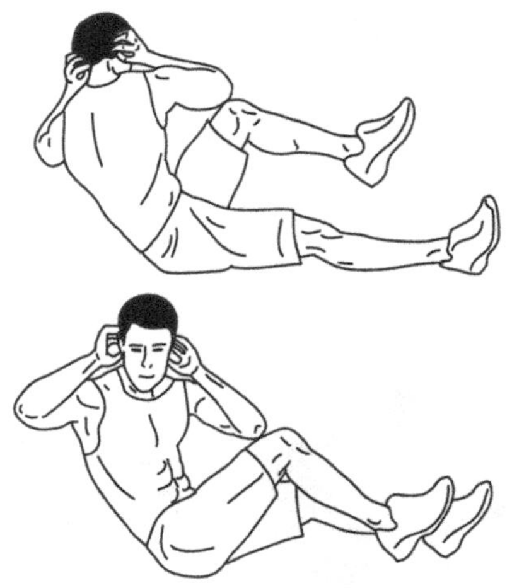

20 knee-to-elbow crunches
x 3 sets in total
20 seconds rest between sets

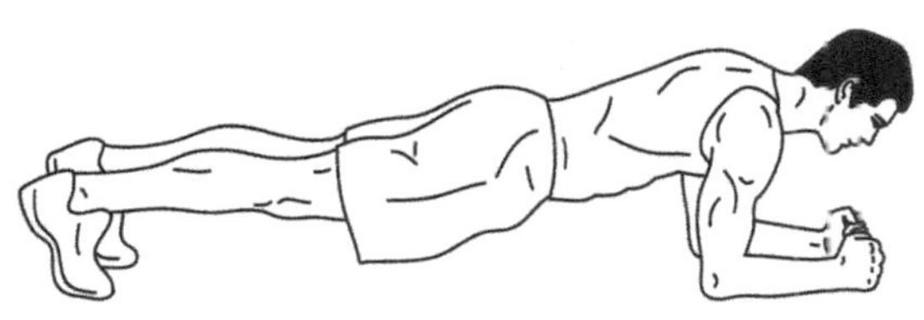

1 minutes elbow plank

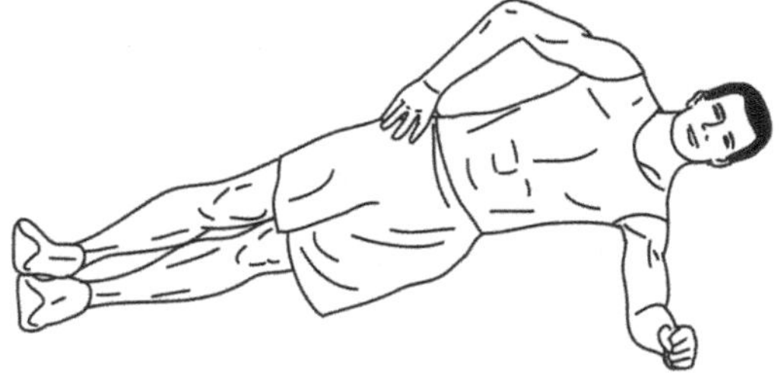

1 minutes side elbow plank
30 seconds per side

38 Express Abs

There are four main muscle groups that make up the ab wall in its totality and Abs Express is designed to help you test each one of them for better, faster results. When it comes to building quality abs there really is no shortcut. This set of exercises will help you get there, all you have to do is put in the time and do the work.

express abs

REPEAT ONCE | DAREBEE WORKOUT © darebee.com

LEVEL I 6 reps **LEVEL II** 10 reps each **LEVEL III** 20 reps each

LEVEL I 6-count hold **LEVEL II** 10-count hold **LEVEL III** 20-count hold

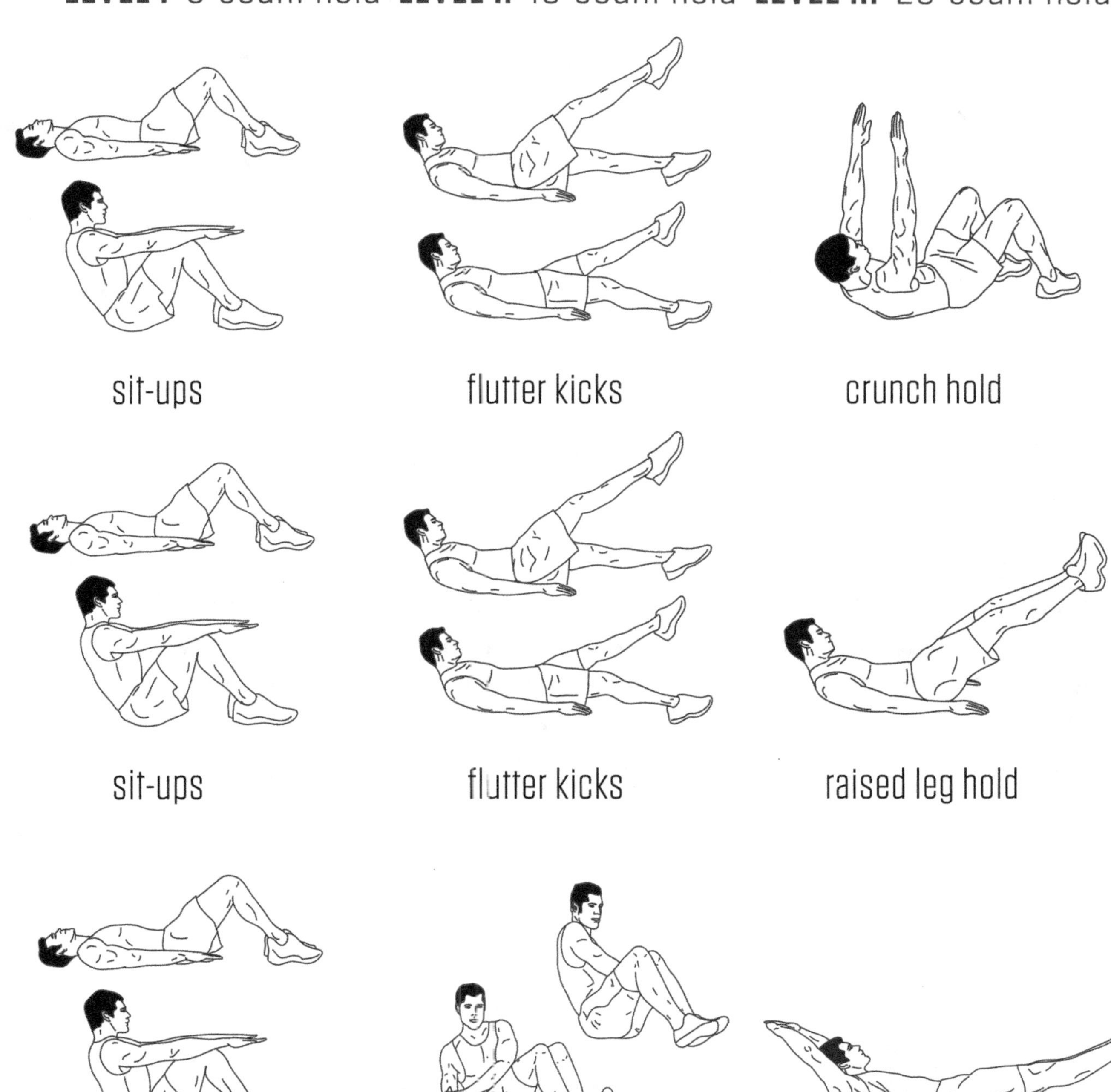

sit-ups | flutter kicks | crunch hold

sit-ups | flutter kicks | raised leg hold

sit-ups | sitting twists | hollow hold

39 Extreme Abs

Abs power everything. They facilitate every movement. They amplify the power the body can generate. Extreme Abs is a difficulty Level V workout that will make you say "ouch!". It is worth it in terms of the results it delivers not just in the way you feel, but in the way you do anything!

extreme **abs**

DAREBEE WORKOUT © **darebee.com**

30 seconds each exercise | no rest between exercises

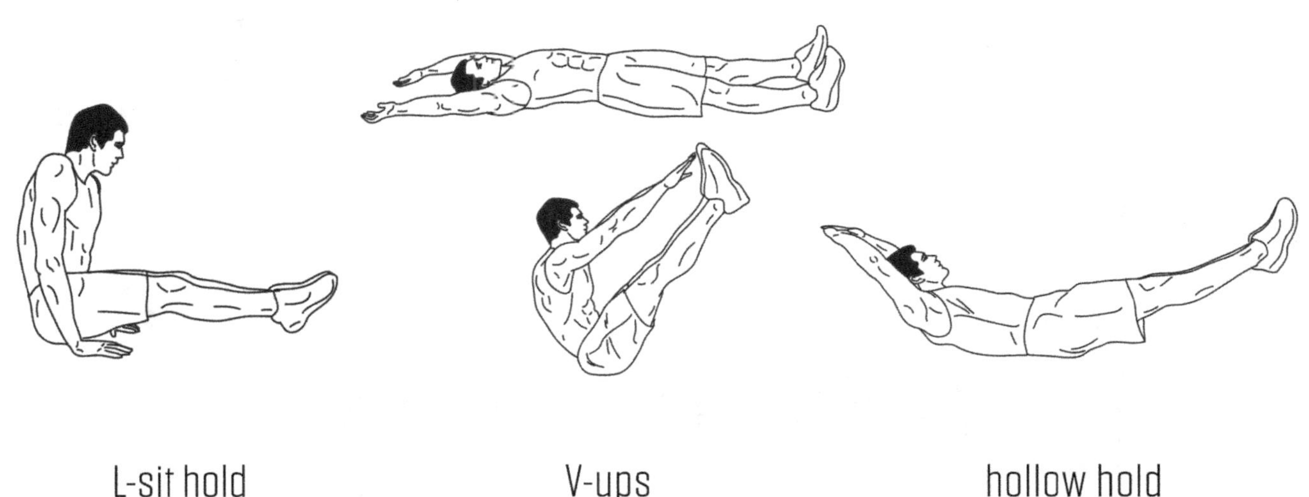

L-sit hold

V-ups

hollow hold

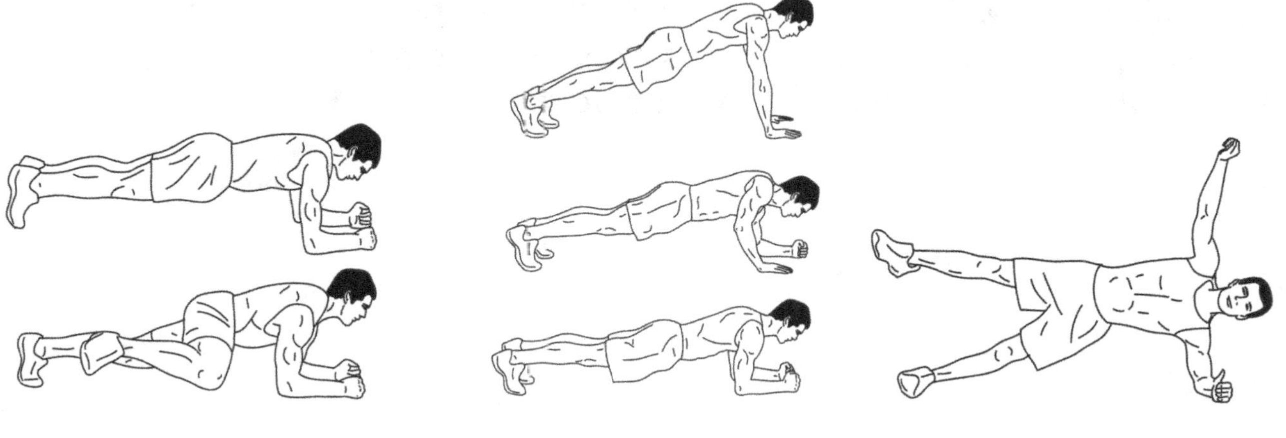

elbow plank crunches

up and down planks

side star plank

40 Five Minute Plank

Training the abdominal muscle group is no easy task. The muscles do not all respond to training at the same rate and there is a core group of abdominal s, running beneath the external ones with muscle fibres pointing the opposite way. This makes for a core picture which no single exercise can adequately address which helps explain why strong abs are hard to attain, which makes them an aim to strive for.

FIVE MINUTE PLANK

DAREBEE WORKOUT © darebee.com

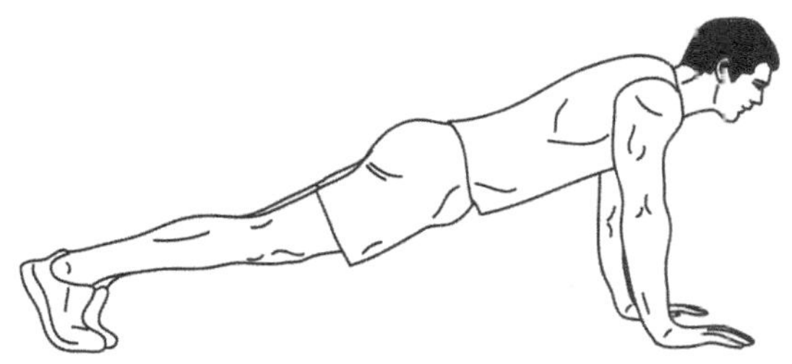

60sec full plank

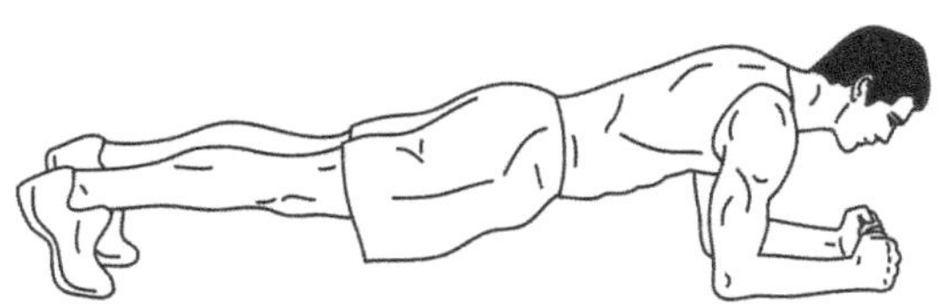

30sec elbow plank

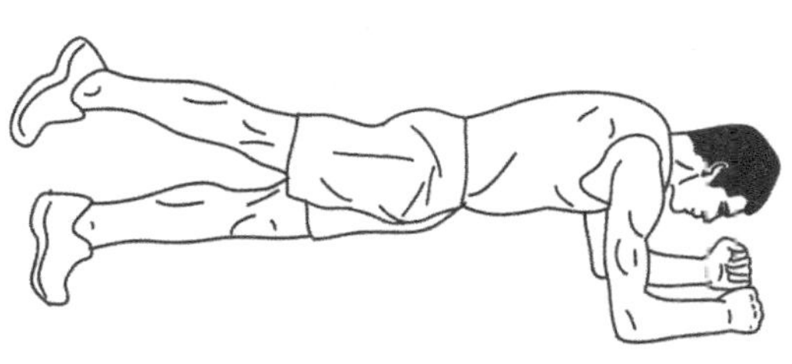

60sec raised leg plank
30 seconds - each leg

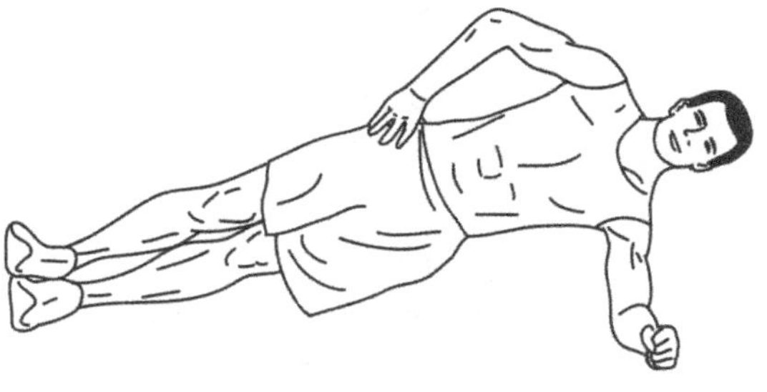

60sec side plank
30 seconds - each side

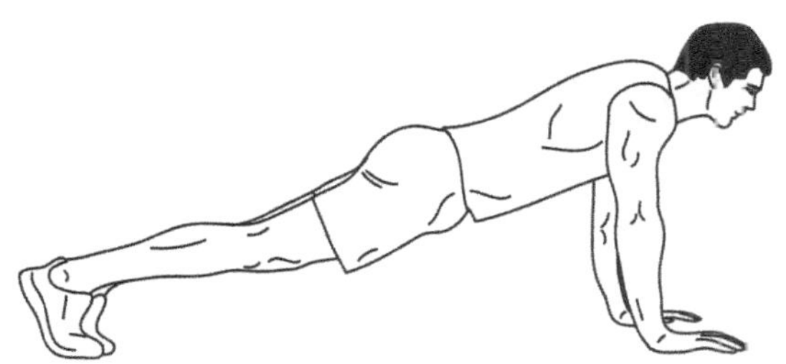

30sec full plank

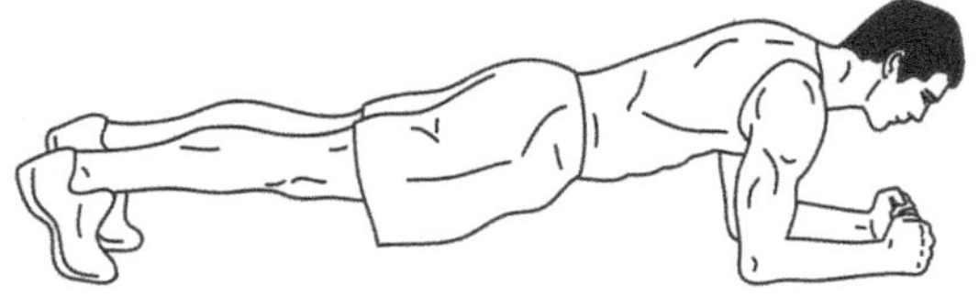

60sec elbow plank

41 Good Morning, Abs

Abs are core to any kind of workout and this Morning abs routine can be performed first thing int he day before you get out of bed or last thing at night before you close your eyes and unplug from the conscious world. Ok, you can't be cozily tucked in under the blankets and do it, but you've worked that bit out already.

Good morning, abs

DAREBEE WORKOUT © darebee.com

LEVEL I 3 sets **LEVEL II** 4 sets **LEVEL III** 5 sets **REST** up to 2 minutes

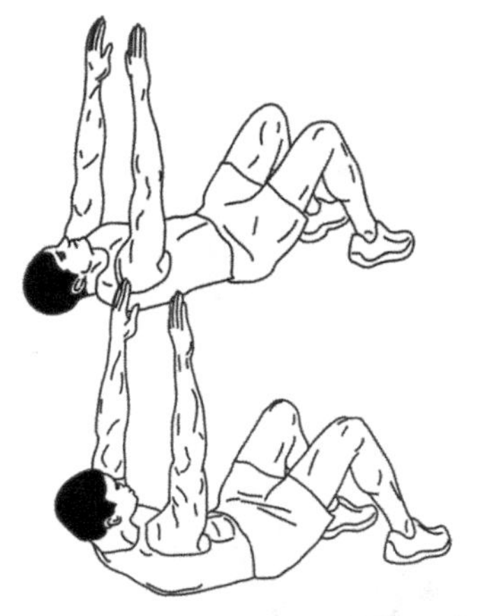

10 high crunches

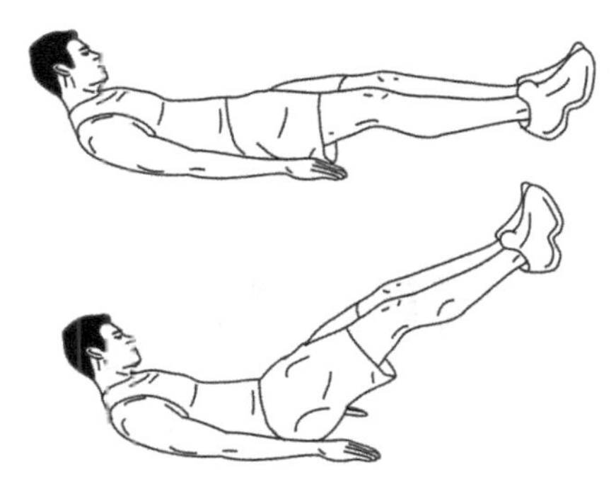

10 leg raises

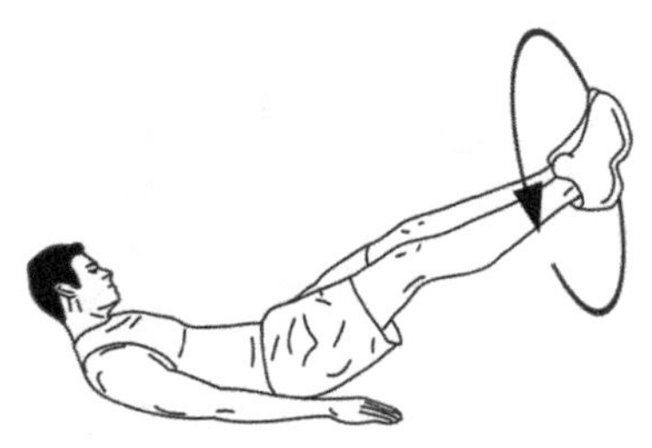

10 raised leg circles

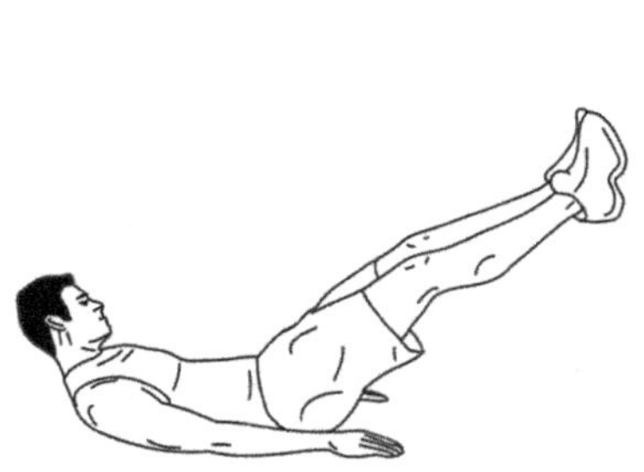

10-count raised leg hold

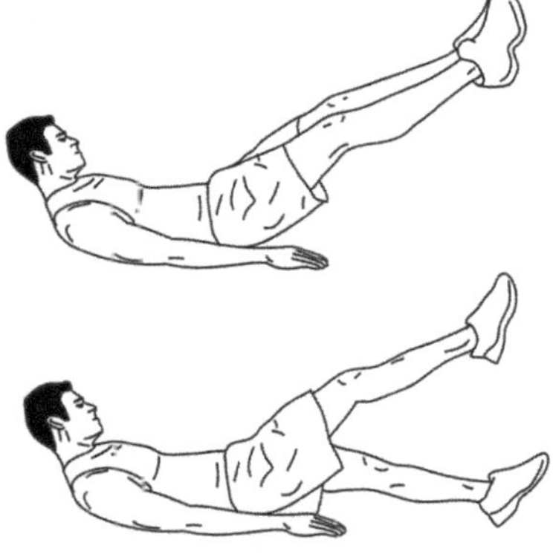

10 flutter kicks

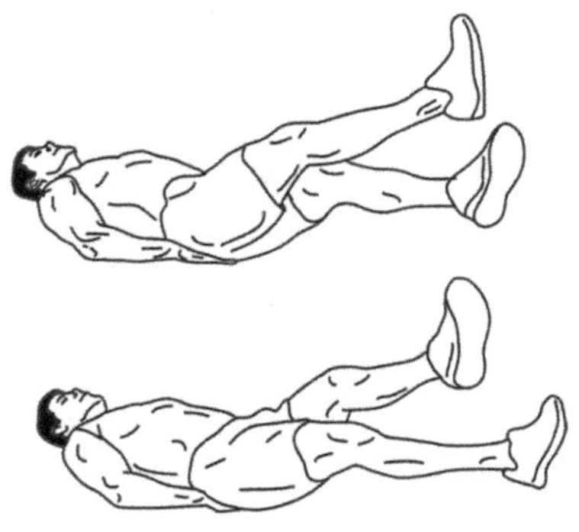

10 scissors

42 Hardcore

A good core will always come in handy. Whether it comes to balancing on the deck of a boat in high seas or performing the latest exercise at home a strong core helps make the task easier. Plus it's great for your posture.

HARD CORE

DAREBEE WORKOUT © darebee.com

LEVEL I 3 sets **LEVEL II** 5 sets **LEVEL III** 7 sets **REST** up to 2 minutes

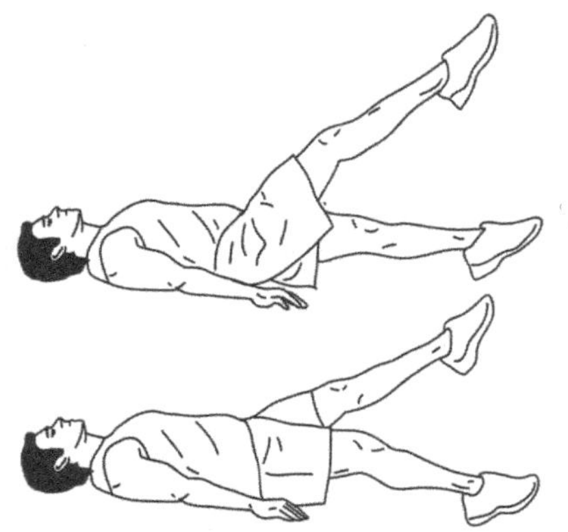

20 flutter kicks

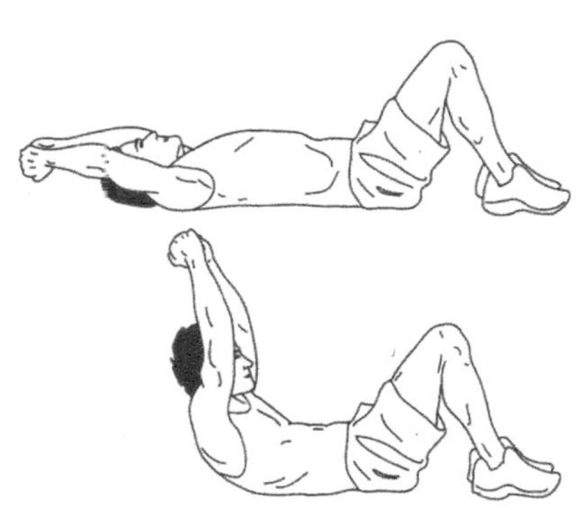

12 long arm crunches

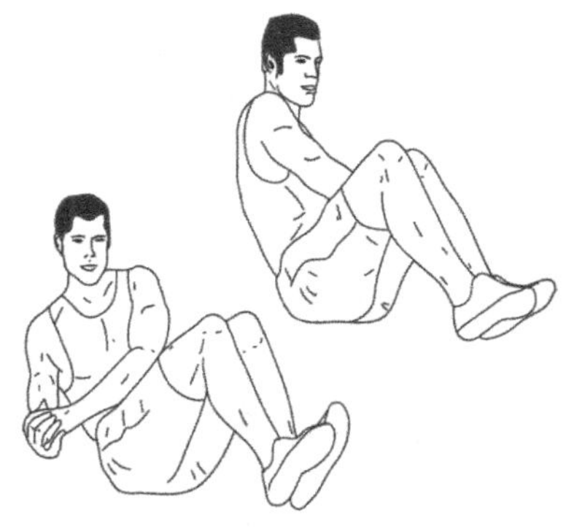

14 sitting twists

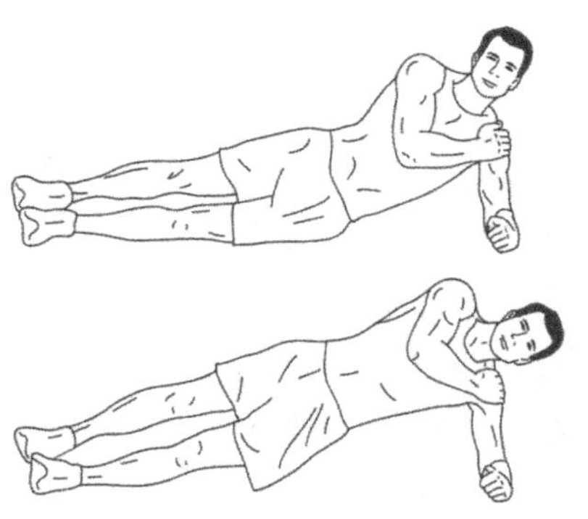

10 side bridges

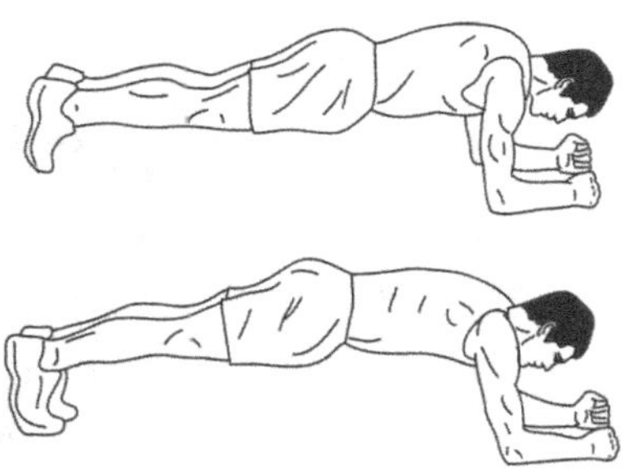

10 body saw

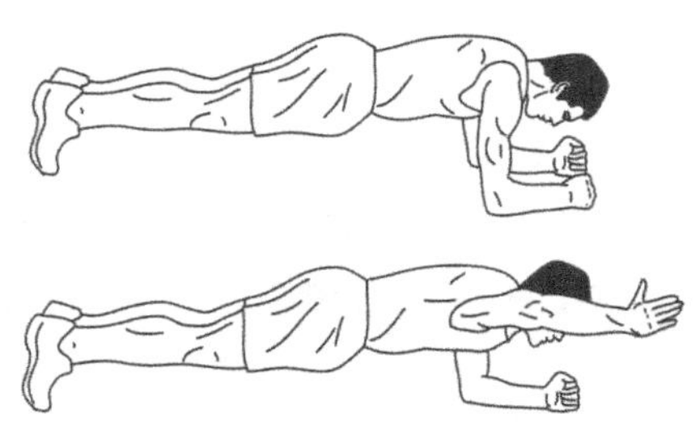

20 plank arm raises

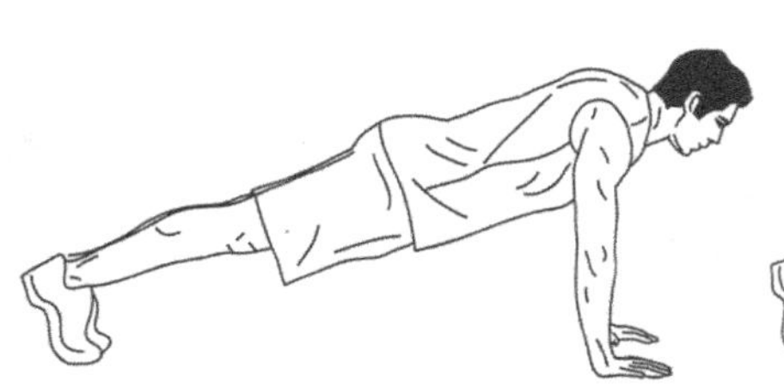

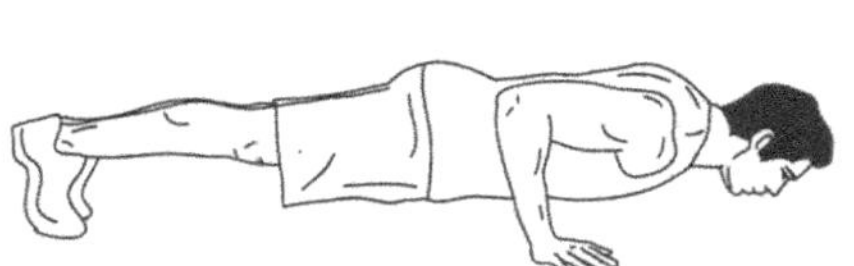

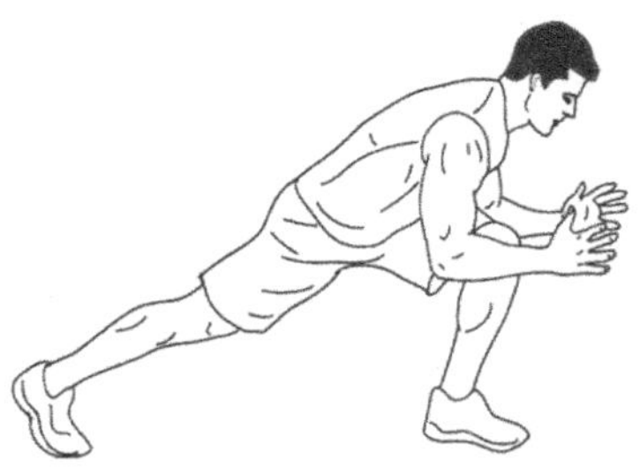

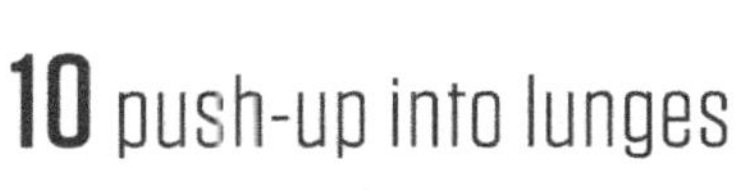

10 push-up into lunges

43 Hello, Abs!

Strong abs change the performance of every physical activity. They facilitate and preserve power transfer from the lower body to the upper one and vice versa. They affect the way we sit and walk, how quickly we tire and even how explosively we can move. Strong abs require almost daily exercise to develop and maintain. The Hello, Abs! workout is your go-to workout for daily abs exercises. You'll be pleasantly surprised by the results.

Hello, abs!

DARBEE WORKOUT © darebee.com

LEVEL I 3 sets **LEVEL II** 4 sets **LEVEL III** 5 sets **REST** up to 2 minutes

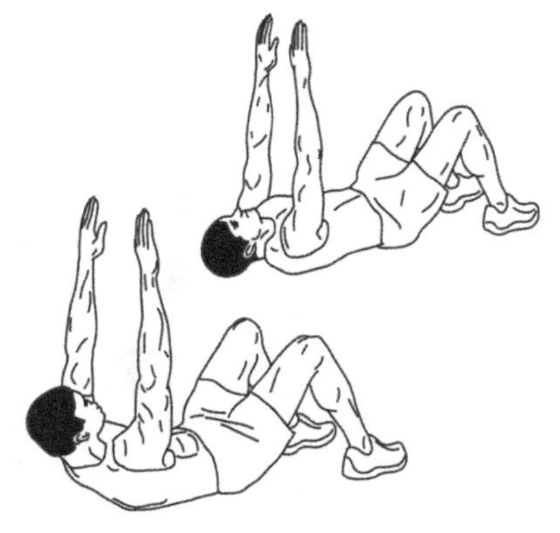

20 high crunches

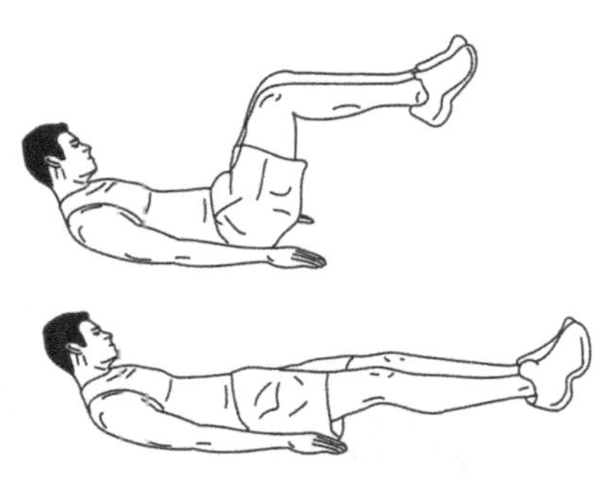

20 crunch kicks

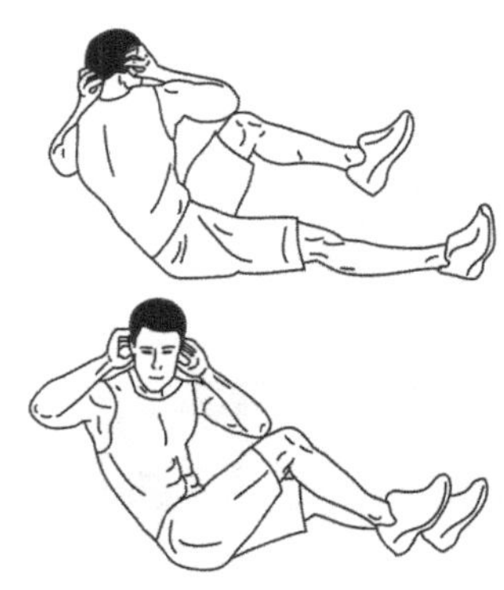

20 knee-to-elbow crunches

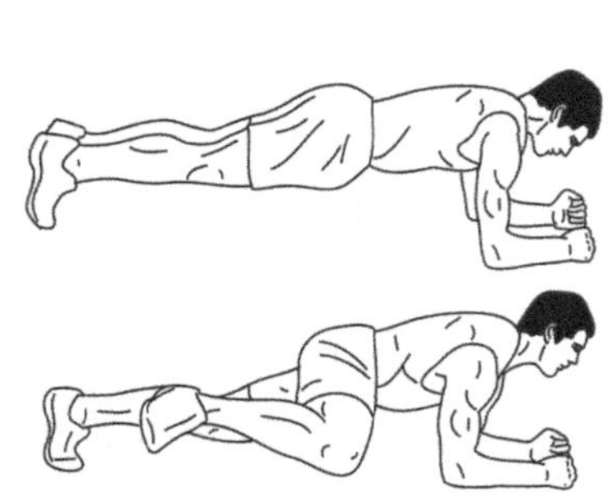

20 plank crunches

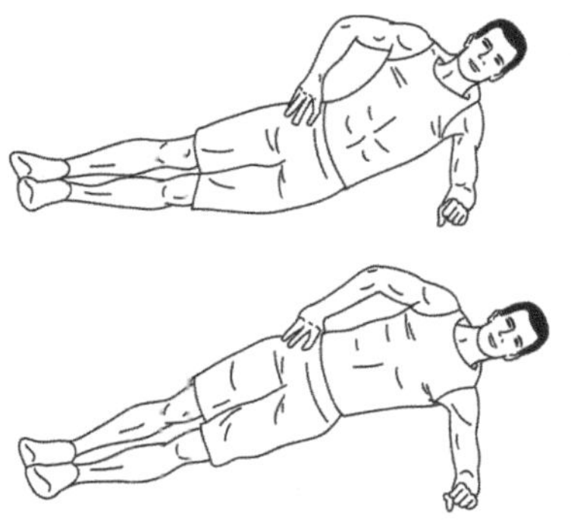

20 side bridges

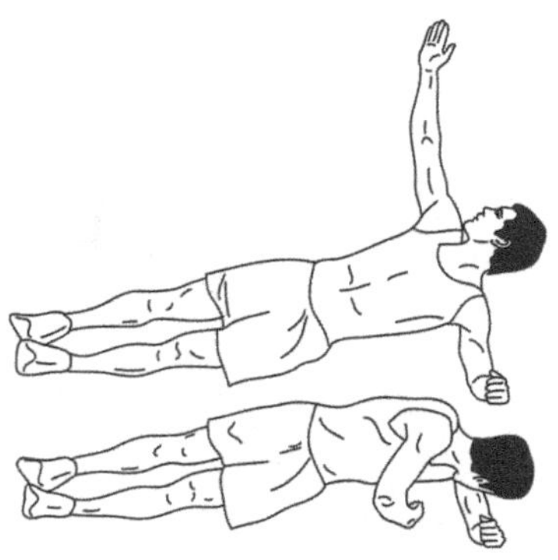

20 side plank rotations

44 Homemade Abs

Abs need constant work in order to be strong, supple and well-defined. The Homemade Abs workout helps you keep your abs in shape by targeting the four major abdominal muscle groups.

homemade abs

DAREBEE WORKOUT © darebee.com

LEVEL I 3 sets **LEVEL II** 4 sets **LEVEL III** 5 sets **REST** up to 2 minutes

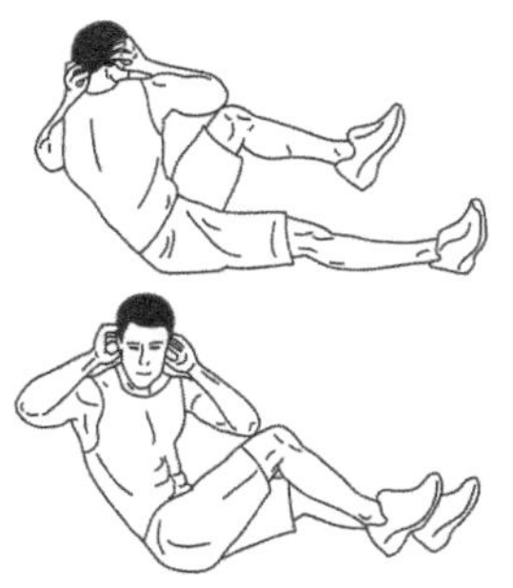

4 knee-to-elbows

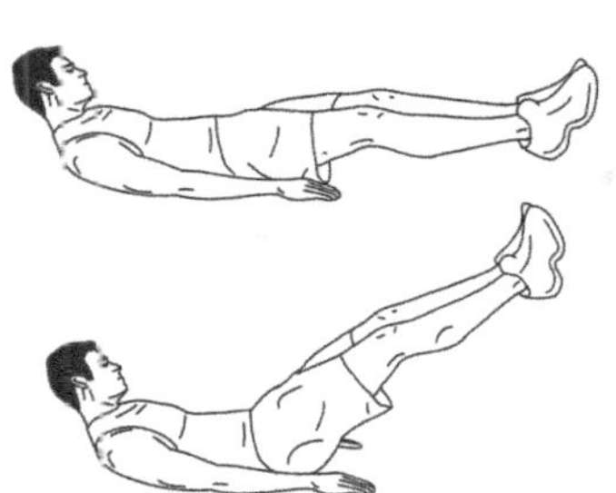

10 leg raises

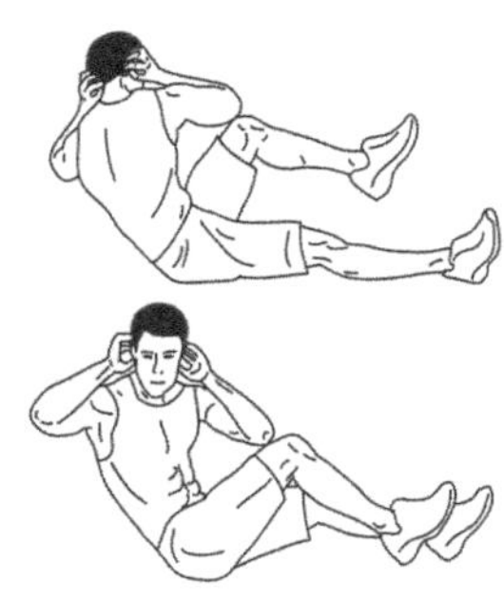

4 knee-to-elbows

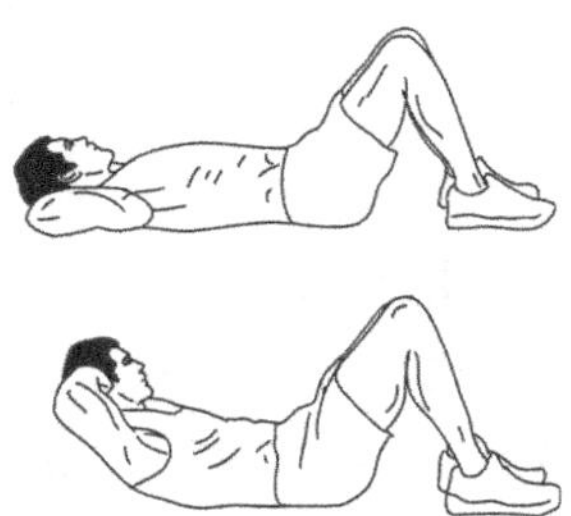

10 crunches

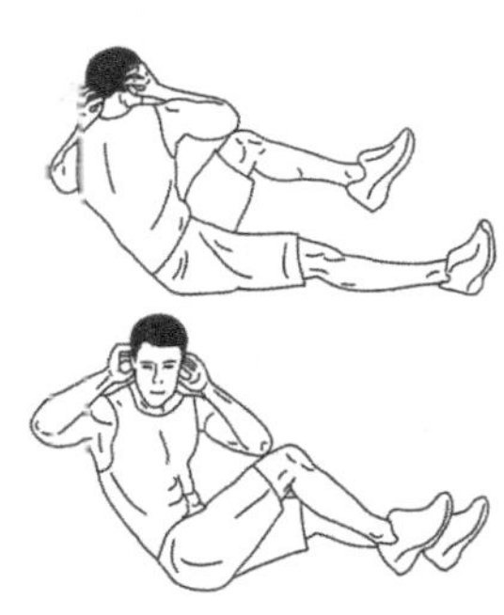

4 knee-to-elbows

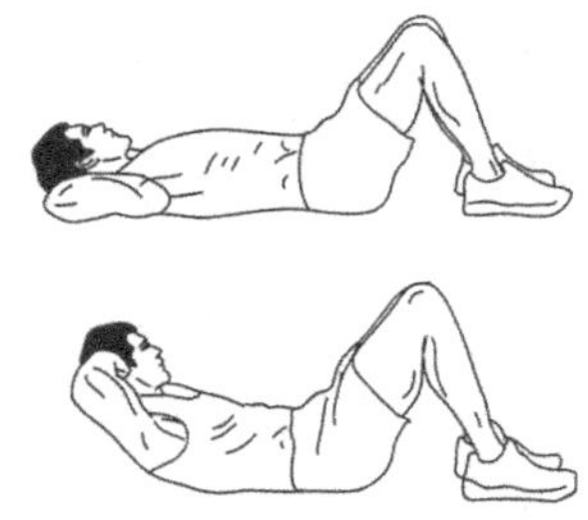

10 crunches

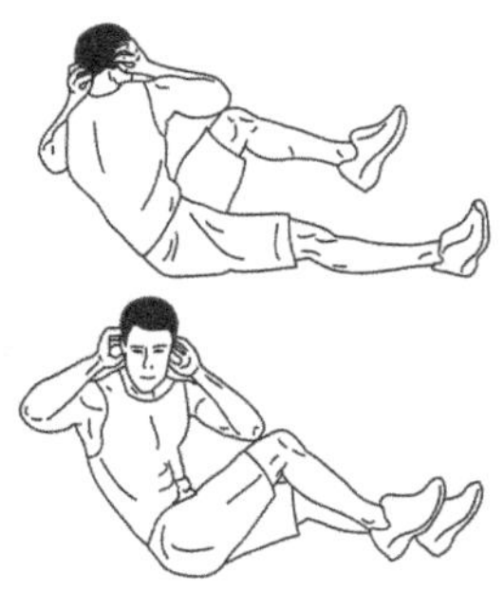

4 knee-to-elbows

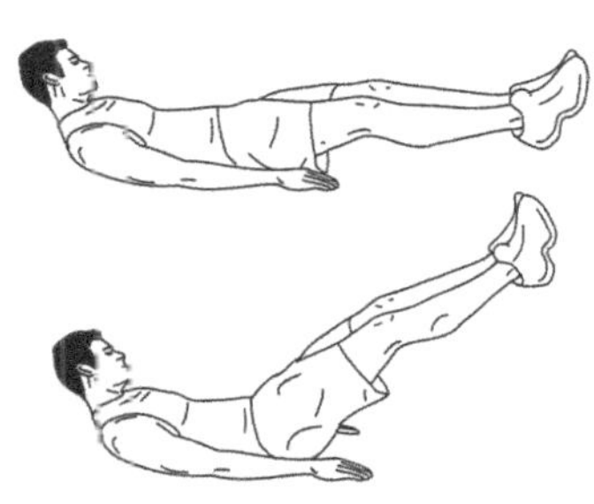

10 leg raises

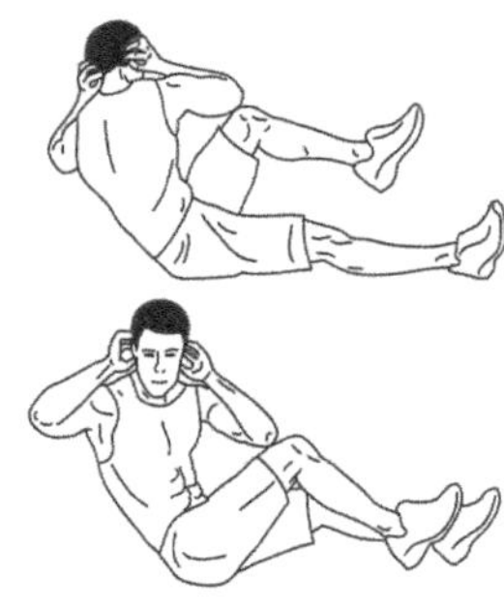

4 knee-to-elbows

45 Ironclad Abs

What you really want to do with your abs is transform them into a wall of protective, empowering muscle. There is no real shortcut you can take here. You need to do the work and feel the results. The Ironclad abs workout is perfect for giving you the results you need.

ironclad abs

BUILD

DARECBEE WORKOUT © darebee.com

LEVEL I 3 sets **LEVEL II** 4 sets **LEVEL III** 5 sets **REST** up to 2 minutes

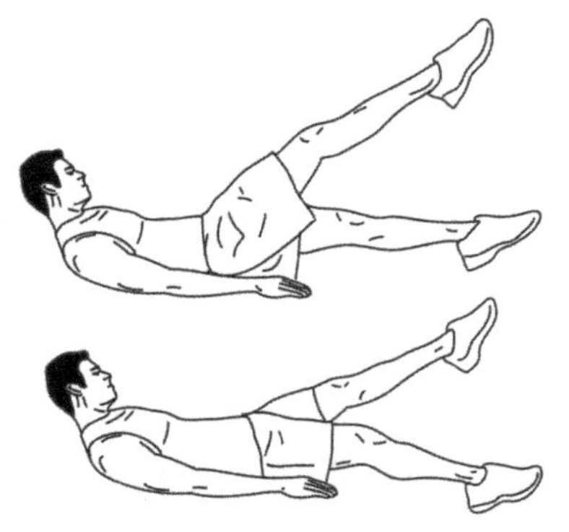

10 flutter kicks

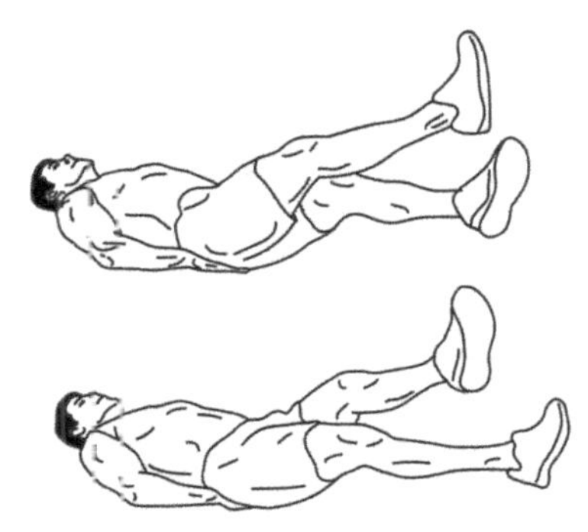

4 scissors

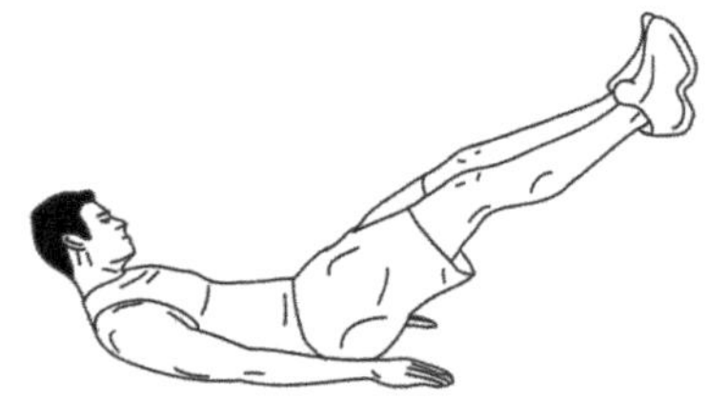

10-count hold

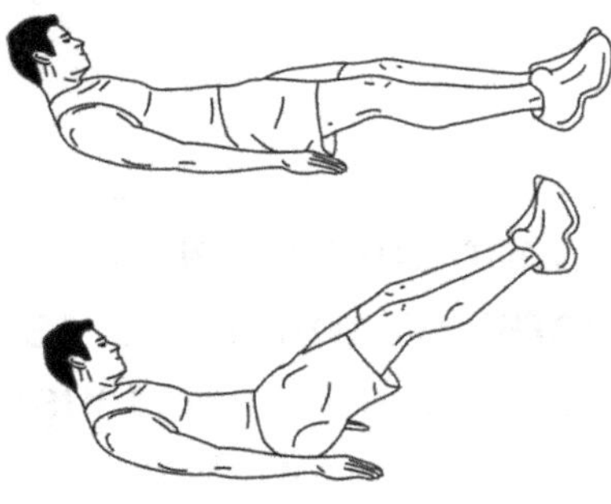

10 leg raises

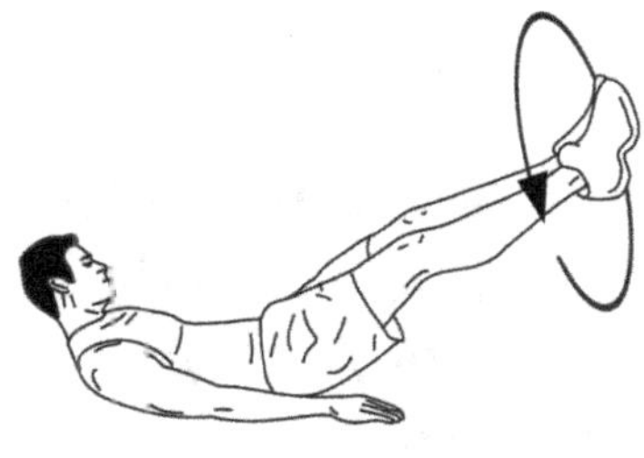

4 raised leg circles

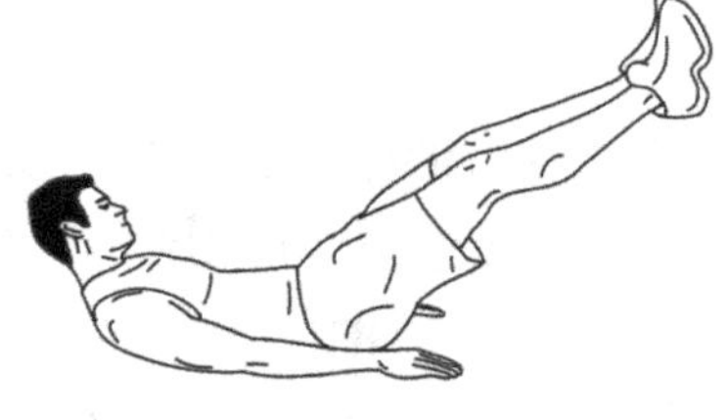

10-count hold

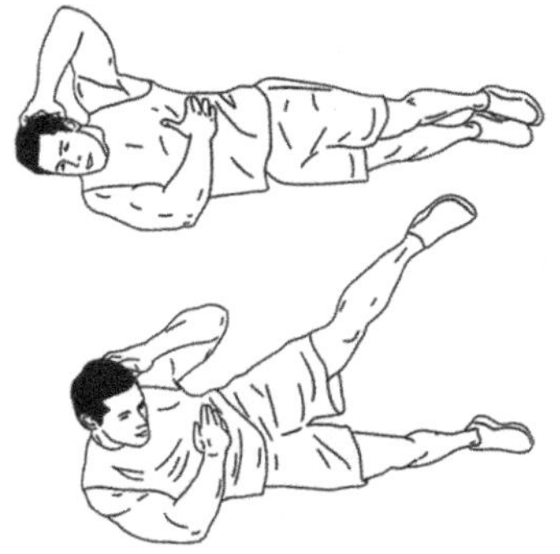

10 jackknives

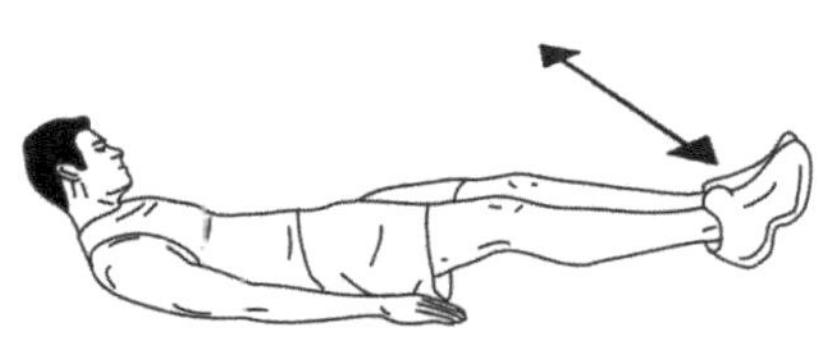

4 raised leg swings

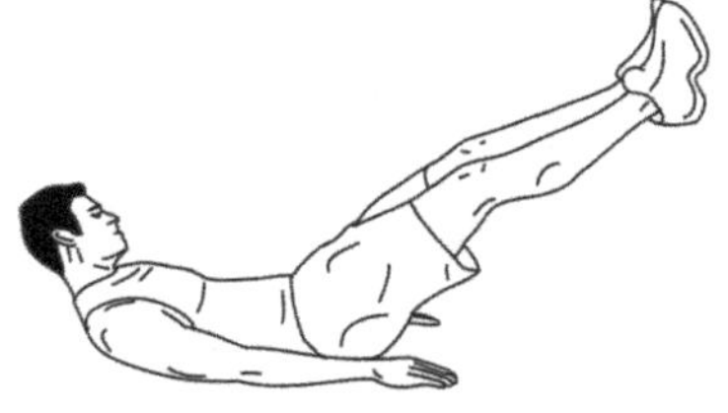

10-count hold

46 Killer Abs

The abdominal muscle groups form one of the most important power cores of the body. Training them has to be a steady, incremental job that requires patience and persistence. The Killer Abs workout is here to help you do just that. Follow each exercise, pay attention to form. Add perspiration. Your recipe for killer abs is then ready.

killer abs

DAREBEE WORKOUT © darebee.com

LEVEL I 3 sets **LEVEL II** 4 sets **LEVEL III** 5 sets **REST** up to 2 minutes

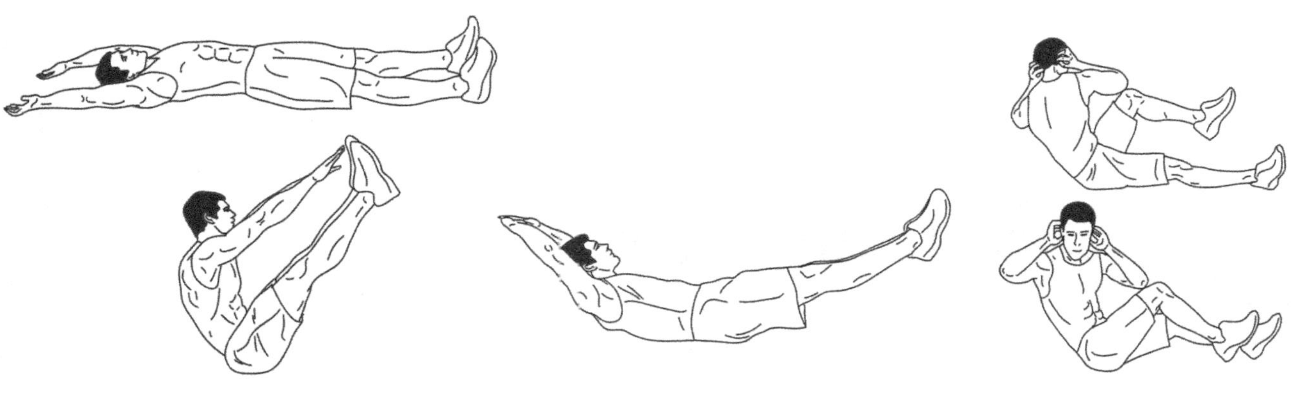

20sec V-ups **20sec** hollow hold **20sec** knee-to-elbow

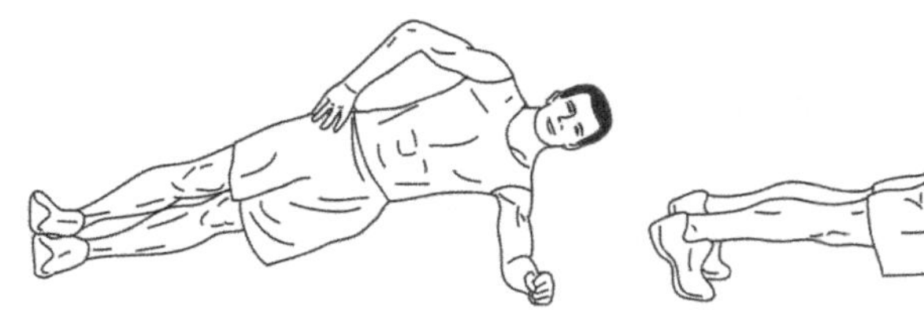

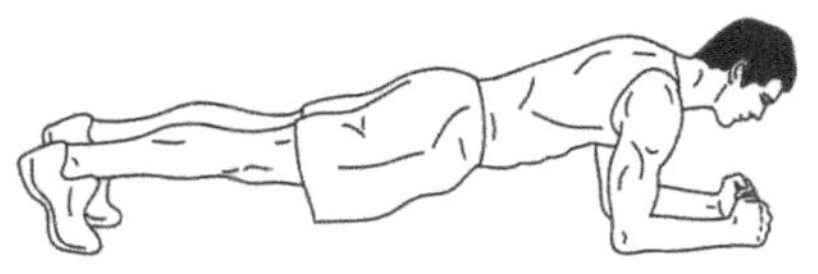

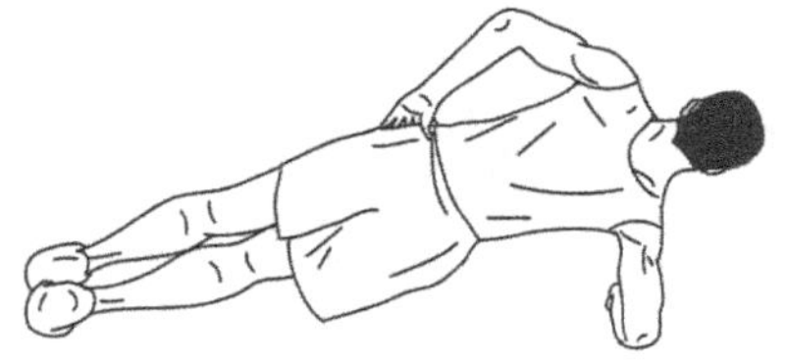

20sec side plank (left) **20sec** elbow plank **20sec** side plank (right)

47 Killer Core

A strong core enables you to do anything that requires balance, distributed load, explosive move or rotational motion, better. This pretty much includes everything. Killer core is a workout that targets your core. You should do it as often as you can. It will change the way your body generates power and then distributes it to the muscles that need it most.

killer core

DAREBEE WORKOUT © darebee.com

LEVEL I 3 sets **LEVEL II** 4 sets **LEVEL III** 5 sets **REST** up to 2 minutes

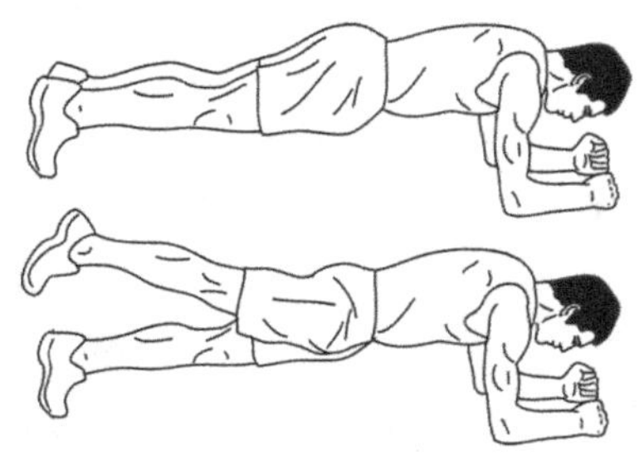

10 plank leg raises

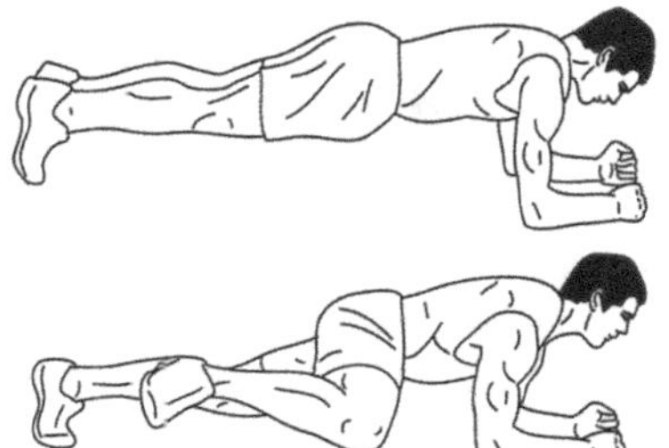

10 plank side crunches

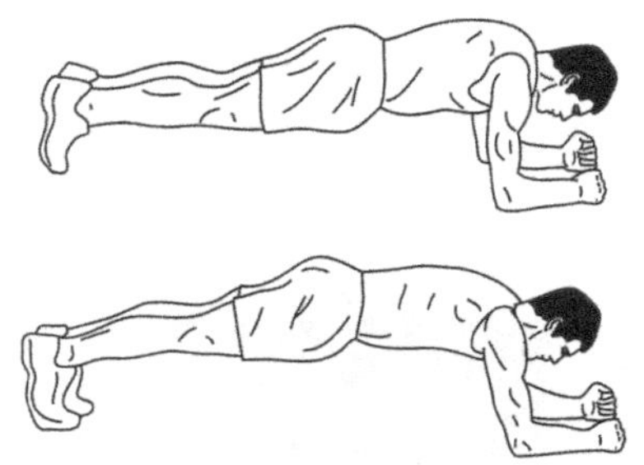

10 body saw

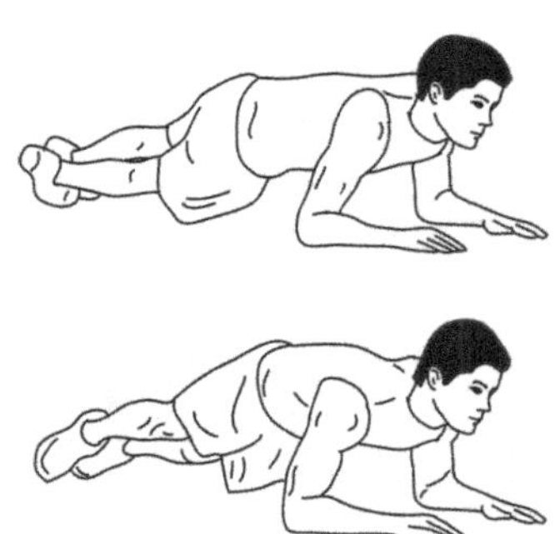

10 plank rolls

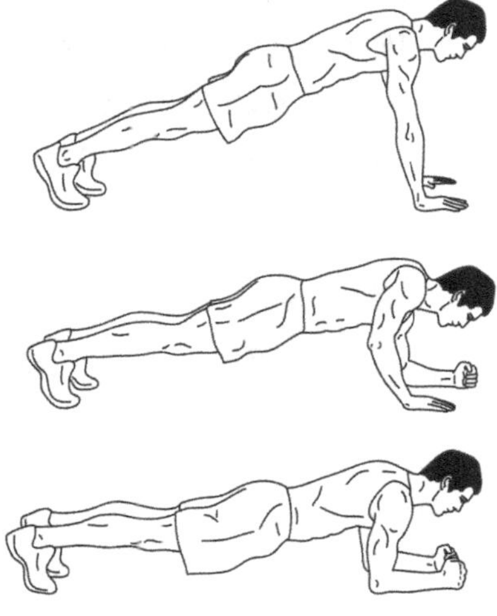

10 up and down planks

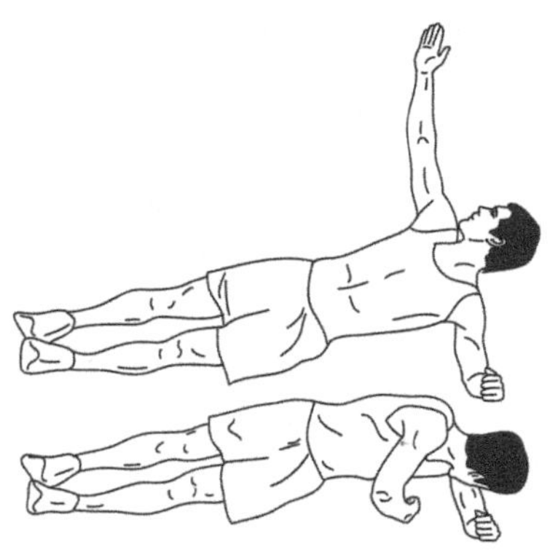

10 side plank rotations

48 Master Pack

When you're talking six-pack you're really talking about more muscle groups than one. The abdominals are made up of four distinct muscle groups: the Transverse Abdominis (also called core), the External Abdominal Obliques, the Internal Abdominal Obliques, the Rectus Abdominis (which also happen to be handily divided into upper and lower abdominals). The Master Pack workout takes care of them all.

Master Pack

LEVEL I 3 sets **LEVEL II** 4 sets **LEVEL III** 5 sets **REST** up to 2 minutes

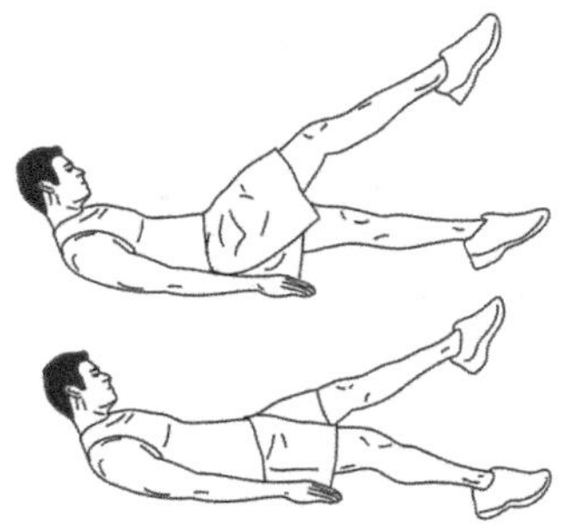

20 flutter kicks

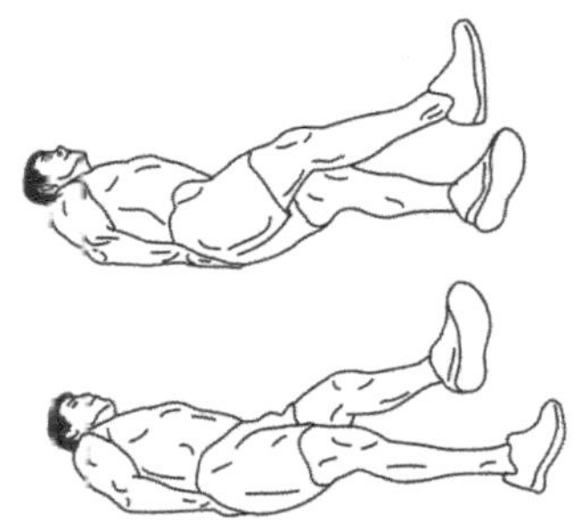

20 scissors

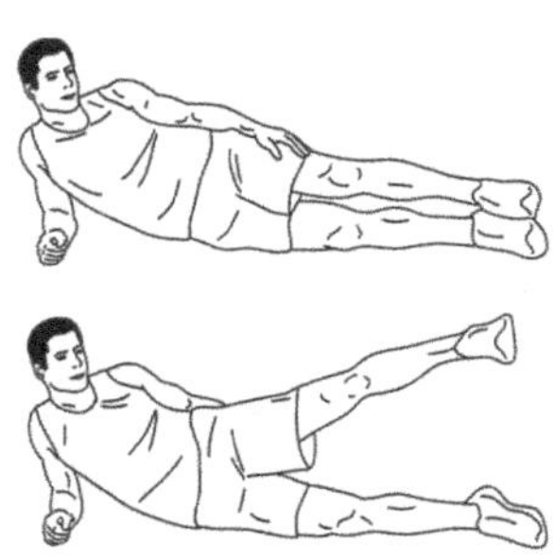

20 side leg raises

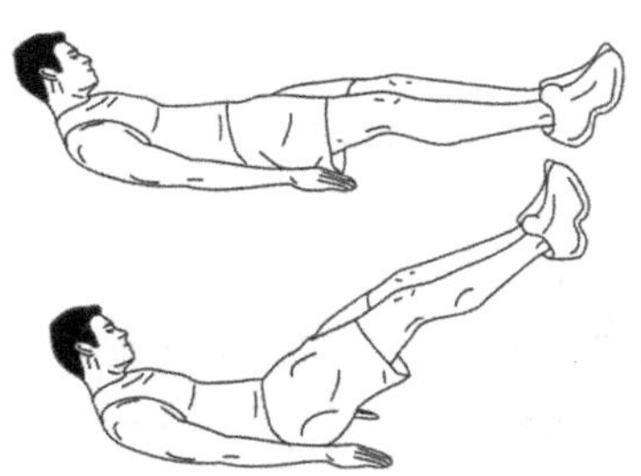

10 leg raises

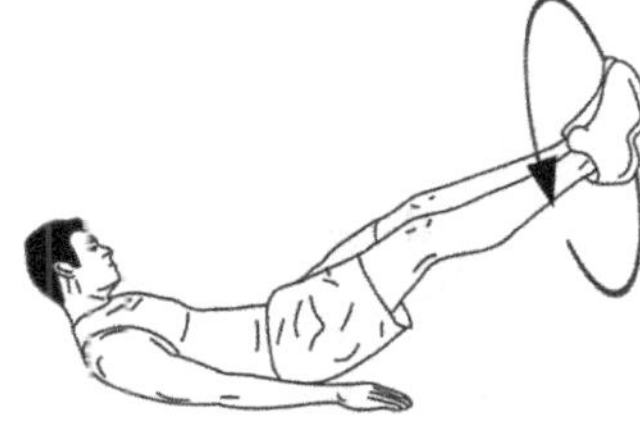

10 raised leg circles

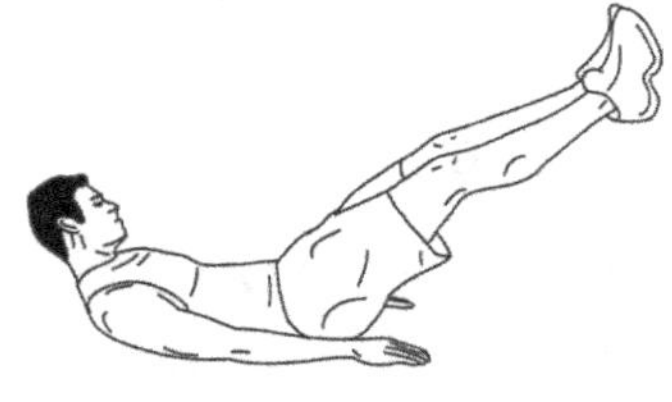

20sec raised leg hold

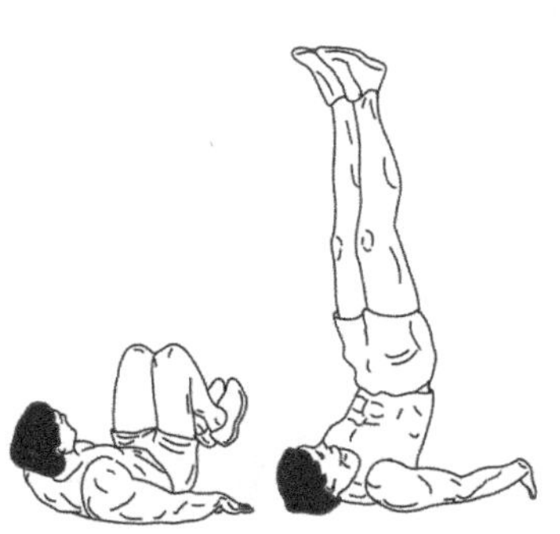

10 butt-ups

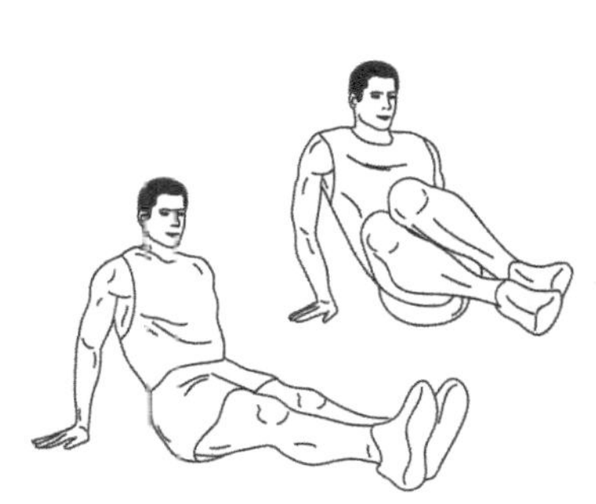

10 knee-in & twist

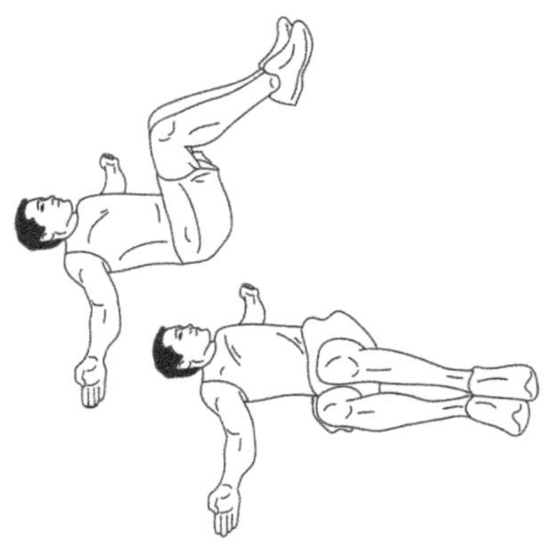

10 half wipers

49 Master Plank

Core work requires time, patience and perseverance. Master Plank is a workout that works the core and abs providing stability and enhanced athletic performance. The Plank, of course, recruits a lot of other muscle groups in a small way which is an additional benefit. It is your core, however, that it will work and it is there that you will feel the benefits of this workout.

MASTER PLANK

DAREBEE WORKOUT © darebee.com

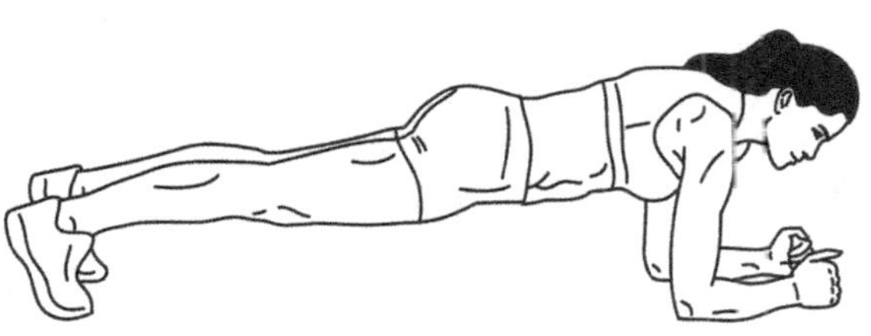

30sec
elbow plank

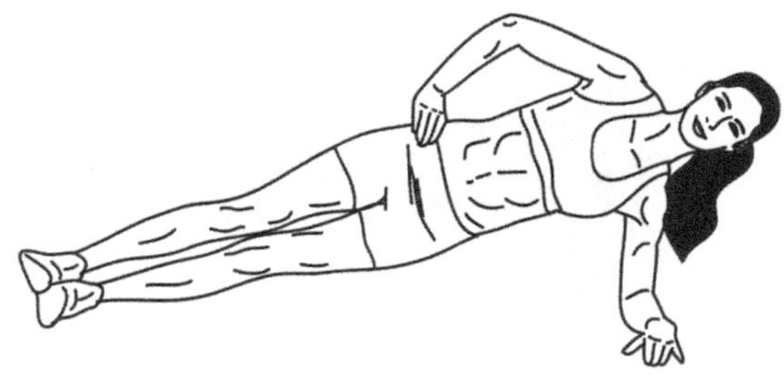

60sec
side elbow plank

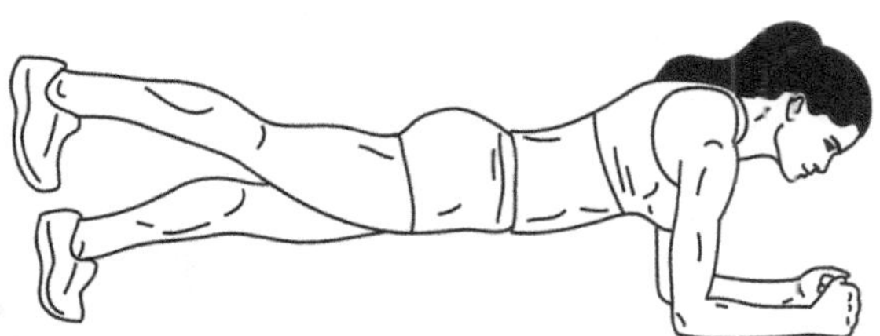

60sec
raised leg elbow plank

30sec
elbow plank

50 Micro Shred

Abs are there to be worked frequently, at an accessible level. Micro Shred is only a difficulty Level II workout but add it to the routines you go to when you're not busy discovering the limits of your physical capability and feel the difference it will make to your basic abs and core strength.

MICRO SHRED

WORKOUT by DAREBEE © darebee.com

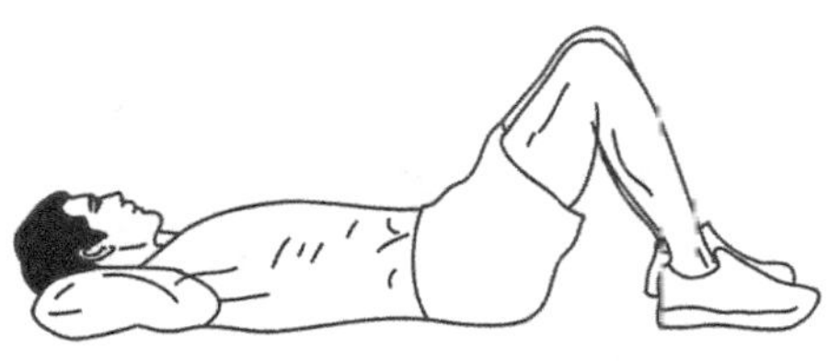

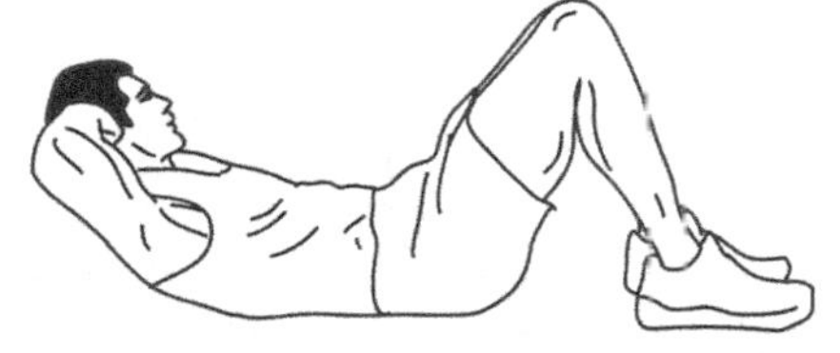

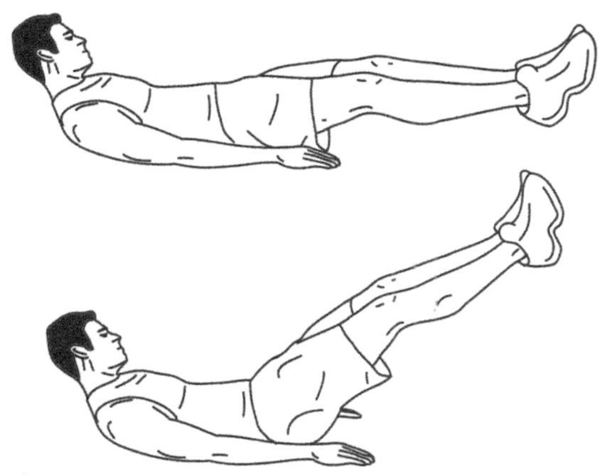

20 crunches

10 leg raises

20 crunches

10 leg raises

20 crunches

10 leg raises

20 crunches

10 leg raises

20 crunches

10 leg raises

done

51 Origami Abs

The abs, really consist of four distinct, inter-related muscle groups of which the frontal abs or Rectus Abdominis is just one and, arguably, the least important (although obviously the most visually pleasing). Origami Abs is the workout that targets all four, giving you the perfect opportunity to improve inside and out, quite literally in this case.

origami abs

DAREBEE WORKOUT © darebee.com

LEVEL I 3 sets **LEVEL II** 4 sets **LEVEL III** 5 sets **REST** up to 2 minutes

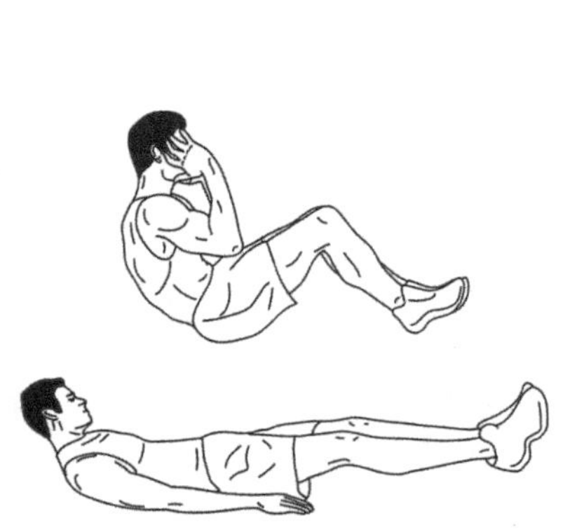

20 sit-up + crunch kick

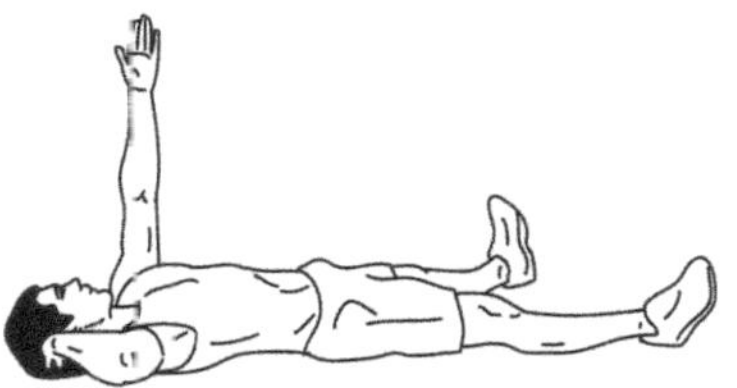

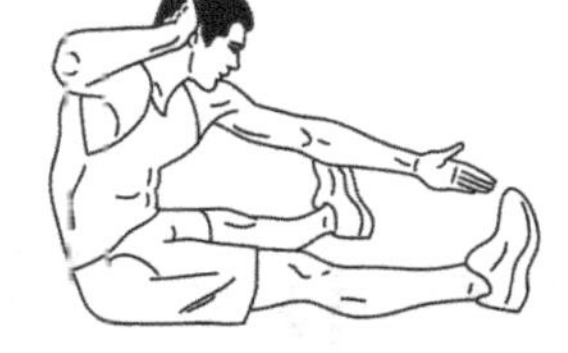

20 sit-up + reach

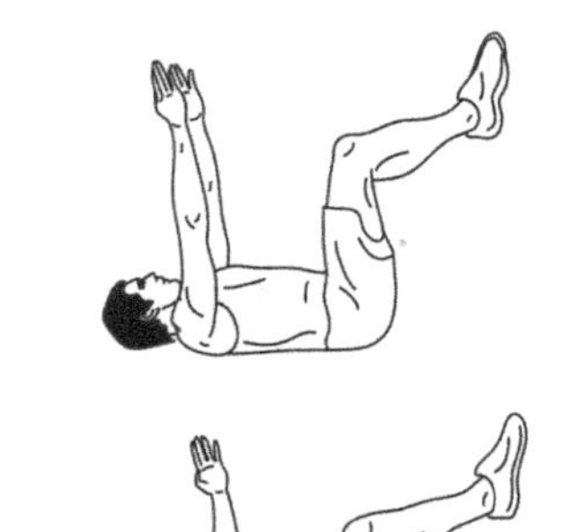

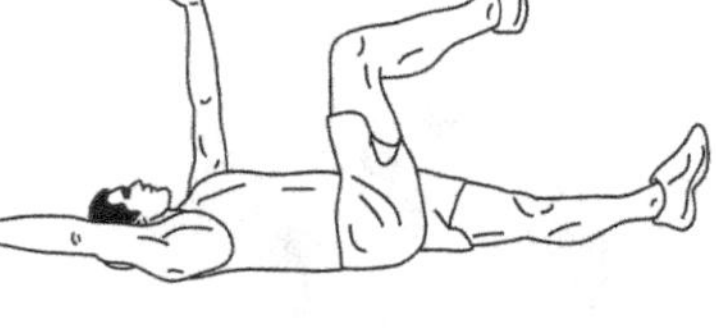

20 dead bug

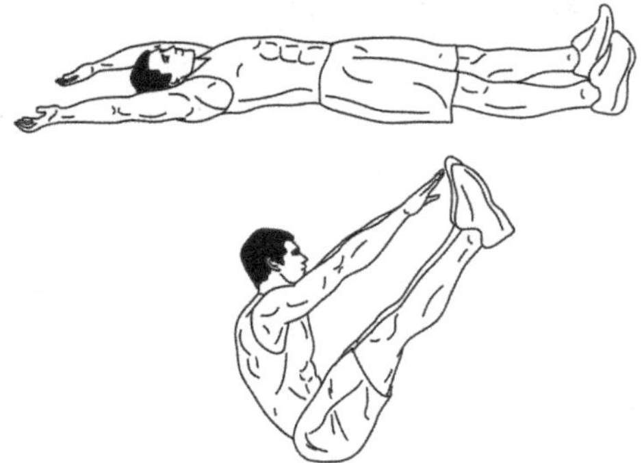

20 V-ups

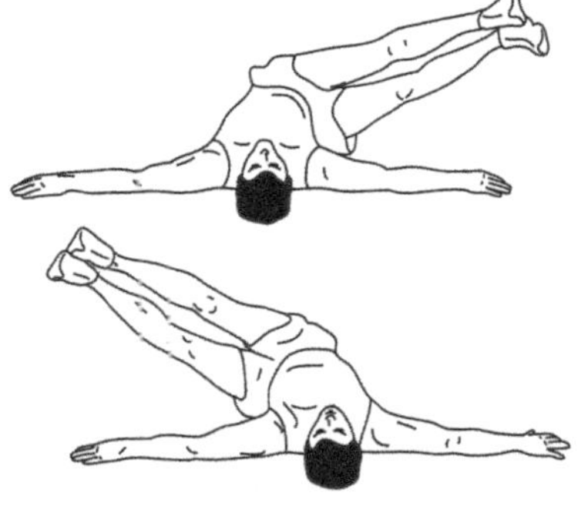

20 windshield wipers

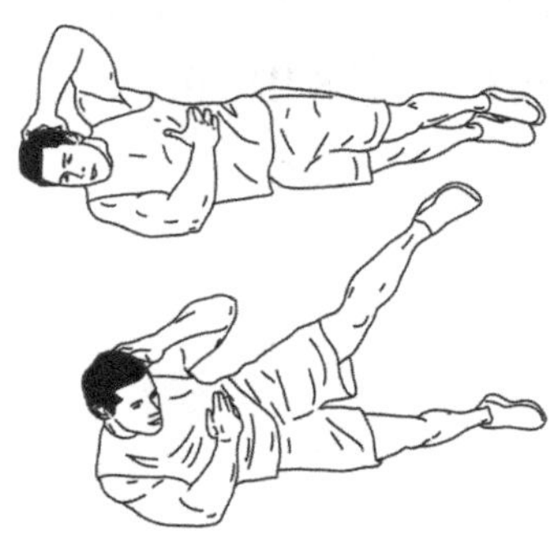

20 side jackknives

52 Shredder Abs

For those days when you really feel like putting your body through some serious ab work, Shredder Ad Edition is the workout you simply wouldn't be able to face yourself in the mirror if you didn't just do it. At least once. In this workout the ab groups are targeted sequentially providing an ever increased load that results in the kind of muscular adaptation response that results in ripped abs.

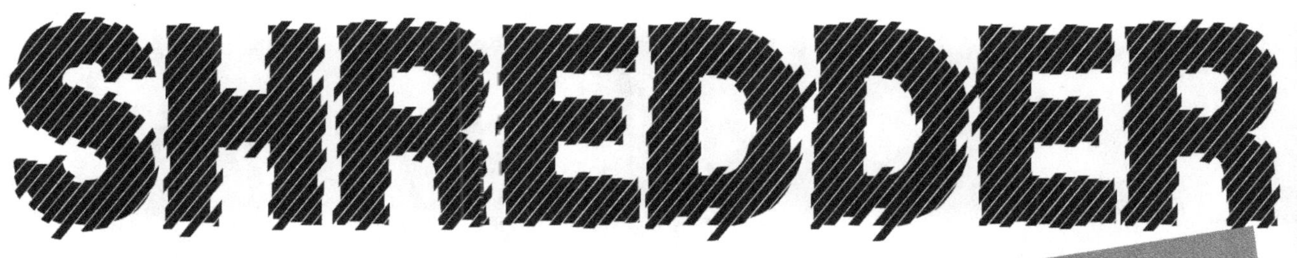

SHREDDER

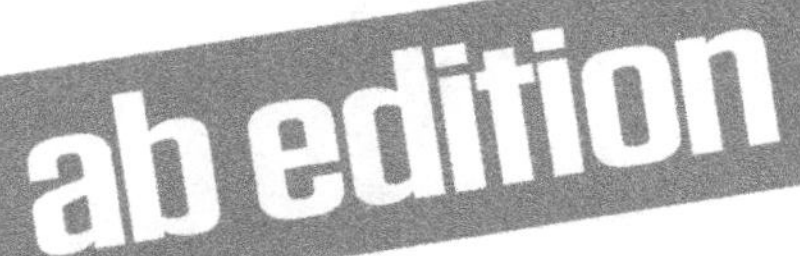

ab edition

DARREBEE WORKOUT © darebee.com
2 minutes rest between exercises

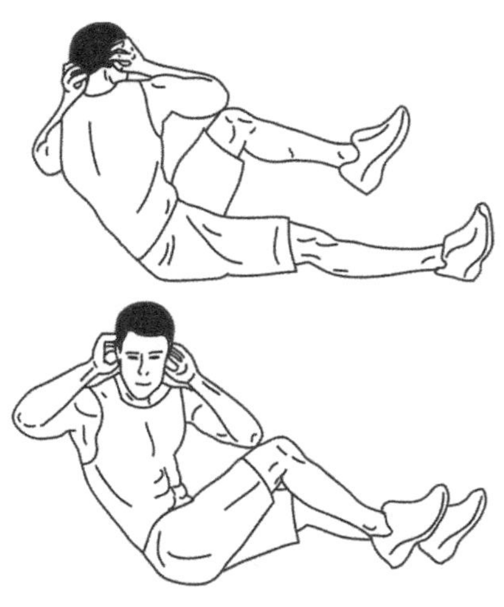

30 knee to elbows **x 3 sets** in total
30 seconds rest between sets

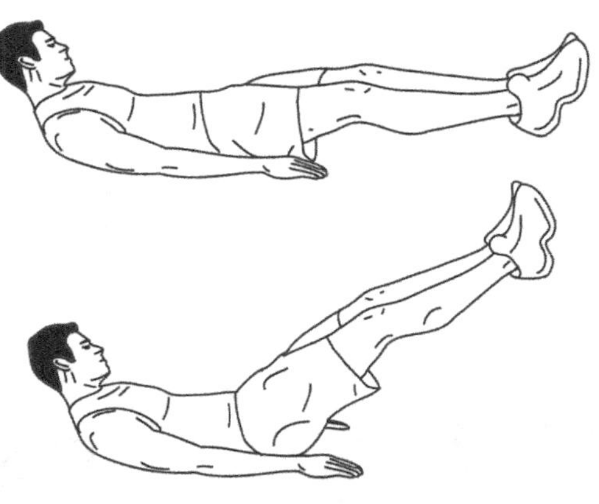

30 leg raises **x 3 sets** in total
30 seconds rest between sets

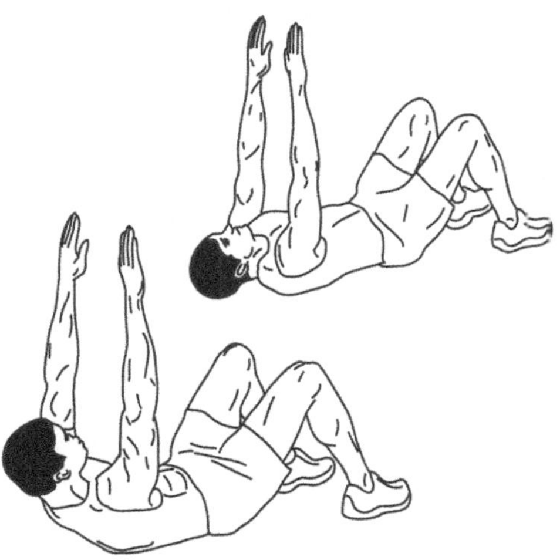

30 high crunches **x 3 sets** in total
30 seconds rest between sets

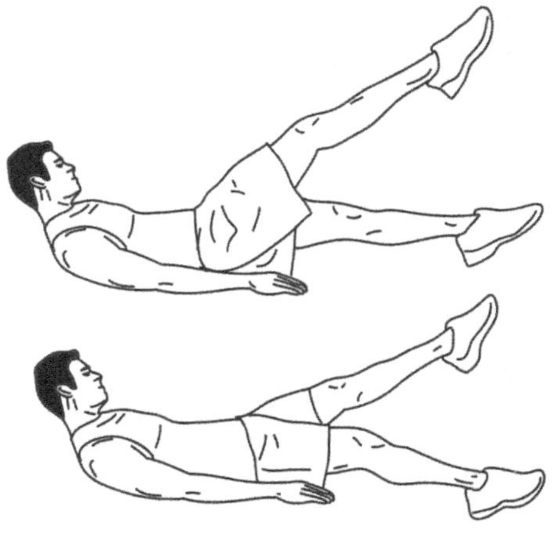

30 flutter kicks **x 3 sets** in total
30 seconds rest between sets

53 Six Pack

The four muscle groups that make up the abdominal muscles help connect the power of the lower body to that of the upper body making us more effective and efficient in just about anything. Six Pack targets just those groups helping make your abs and core stronger.

six pack

DARBEE WORKOUT © darebee.com

LEVEL I 3 sets **LEVEL II** 4 sets **LEVEL III** 5 sets **REST** up to 2 minutes

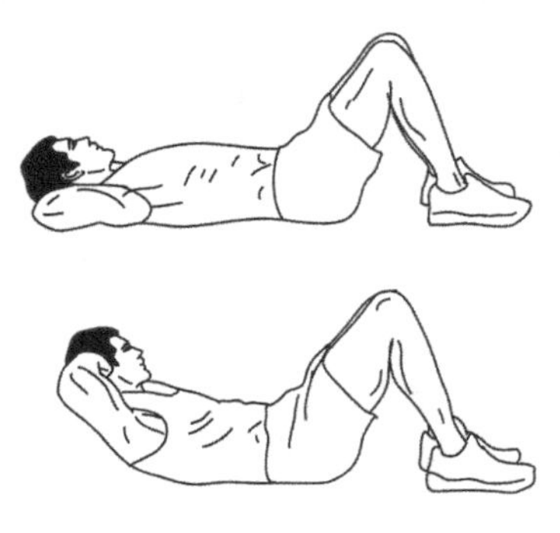

20 crunches

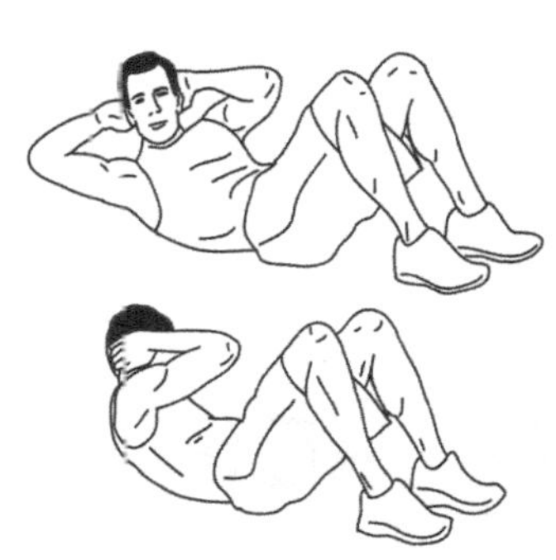

20 cross crunches

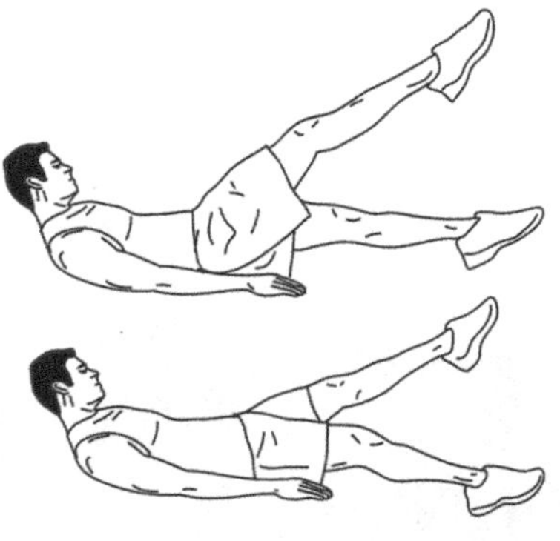

20 flutter kicks

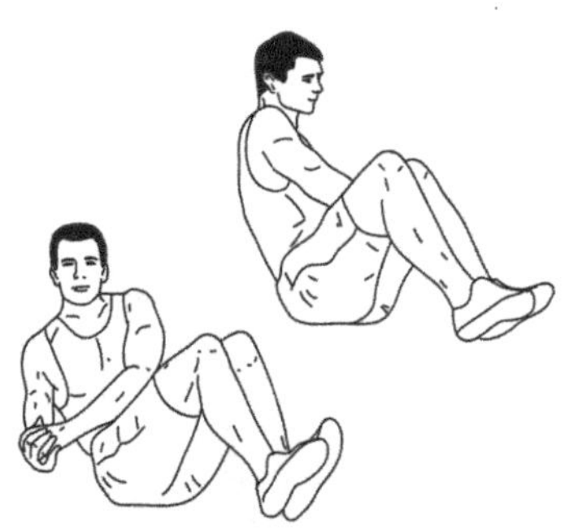

10 sitting twists

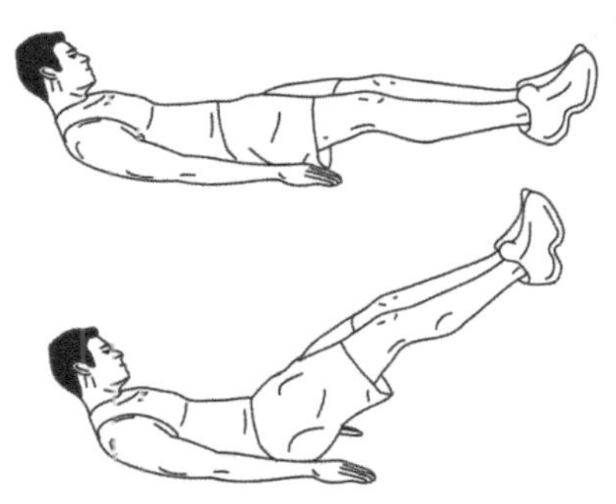

10 leg raises

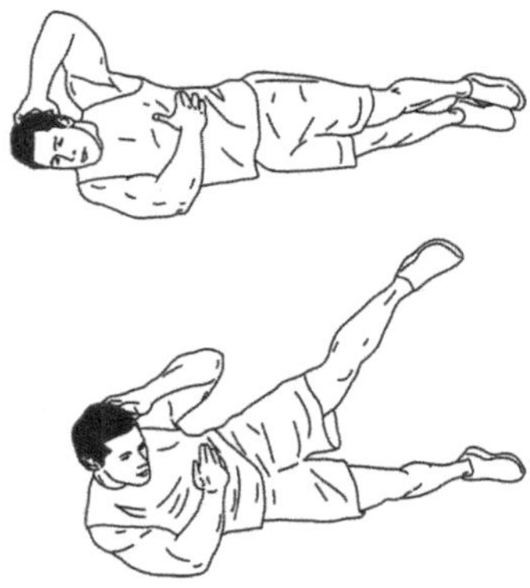

20 side jackknives

54 Sofa Abs

At the end of a busy day, all you want is the chance to put work out of your mind, land on the sofa, turn the telly on and ... work your abs. The sofa's your gym. Your body is your equipment. This is the Sofa Abs workout. If you're on the sofa, it's time to work your abs.

sofa **abs**

BUILD

DARBEE WORKOUT © darebee.com

LEVEL I 3 sets **LEVEL II** 4 sets **LEVEL III** 5 sets **REST** up to 2 minutes

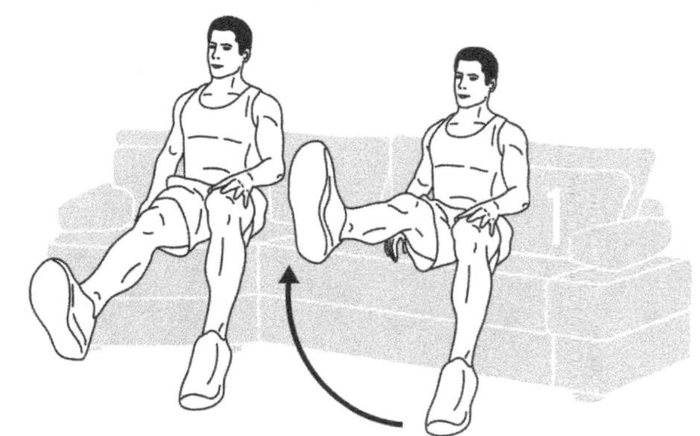

20 leg swings

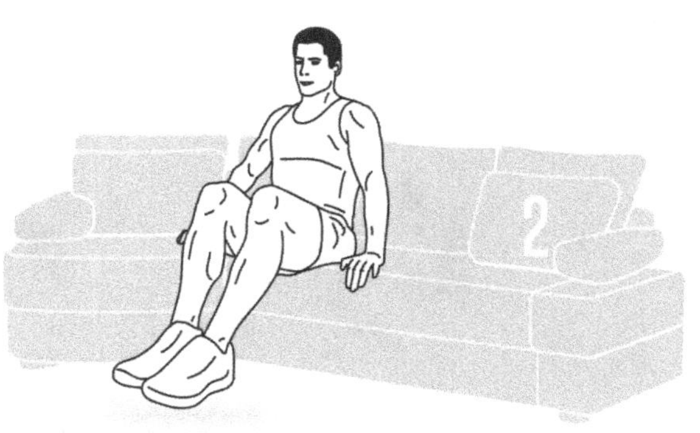

20-count raised knees hold

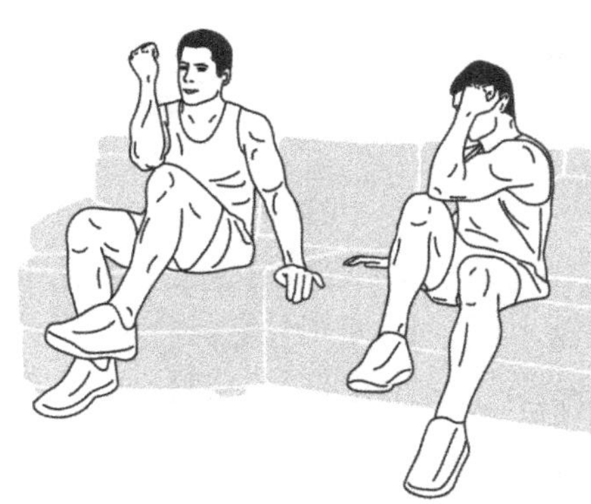

20 knee to elbows

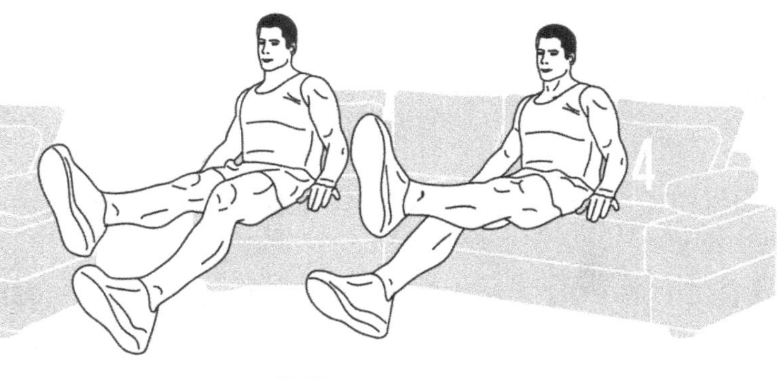

20 flutter kicks

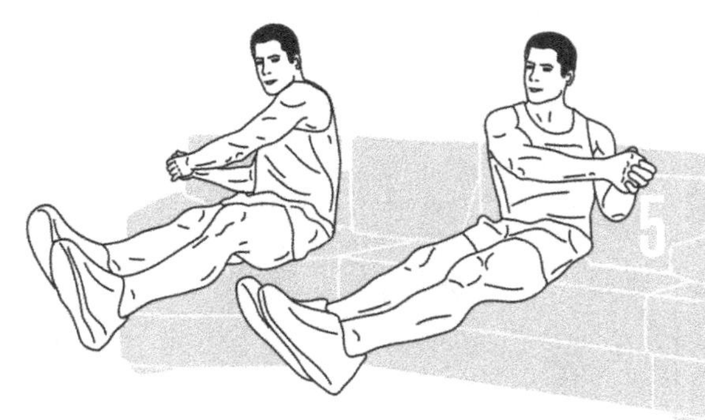

10 raised legs twists

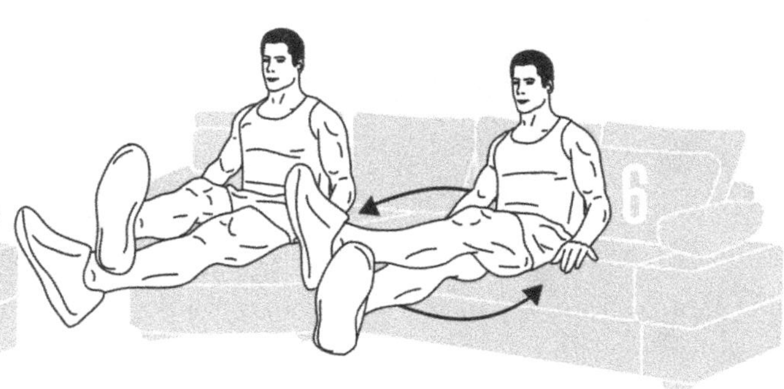

10 scissors

55 Supercut Abs

Supercut Abs targets all four muscle groups of the abdominal muscle wall and it also does not neglect your lower back, arms and shoulders. Do it every time you want to work your abs for strength and endurance. It will also help increase core stability, balance and help with definition. Strong, balanced abs help in generating power in ballistic movements, they better connect the lower and upper body and help improve posture and even increase endurance.

supercut abs

BUILD

DARebee WORKOUT © darebee.com

LEVEL I 3 sets **LEVEL II** 4 sets **LEVEL III** 5 sets **REST** up to 2 minutes

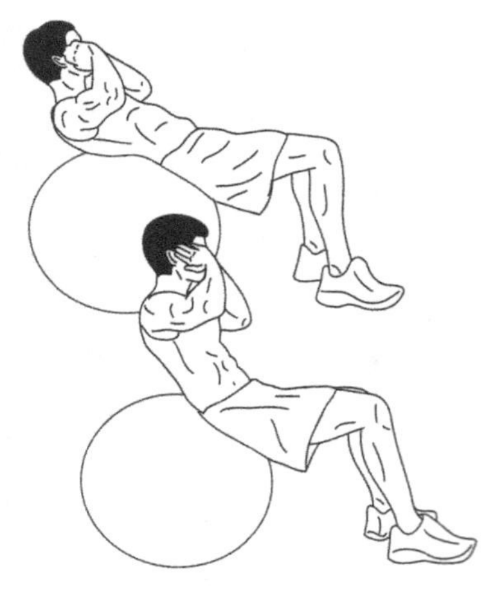

20 crunches

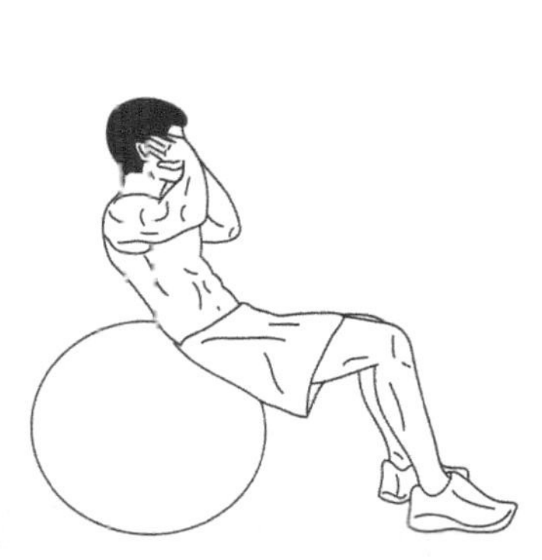

20-count crunch hold

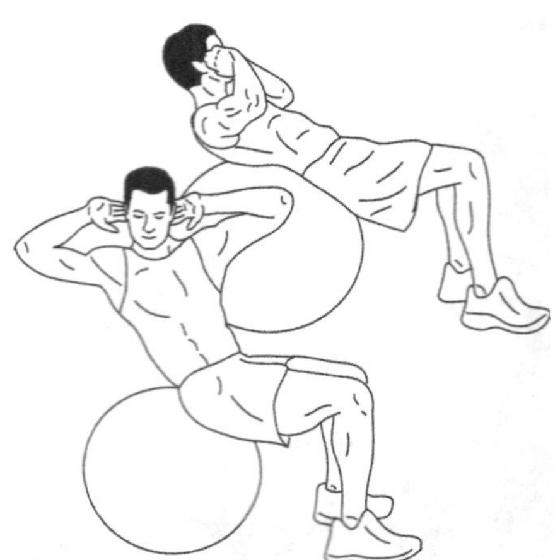

20 cross crunches

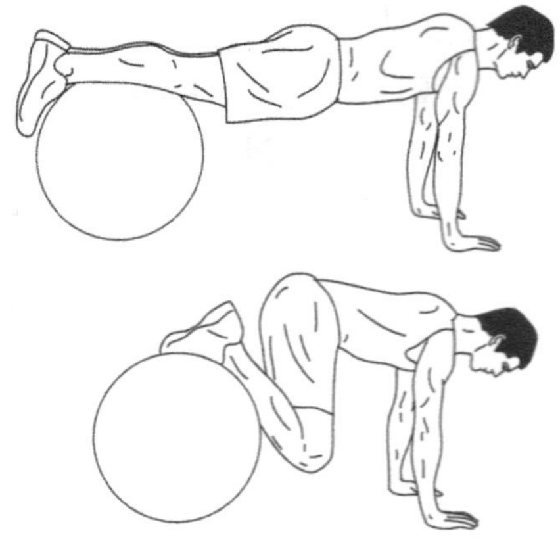

10 reverse crunches

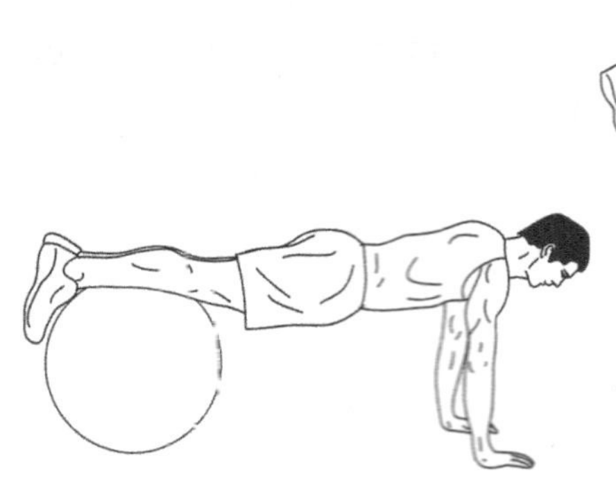

10-count plank

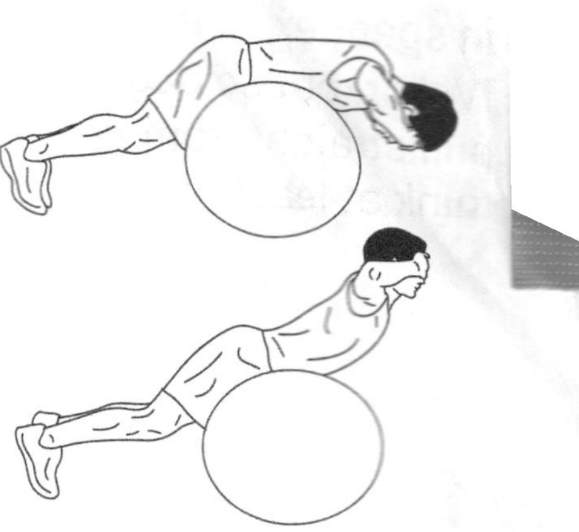

10 back extensions

56 Superhero Abs

Superheroes battle evil and fight for good and it's almost a full-time job, but in their spare time they work on their abs (com'on you must have noticed!). To sport the kind of rippling, taut ab wall look that just pops when dressed in spandex, you need the Superhero Abs workout. This is a difficulty Level IV workout so beginners needn't apply (then again Superhero ranks never pull straight from beginners). Make this part of your regular workouts - think at least once a week, maybe more.

superhero abs

DARεBEE WORKOUT © darebee.com
60 seconds rest between exercises

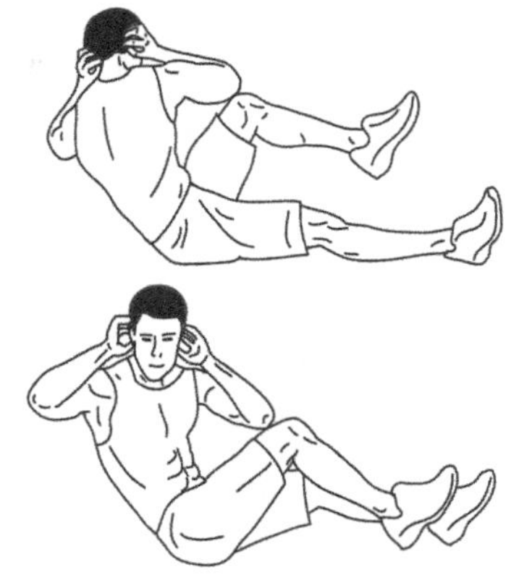

20 knee-to-elbow crunches **x 4 sets**
20 seconds rest between sets

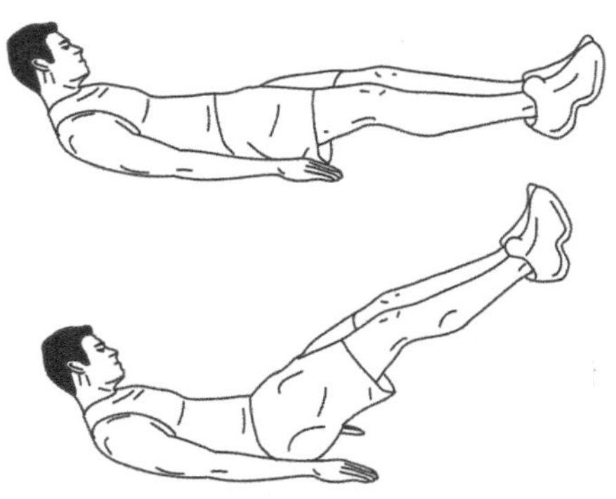

20 leg raises **x 4 sets**
20 seconds rest between sets

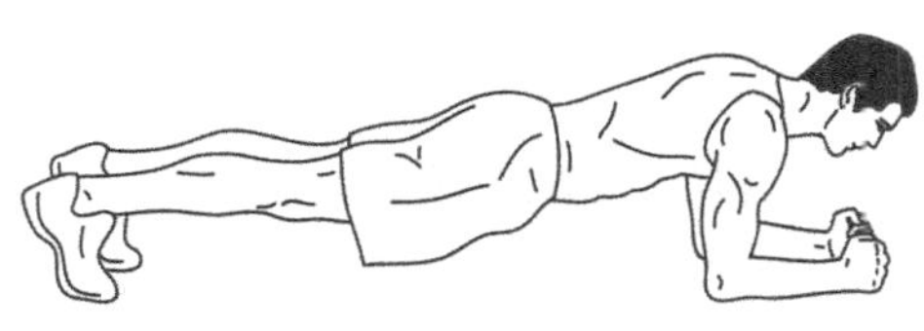

2 minutes elbow plank ho d
repeat once

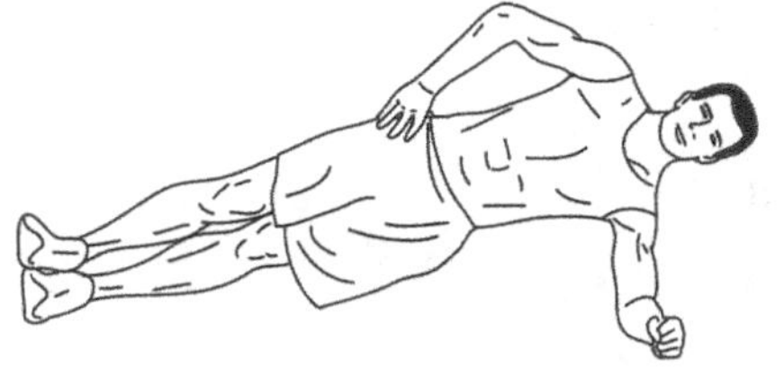

2 minutes side elbow plank
one minute per side | repeat once

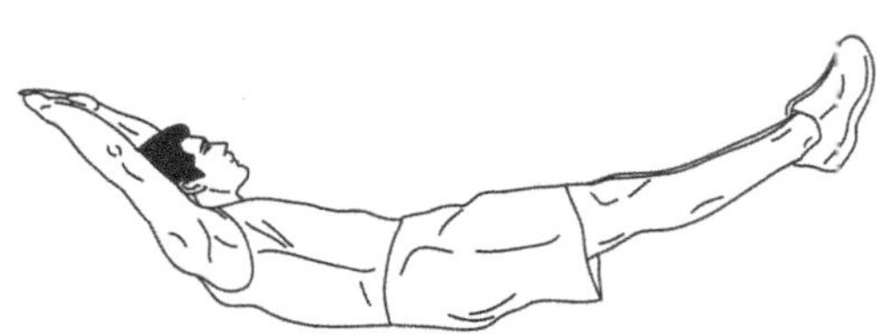

2 minutes hollow hold
repeat once

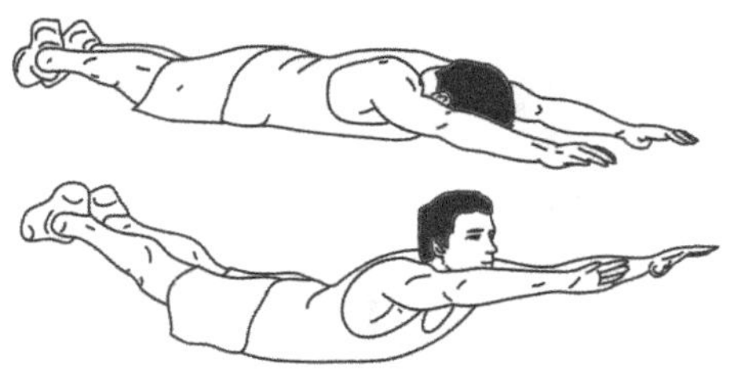

10 superman stretches **x 4 sets**
20 seconds rest between sets

57 Total Abs

A strong abdominal wall is your secret weapon. Not only does it make you feel good and look good but it becomes a performance multiplier in everything you do. Because the abs are used to transfer power from the lower body to the upper body and vice versa, a strong abdominal wall enables this to happen with the minimum amount of loss. When you have ripped abs, therefore, you run faster, lift better, feel stronger and look good naked. Totally unfair, right?

total abs

DAREBEE WORKOUT © darebee.com

LEVEL I 3 sets **LEVEL II** 4 sets **LEVEL III** 5 sets **REST** up to 2 minutes

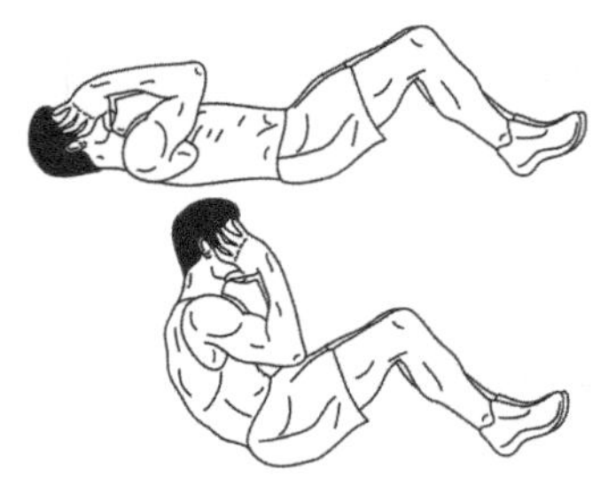

20 sit-ups

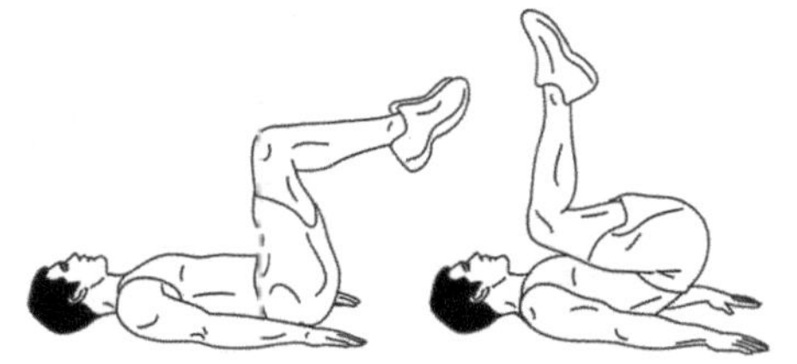

20 reverse crunches

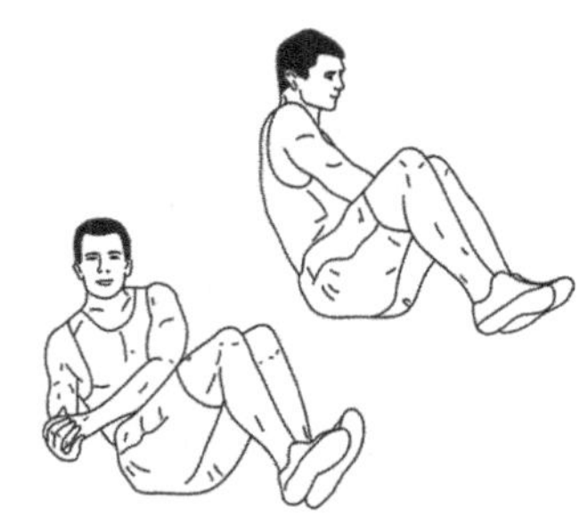

20 sitting twists

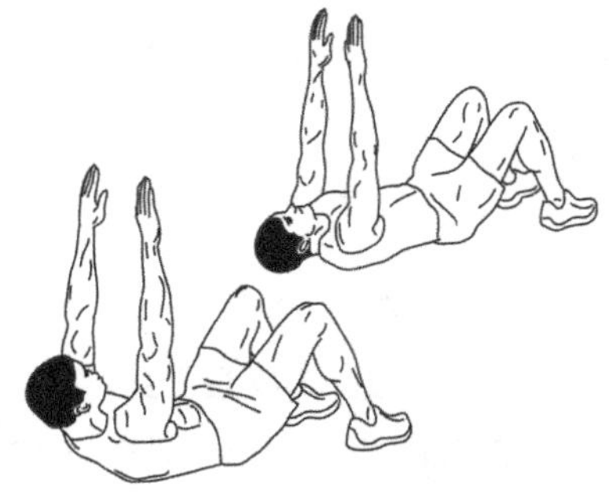

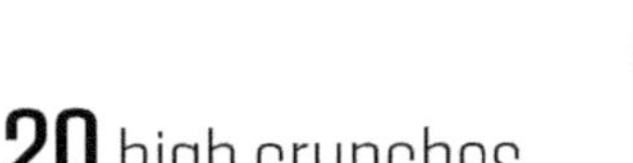

20 high crunches

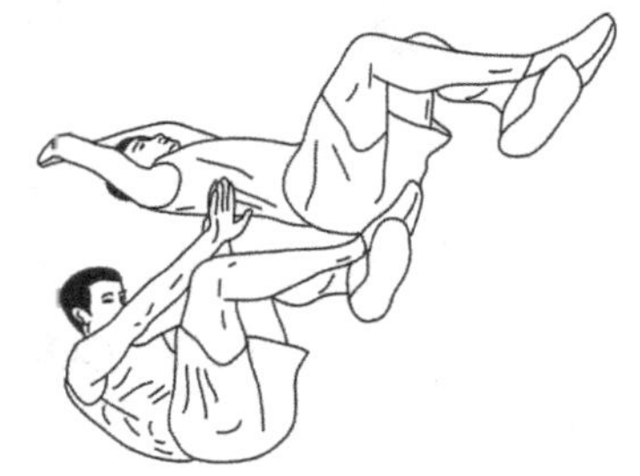

20 knee crunches

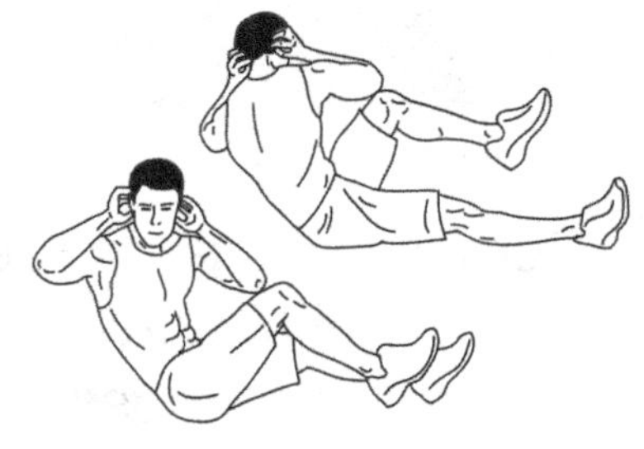

20 knee-to-elbow crunches

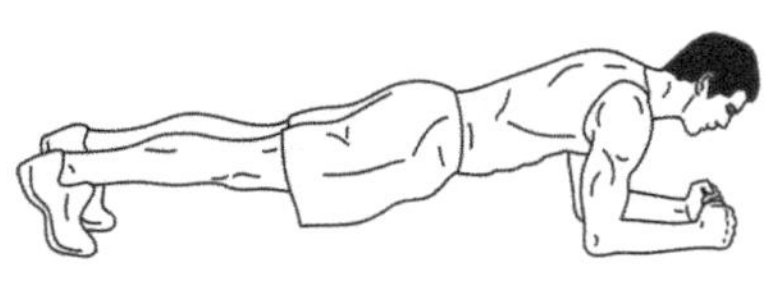

20sec elbow plank

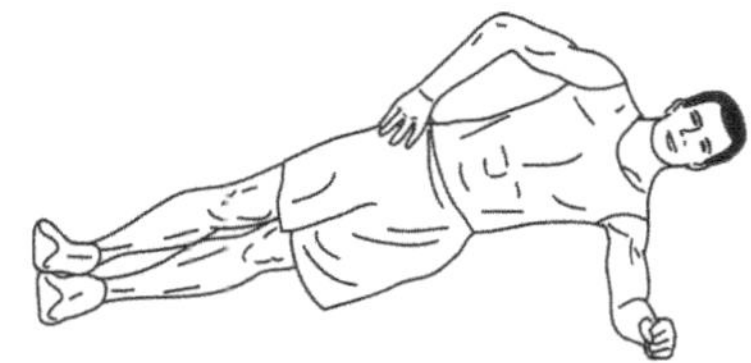

20sec side elbow plank

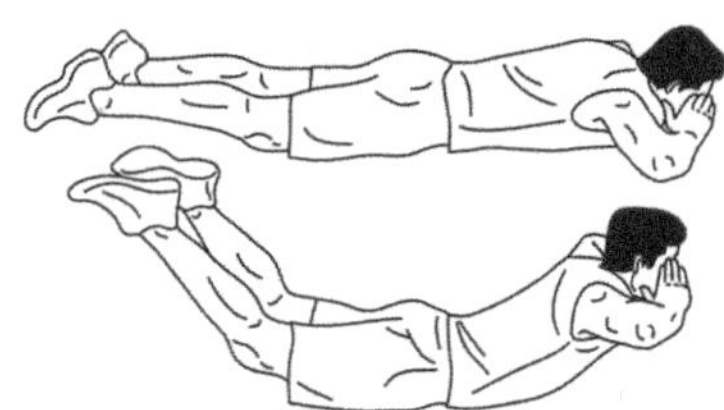

5 back extensions

58 Tough Cookie

Get your abs and core screaming with the Tough Cookie workout. This recipe will require an ton of iron will, ten scoops of resolve and a dash of pure stubbornness. Keep your plank up all the way throughout for the best results.

TOUGH COOKIE

DAREBEE WORKOUT © darebee.com

LEVEL I 3 sets **LEVEL II** 4 sets **LEVEL III** 5 sets **REST** up to 2 minutes

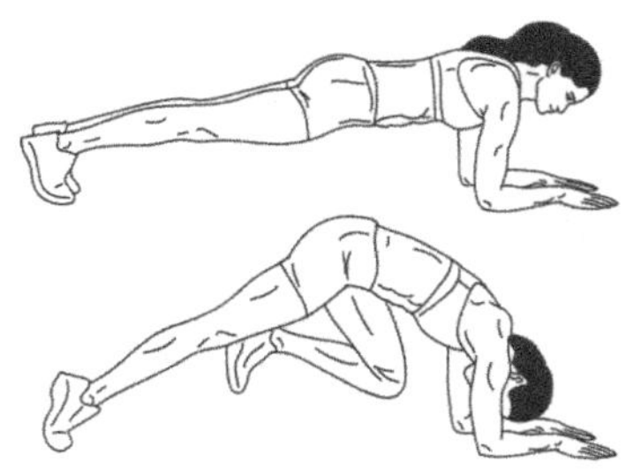

12 plank knee-ins

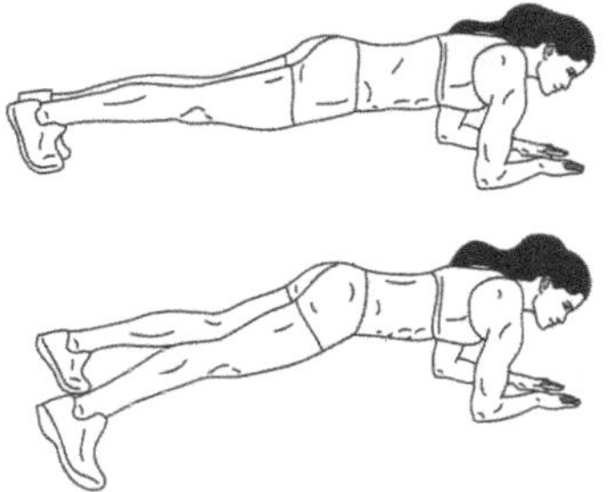

12 plank step-outs

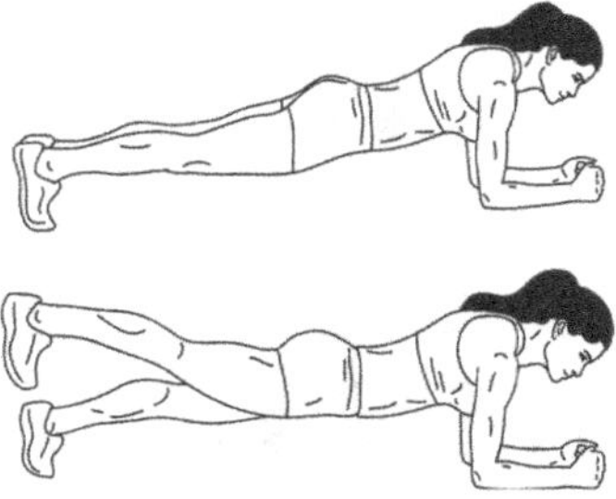

12 plank leg raises

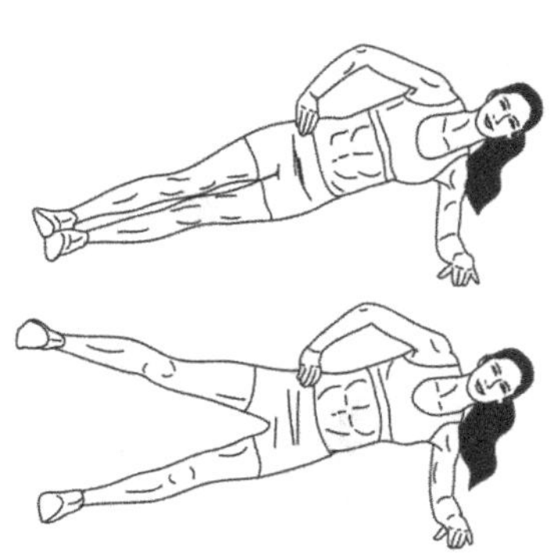

12 side plank leg raises

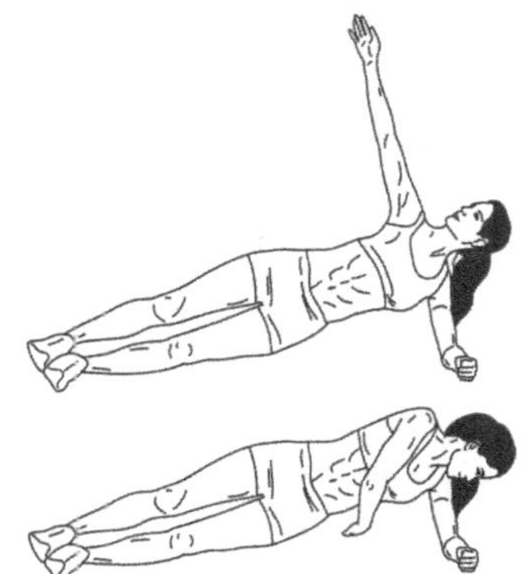

12 side plank rotations

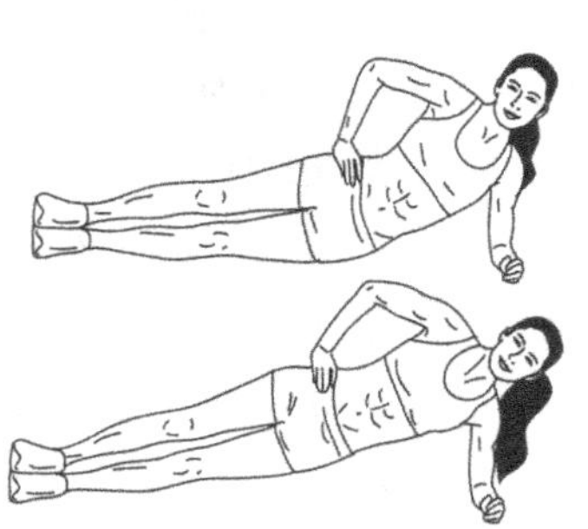

12 side bridges

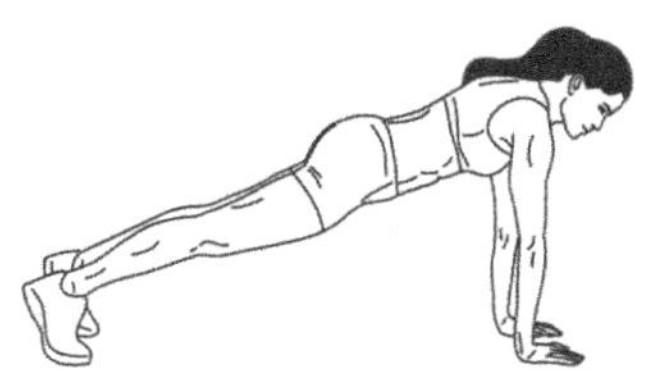

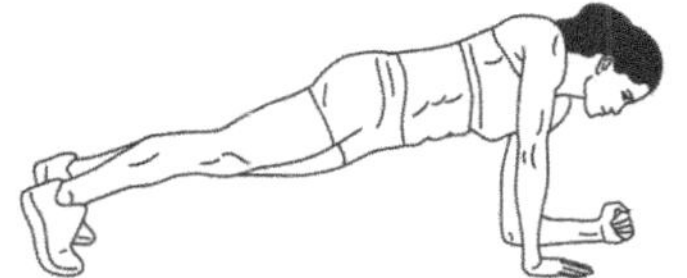

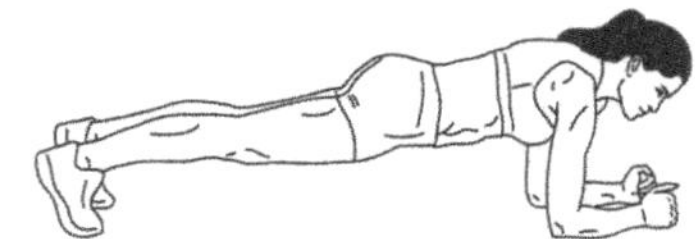

6 up and down planks

59 Washboard Abs

The abs are the body's powerhouse ensuring that energy generated by the lower body is as fully conserved as possible as it is transferred to the upper body. Training them takes time, patience and, of course, perseverance. Washboard Abs is a workout that targets the four distinct muscle groups that make up the ab wall and power the body's performance. Make this one a regular in your workout routines and you will feel the difference.

wash board abs

BUILD

DARBEE WORKOUT © darebee.com

LEVEL I 3 sets **LEVEL II** 4 sets **LEVEL III** 5 sets **REST** up to 2 minutes

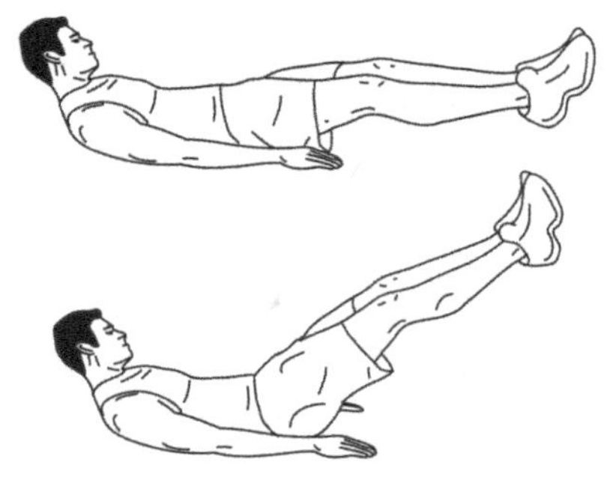

10 leg raises

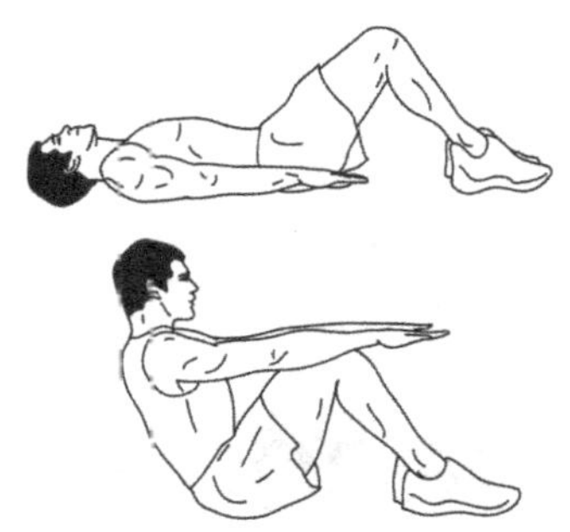

20 sit-ups

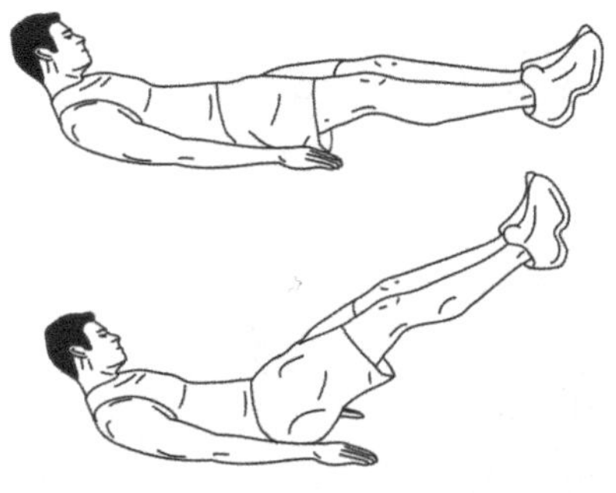

10 leg raises

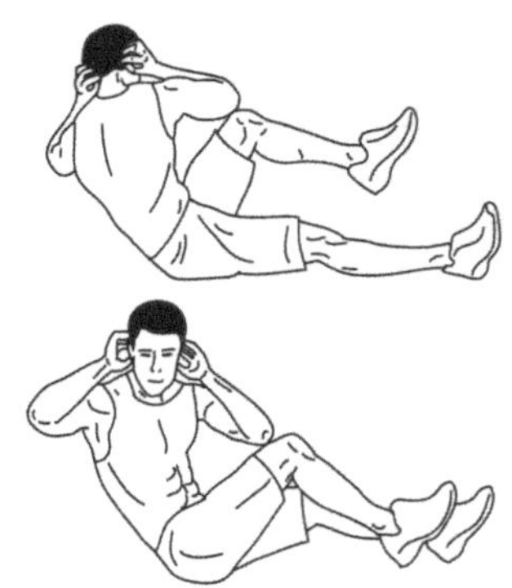

20 knee-to-elbow crunches

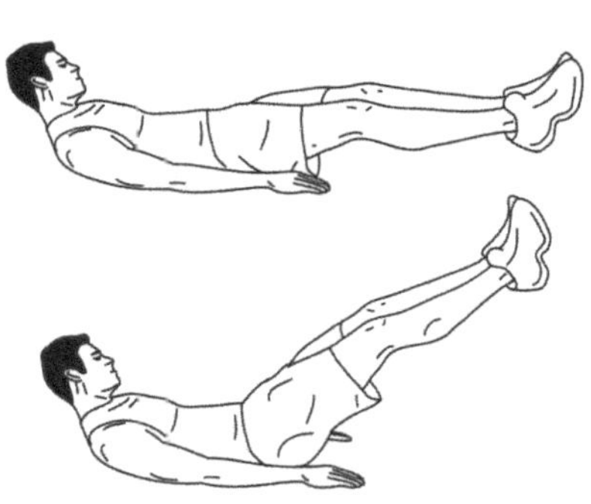

10 leg raises

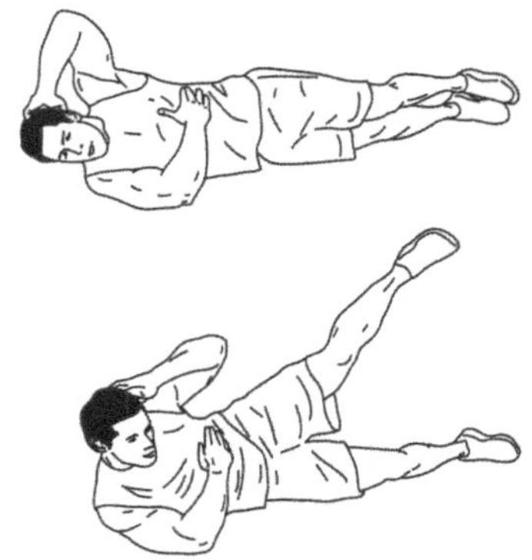

20 side jackknives

60 Ab Decoder

Abs Decoder will work your abs, glutes, quads and calves. It will help make your front hip flexors stronger and also work your side hip flexors. It won't push you to the edge of your abilities but then again you don't need to go there every day to get a good workout done.

ab decoder

DAREBEE CARDIO & ABS WORKOUT © darebee.com

LEVEL I 3 sets **LEVEL II** 4 sets **LEVEL III** 5 sets **REST** up to 2 minutes

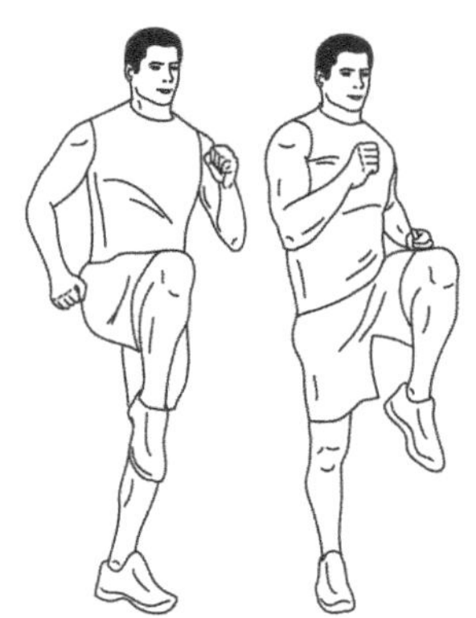

40 high knees

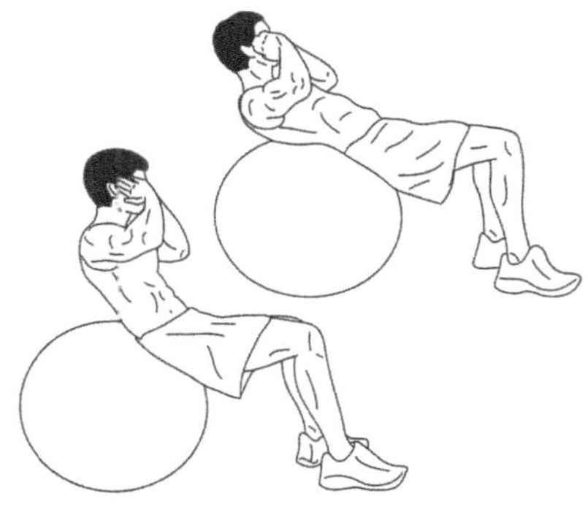

20 crunches

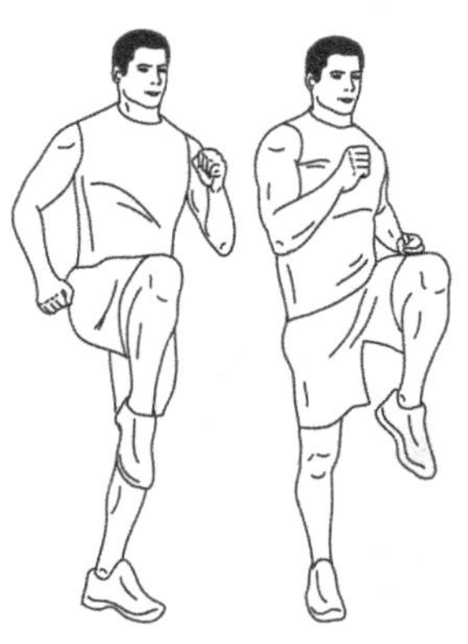

40 high knees

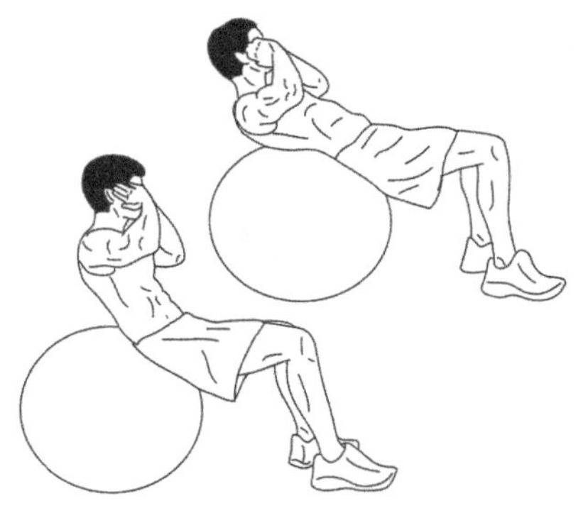

20 crunches

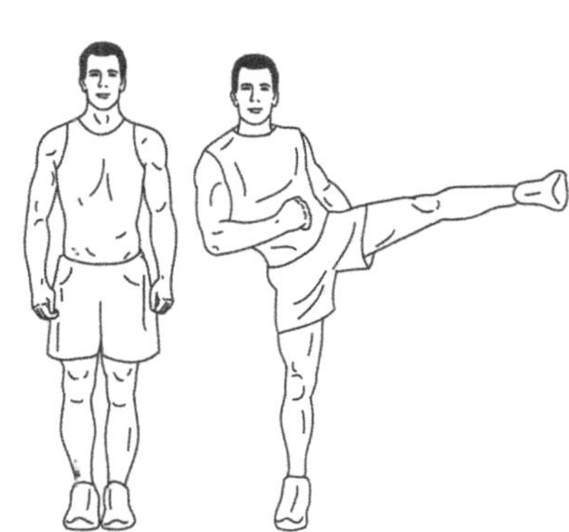

40 side-to-side leg raises

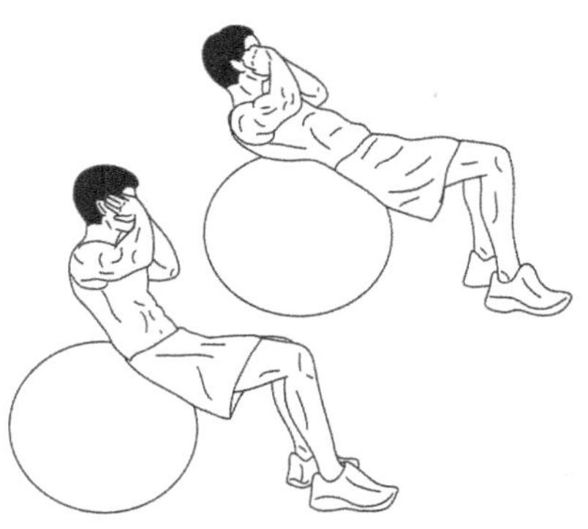

20 crunches

61 Ab Hub

For the days when you need to focus on your abs and core, upper body and shoulders, Ab Hub hits the sweetspot. Geared towards core training, it actually tackles all four ab wall muscle groups for that tightly girdled feel the day after the night before. Do it any time you feel like you don't feel like exercising and you will feel the difference afterwards.

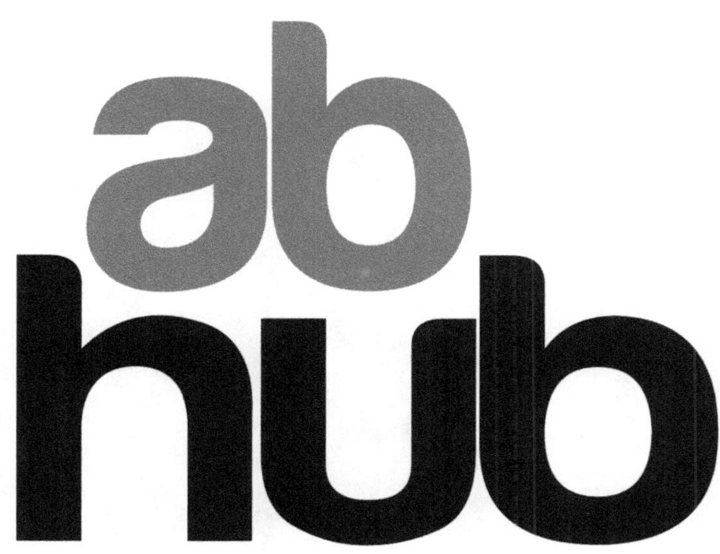

ab hub

DAREBEE WORKOUT
© darebee.com

Level I	3 sets	10 seconds
Level II	4 sets	15 seconds
Level III	5 sets	20 seconds

2 minutes rest between sets

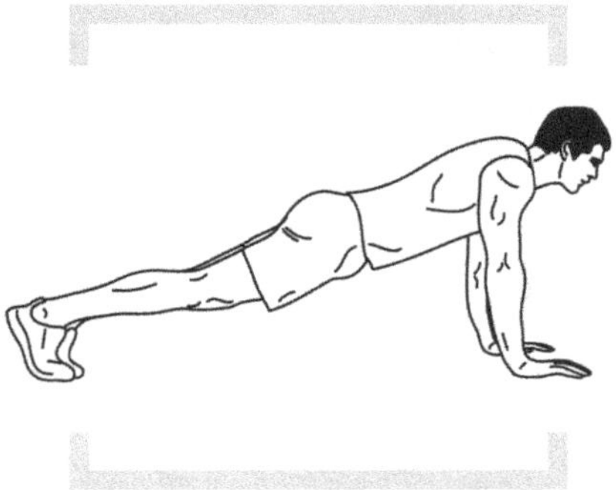

plank hold

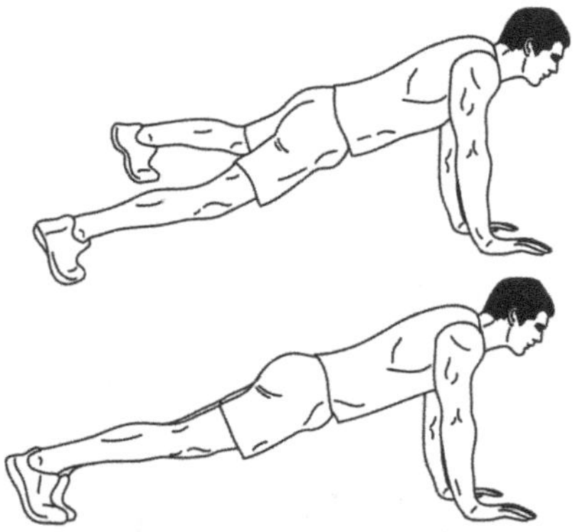

plank jacks

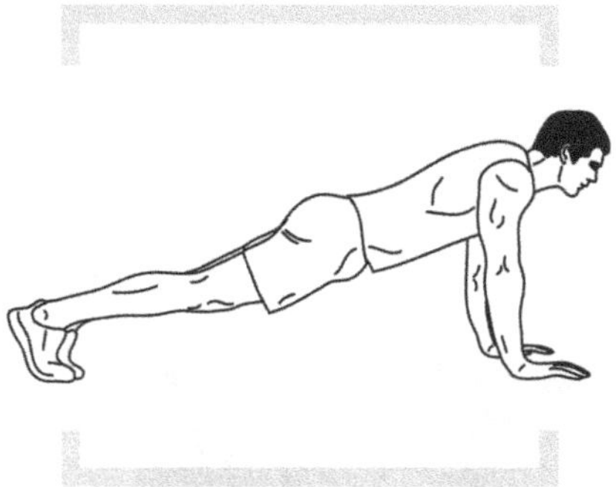

plank hold

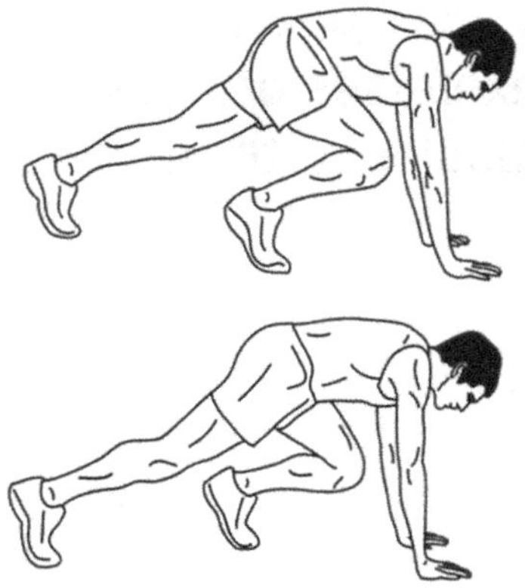

climbers

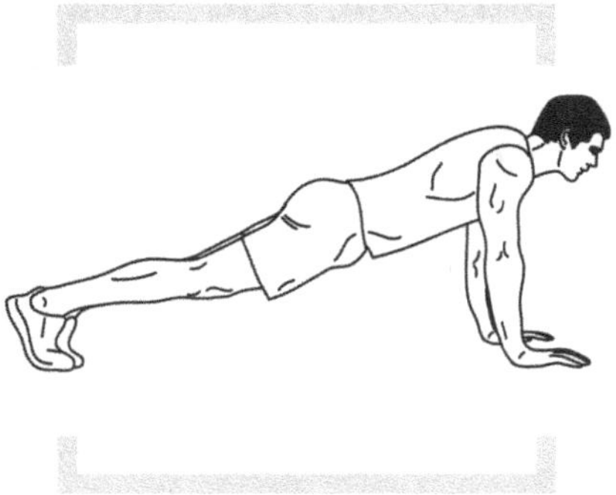

plank hold

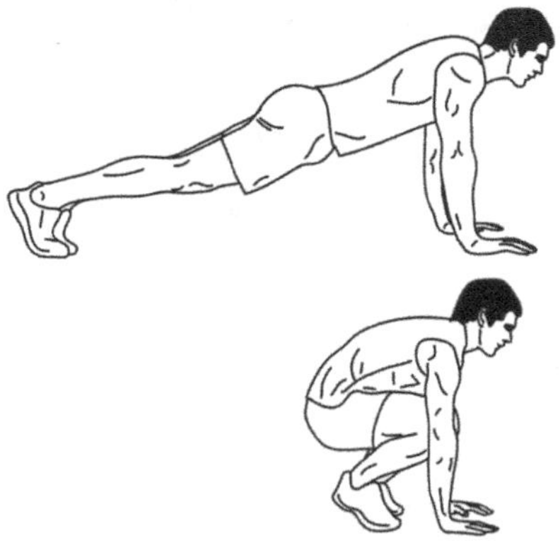

plank jump-ins

extra credit 1 push-up after each exercise

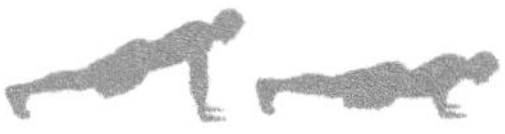

62 Anti-Pooch

Getting rid of belly fat requires some pretty high intensity work and the Anti-Pooch workout totally fits the bill, here. Three solid exercises provide an unrelenting build-up of intensity that will push your muscles to the edge and test your VO2 Max capacity.

ANTI POOCH WORKOUT

by DAREBEE © darebee.com

5 sets | 2 minutes rest in between

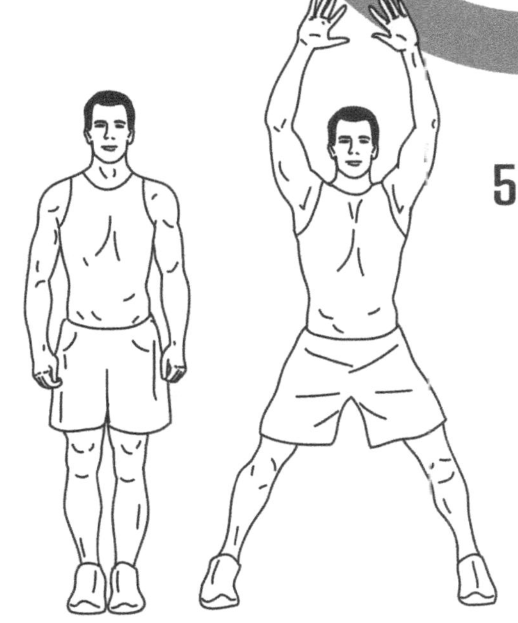

10 jumping jacks

4 sit-ups

10 jumping jacks

4 sit-ups

10 jumping jacks

4 sit-ups

10 jumping jacks

4 sit-ups

10 jumping jacks

4 sit-ups

done

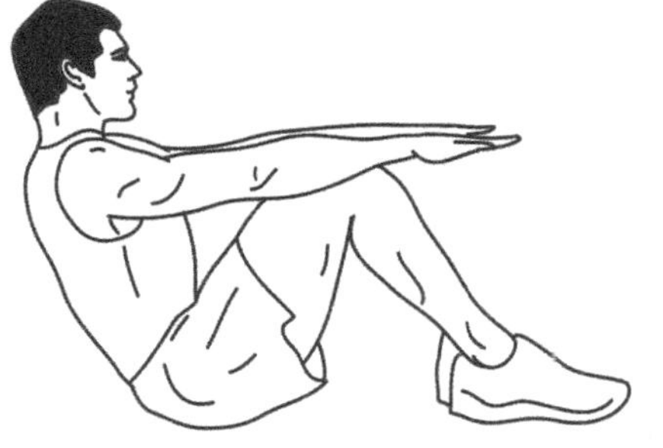

63 Beer Belly

While there is no workout routine, set of exercises or program that will allow you to lose weight locally, there are exercise routines that will tighten your abs, work your core and raise your body temperature putting you, squarely, in the sweatzone. The Beer Belly workout is one of them.

BEER BELLY

DAREBEE WORKOUT © darebee.com

LEVEL I 3 sets **LEVEL II** 5 sets **LEVEL III** 7 sets **REST** up to 2 minutes

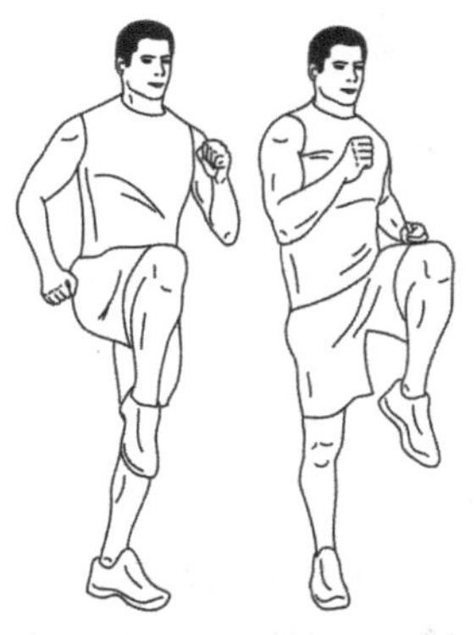

20 high knees

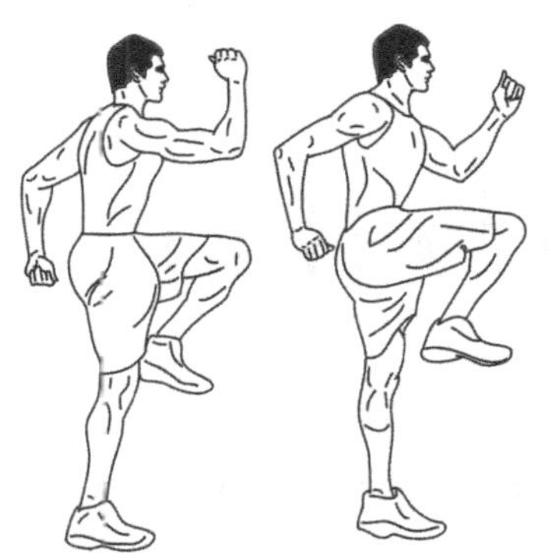

20 march steps

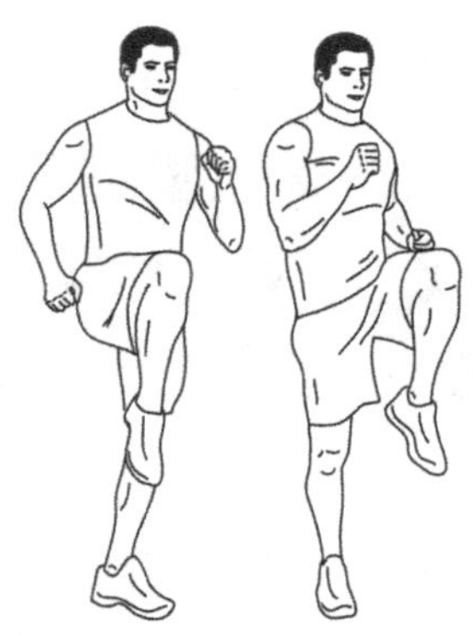

20 high knees

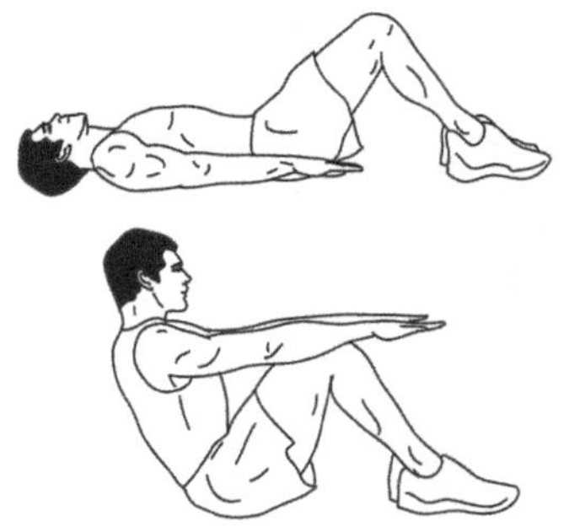

20 sit-ups

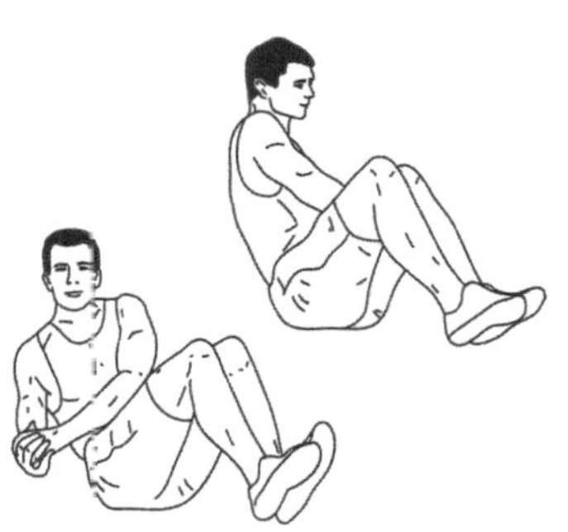

20 sitting twists

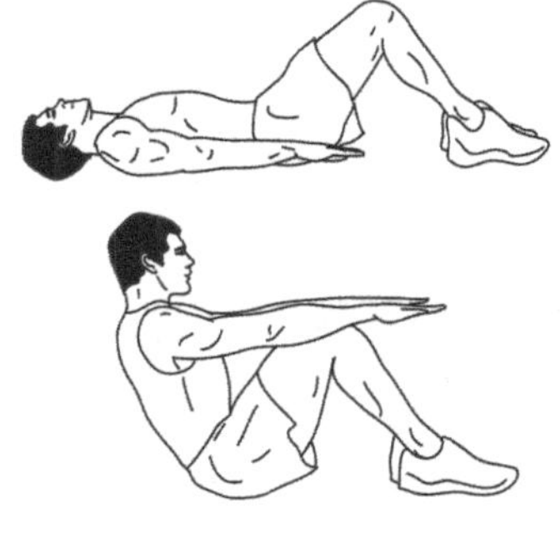

20 sit-ups

64 Belly Burner

For those looking for a workout that can help shift those extra few pounds Belly Burner does the trick. Get those knees past your waist each time you do High Knees and make sure you always land on the ball of the foot when you bring your foot down. Go high and fast on the burpees, working your legs to cram in as many reps each time as possible. Recover on the go in-between with elbow plank.

BELLY BURNER

DAREBEE HIIT WORKOUT © darebee.com

Repeat 7 times in total | 2 minutes rest between sets

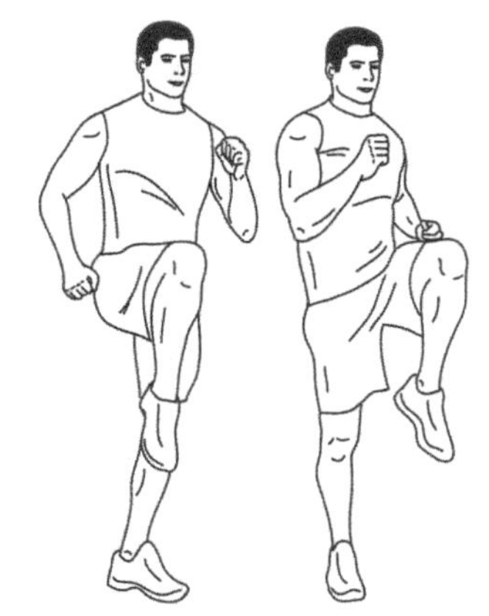

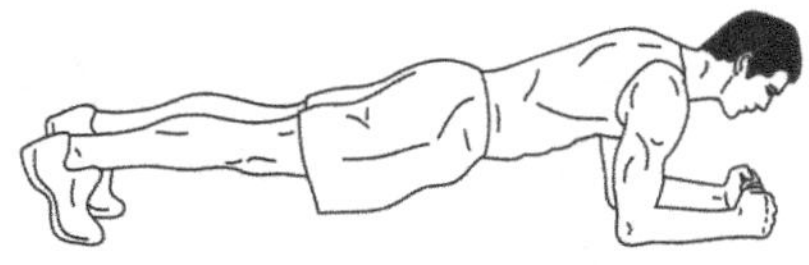

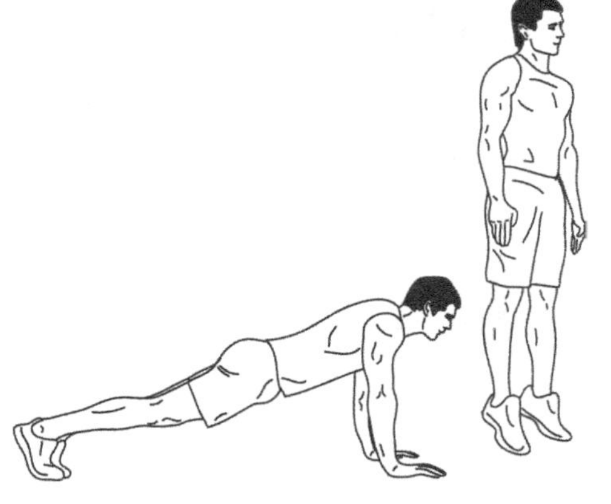

20sec high knees

20sec elbow plank

10sec basic burpees

20sec high knees

20sec elbow plank

10sec basic burpees

20sec high knees

20sec elbow plank

10sec basic burpees

done

65 Belly Melt

Fascial fitness is achieved incrementally. Side Jacks and Jumping Jacks are key to developing the kind of fascial fitness that makes it harder to feel fatigue. This is only a difficulty Level II workout yet, as with so many of the workouts we create, execution is key to success. Keep your arms perfectly straight as the fingertips meet overhead for Jumping Jacks and stay on the balls of your feet while you execute them. Arch your body as you stretch for Side Jacks. Be precise and be controlled and you will reap the benefits.

BELLY MELT

DAREBEE WORKOUT © darebee.com

5 sets | 2 minutes rest between sets

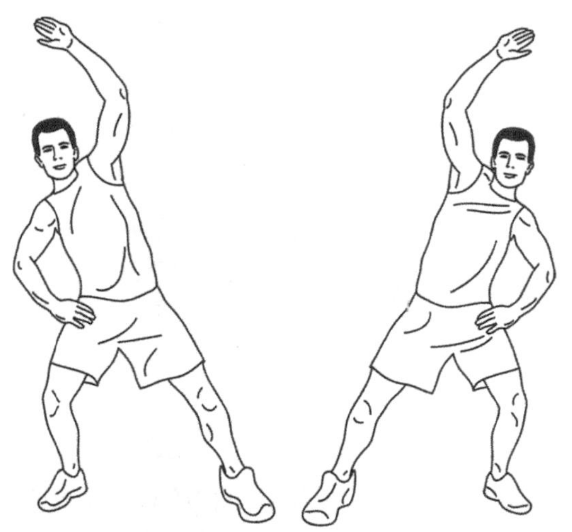

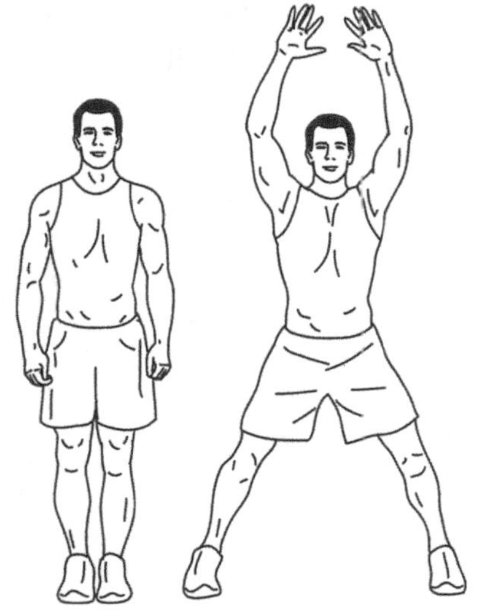

4 side jacks

10 jumping jacks

4 side jacks

10 jumping jacks

4 side jacks

10 jumping jacks

4 side jacks

10 jumping jacks

4 side jacks

10 jumping jacks

done

66 Bulletproof Abs

Bulletproof Abs is a workout that relentlessly piles up pressure on all major ab wall muscle groups. Perform High Knees by bringing your knee up to waist height each time. Make sure you're on the ball of the foot as you land to absorb the impact from each step. This is a difficulty Level IV workout which means you will definitely feel the burn while doing it.

bulletproof abs

HIIT WORKOUT
BY DARERBEE
© darebee.com

Level I 3 sets
Level II 5 sets
Level III 7 sets
2 minutes rest

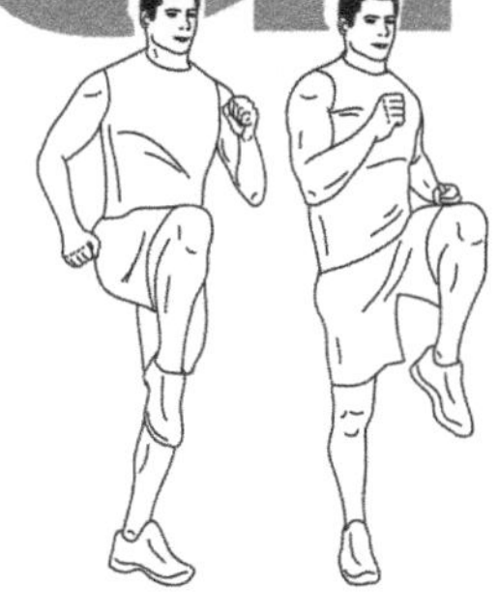

40sec high knees

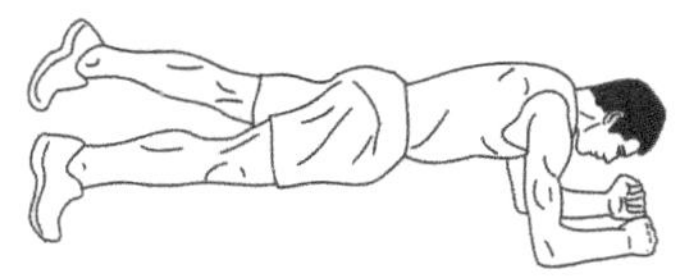

20sec raised leg plank hold (left leg)

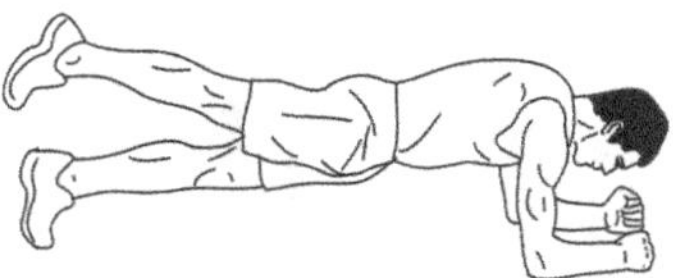

20sec raised leg plank hold (right leg)

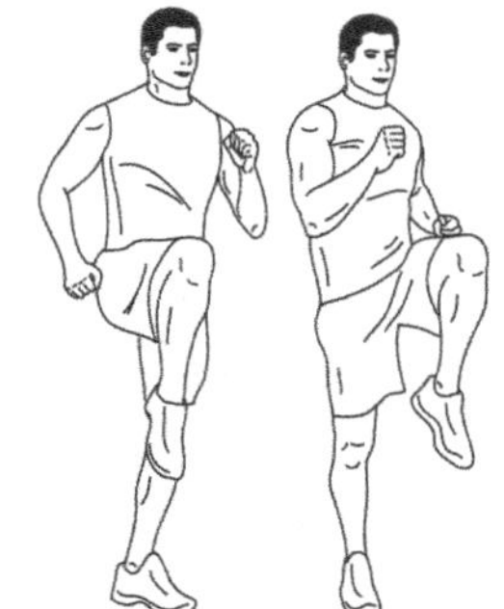

40sec high knees

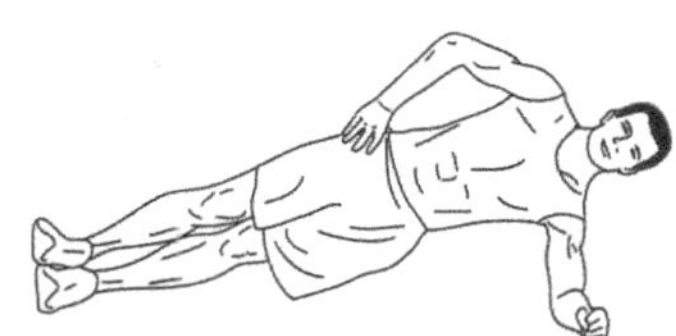

20sec side plank hold (left side)

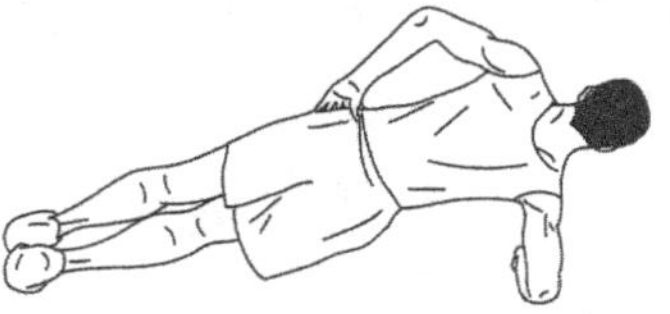

20sec side plank hold (right side)

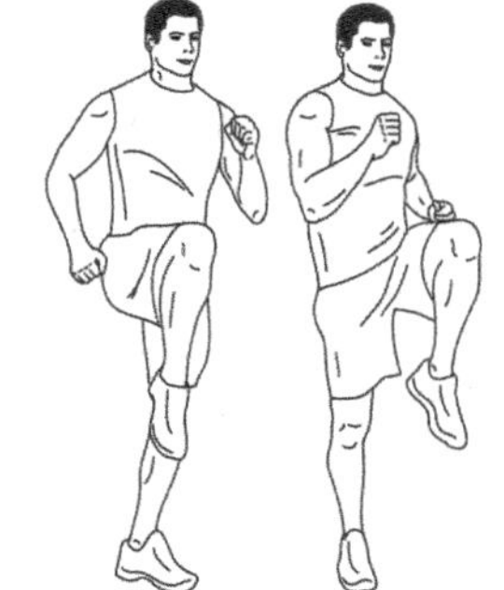

40sec high knees

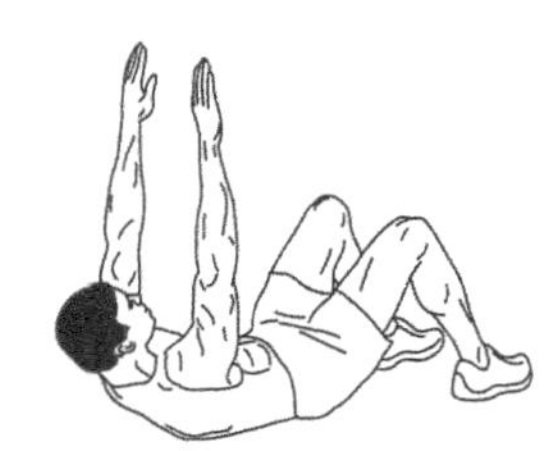

20sec crunch hold

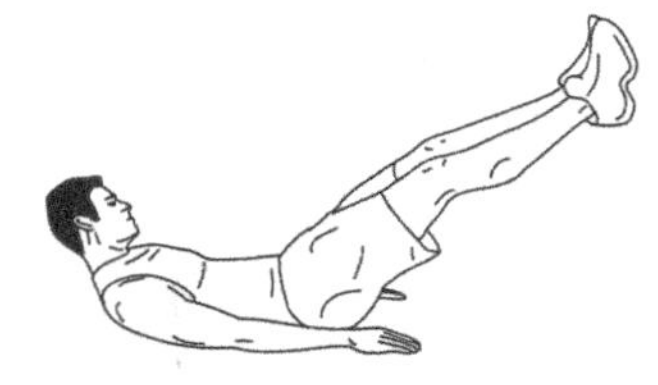

20sec raised leg hold

67 Burn Mode

Jumping Jacks may seem an unlikely exercise to seriously challenge our VO2 Max levels, but performed fast, with perfect form, the heels of the feet never touching down and hands meeting overhead, it becomes key to developing fast, tight, arms/legs coordination and great fascial fitness.

BURN MODE

HIIT WORKOUT
BY DAREBEE

Level I 3 sets
Level II 5 sets
Level III 7 sets
2 minutes rest

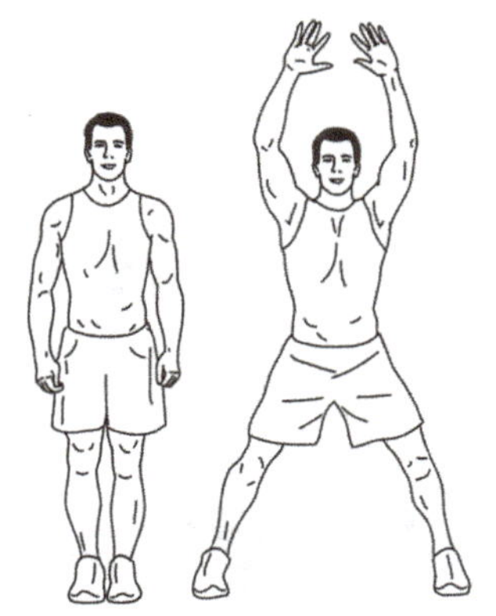

30sec jumping jacks

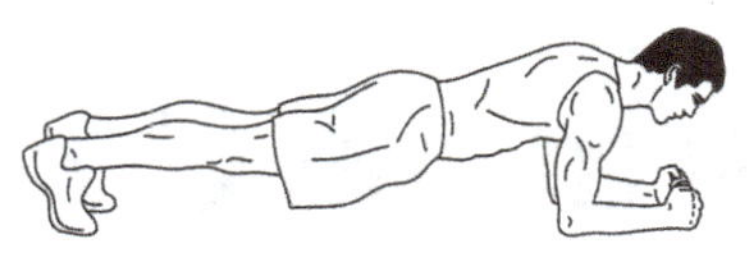

30sec elbow plank

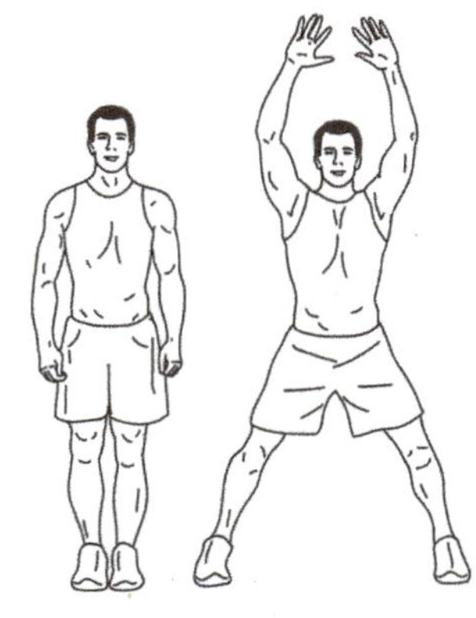

30sec jumping jacks

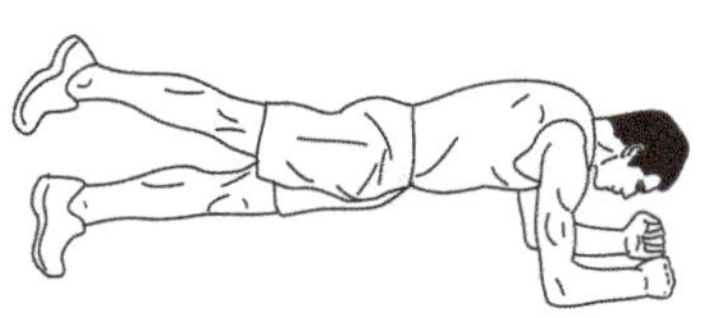

30sec raised leg plank

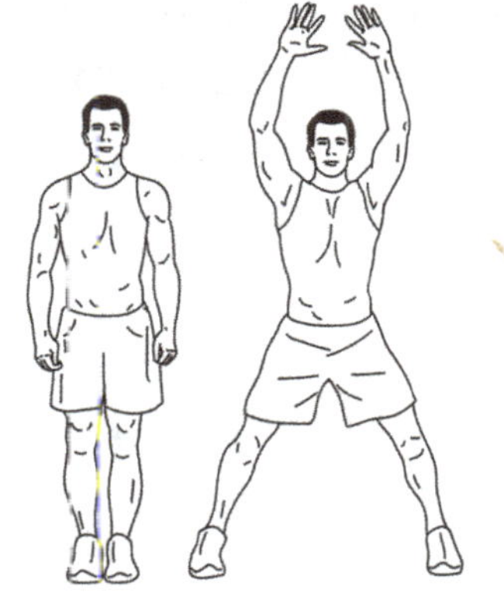

30sec jumping jacks

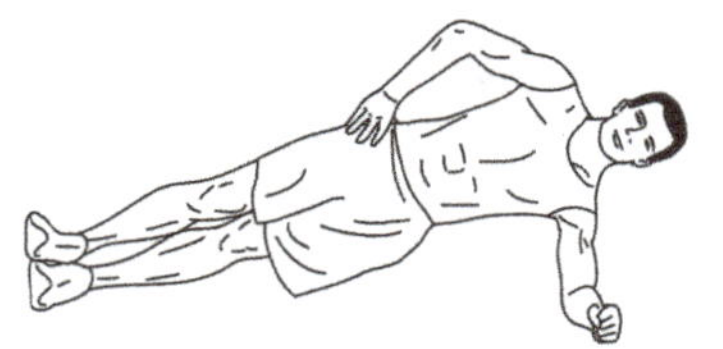

30sec side plank

68 Cardio & Core Express

Speed, agility, better fascial fitness, a stronger core, better abs and better overall aerobic performance are the building blocks of fitness. Cardio & Core Express has all of that. Bounce on the balls of your feet throughout. Raise your knee to waist height during Knee-to-Elbow exercises and make sure you employ a full length straight-arm movement during Jumping Jacks and you have the kind of workout that jumpstarts your fitness every time you do it.

Cardio & Core

EXPRESS

DAREBEE
WORKOUT
© darebee.com
3 sets | 2 minutes rest

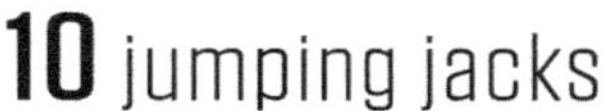

10 jumping jacks

4 knee-to-elbows

10 jumping jacks

4 knee-to-elbows

10 jumping jacks

4 knee-to-elbows

10 jumping jacks

4 knee-to-elbows

10 jumping jacks

4 knee-to-elbows

done

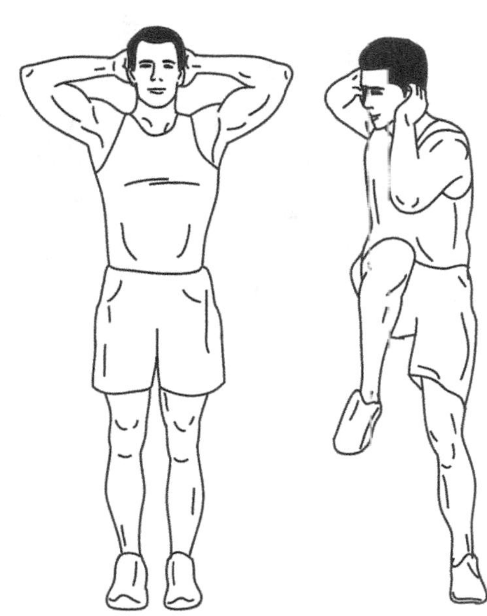

69 Cardio & Core

At the core of every great athletic performance lies a strong core (pun unintended) and great cardiovascular conditioning. While aerobic performance determines just how much oxygen in each breath you take is really absorbed by the lungs and transferred into the bloodstream to be taken to the organs that need it, cardiovascular fitness is the ability of the heart and lungs to get all the blood circulating quickly enough through the body to supply oxygen to the organs and tissues that need it most. The Cardio & Core workout puts your body through its paces testing your core and challenging your cardiovascular fitness. All you have to do now is supply the great athletic performance.

Cardio & Core

DAREBEE WORKOUT © darebee.com

LEVEL I 3 sets **LEVEL II** 5 sets **LEVEL III** 7 sets **REST** up to 2 minutes

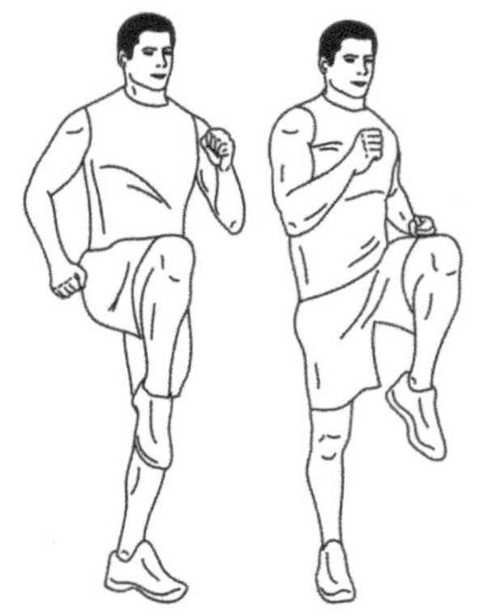

60 high knees

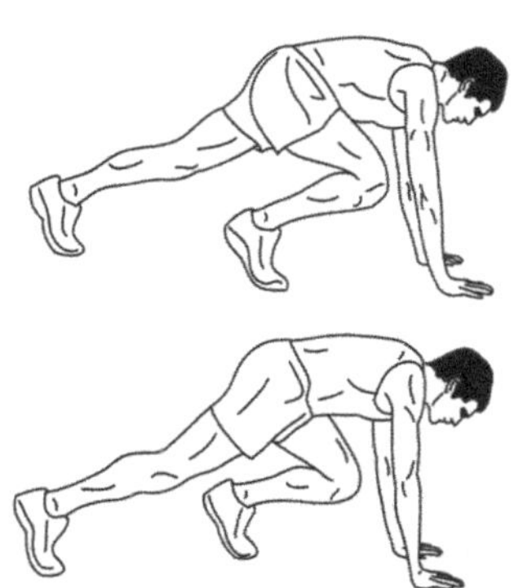

10 climbers

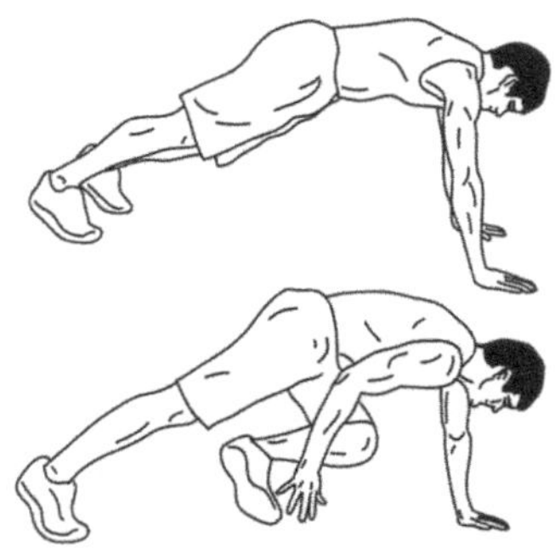

10 climber taps

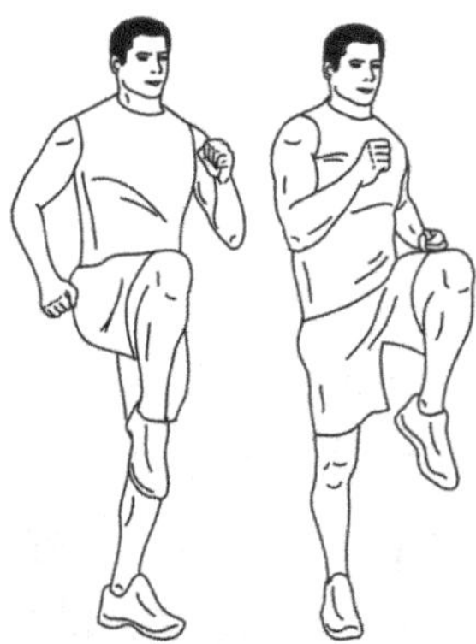

60 high knees

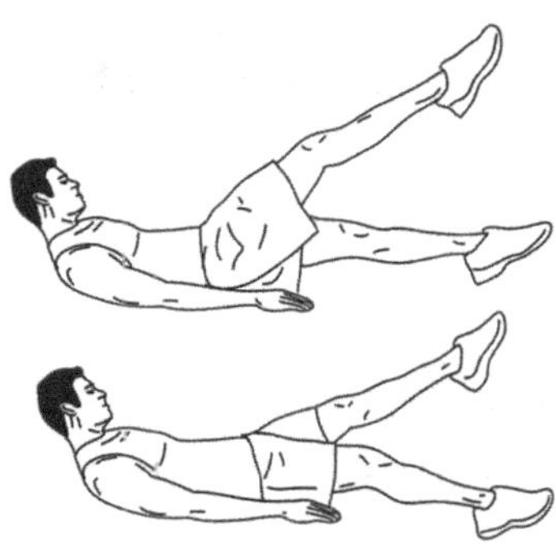

10 flutter kicks

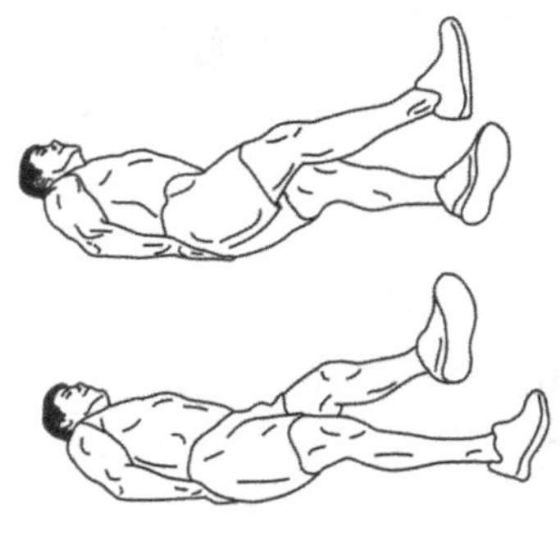

10 scissors

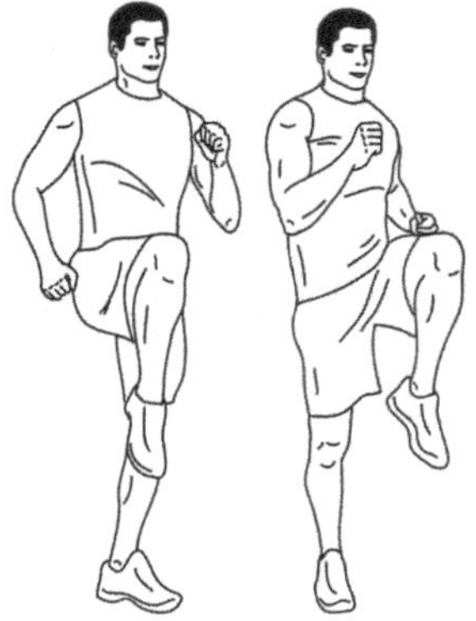

60 high knees

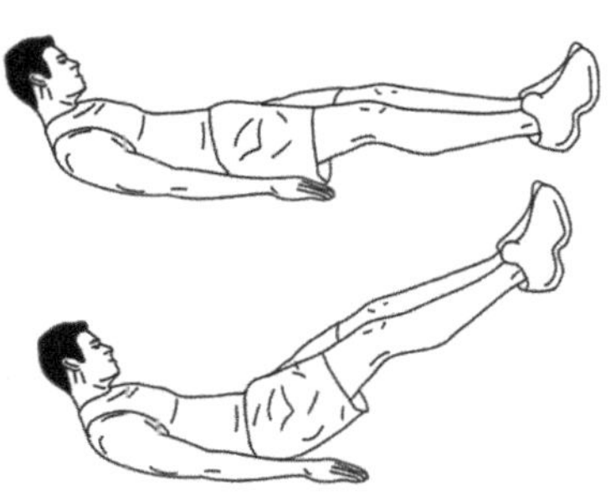

10 leg raises

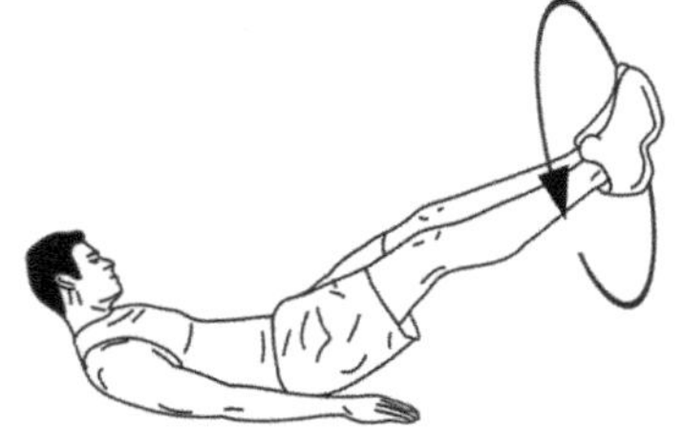

10 raised leg circles

70 Cardio Crunch

The quads, calves and abs are amongst the strongest and largest muscle groups in the body. This makes them critical to posture, overall strength and, of course, athletic performance. Cardio Crunch doesn't just train them, it also loads your cardiovascular system and your lungs, expanding your VO2 range so that you can then also become capable of working out longer, without getting tired.

Cardio Crunch

DAREBEE WORKOUT © darebee.com

LEVEL I 3 sets **LEVEL II** 5 sets **LEVEL III** 7 sets **REST** up to 2 minutes

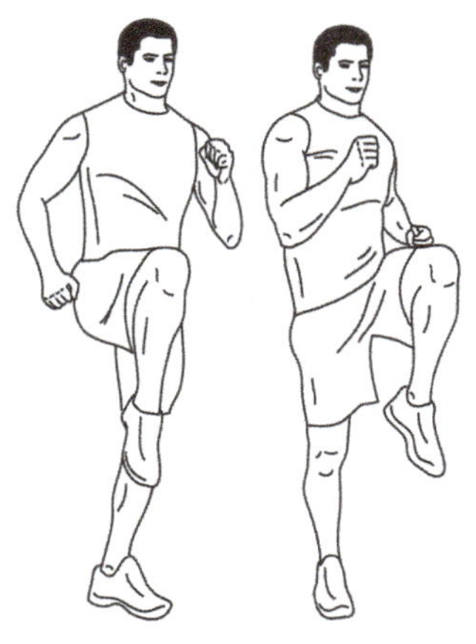

20 high knees

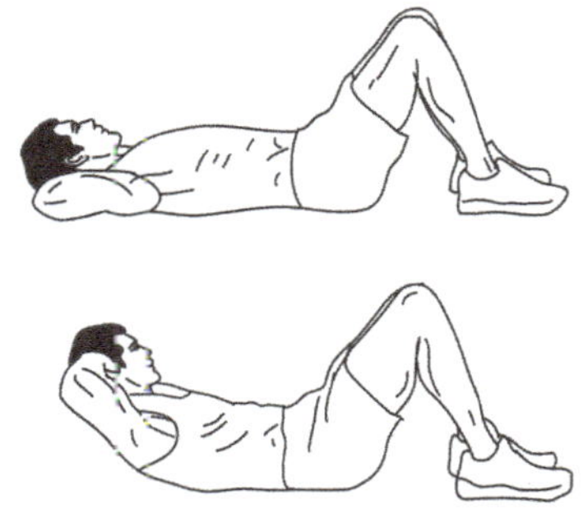

10 crunches

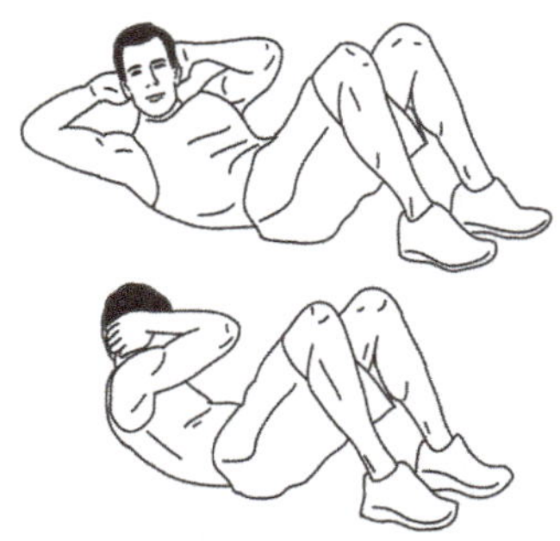

10 cross crunches

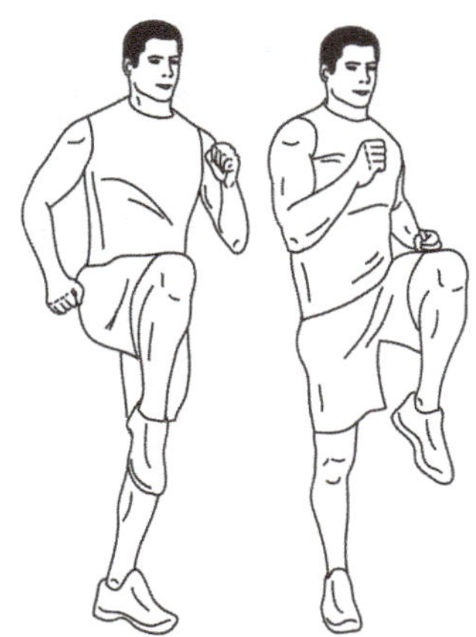

20 high knees

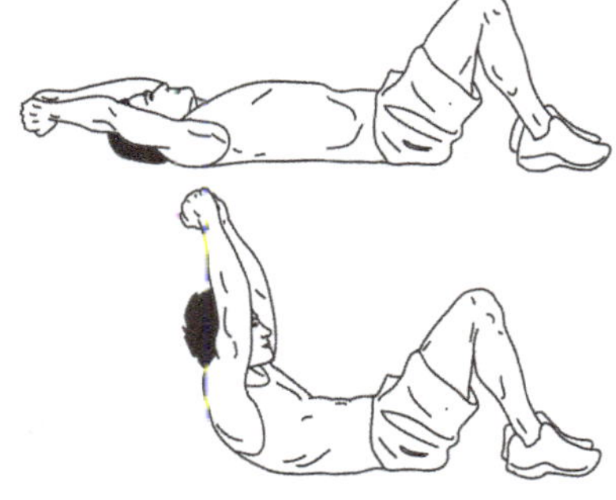

10 long arm crunches

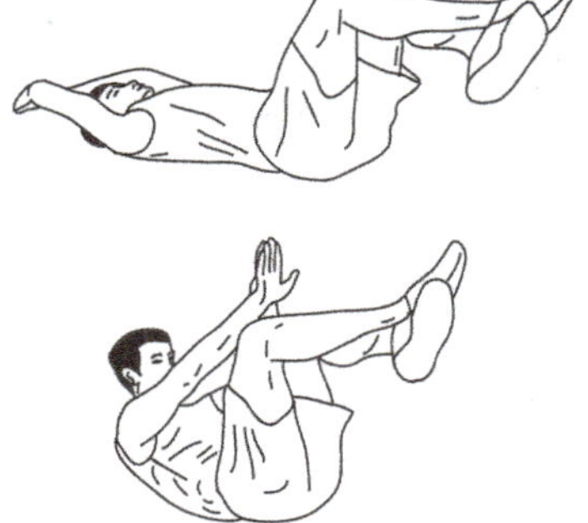

10 knee crunches

71 Cardio Sofa

The Cardio Sofa workout uses your sofa for something decidedly different to couching out. A lower body workout with a strong aerobics component Cardio Sofa is perfect for that rainy day when you feel like going for a run but the weather is against you or when you really don't want to go into all the trouble associated with tidying yourself up so you can go outdoors. Get into the sweatzone fast by making sure your knees are waist height during High Knees and you are really pumping your arms.

cardio sofa

DAREBEE WORKOUT © darebee.com

LEVEL I 3 sets **LEVEL II** 5 sets **LEVEL III** 7 sets **REST** 2 minutes

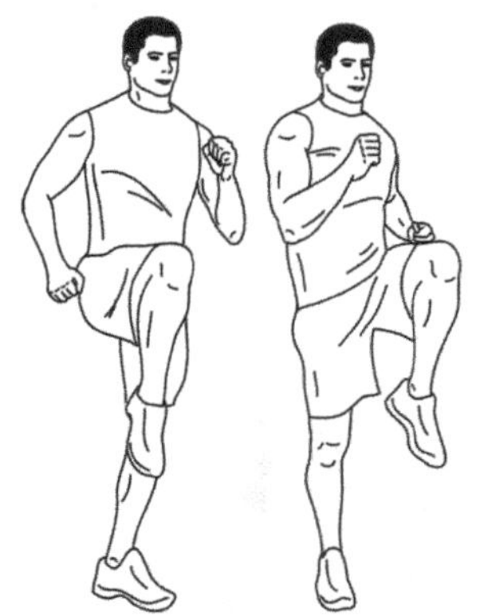

40 high knees

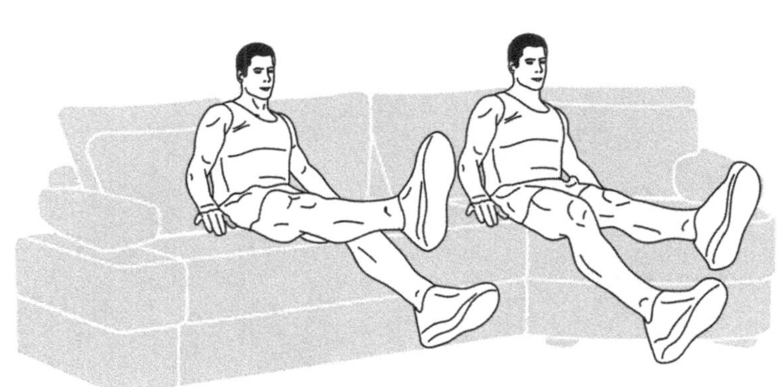

20 flutter kicks

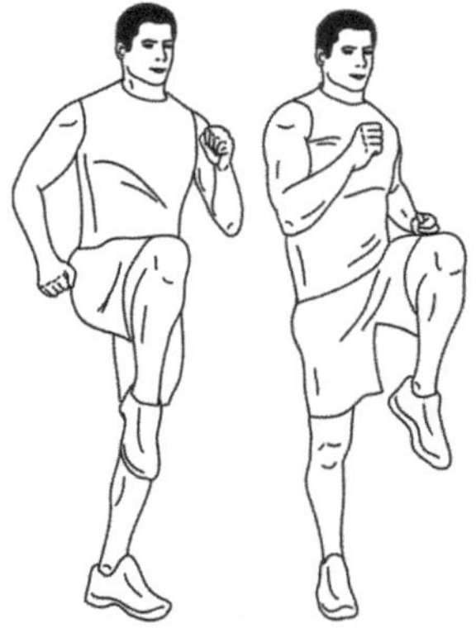

40 high knees

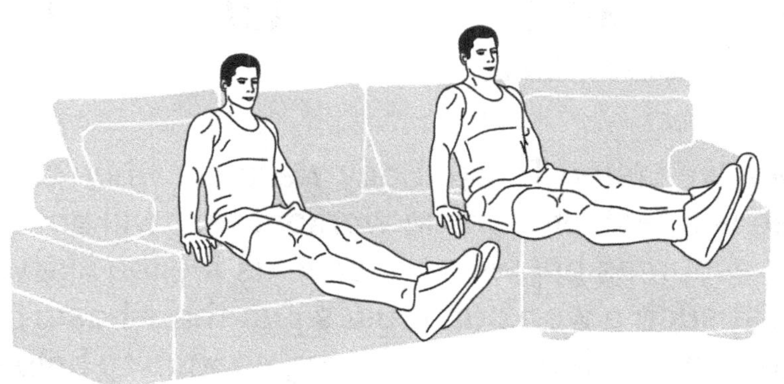

20 leg raises

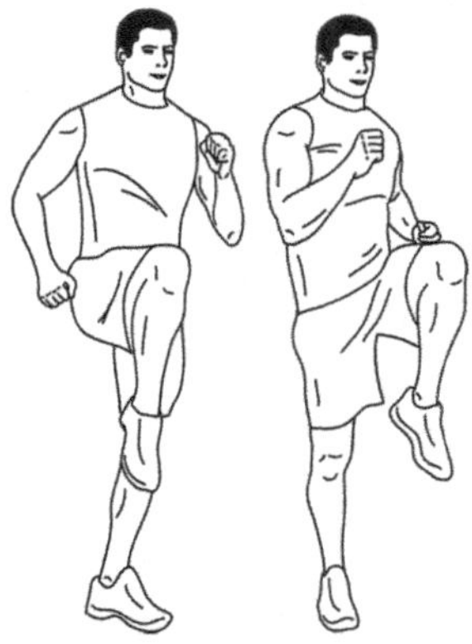

40 high knees

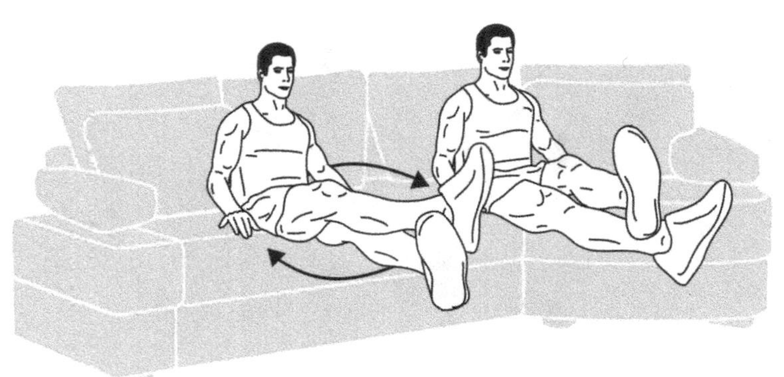

20 scissors

72 Chisel Express

When we Listen To Our Body we know when there are days when all we need is a fast, energizing workout that will not take us to the very brink of our resources but will still leave us feeling like we've worked out. Chisel is just such a workout. It uses just three basic bodyweight exercises in a combination that is challenging enough to help us shape our body and see results. Being a Level II workout however this is the one you do when you are "building up" to greater things or "powering down" and maintaining your edge on days when you're not in your top form.

CHISEL EXPRESS

DAREBEE HIIT WORKOUT © darebee.com

Level I 3 sets **Level II** 5 sets **Level III** 7 sets | 2 minutes rest rest

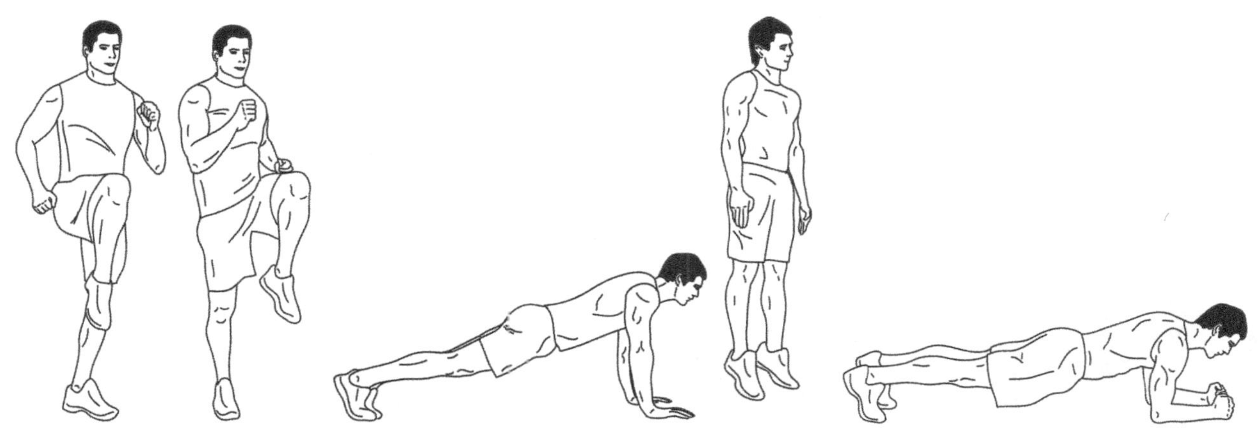

20sec high knees

10sec basic burpees

20sec high knees

10sec basic burpees

20sec high knees

10sec basic burpees

30sec elbow plank

done

73 Codex

Stay glued to the ground and see just how much you can challenge your body. This is a set of exercises that takes a traditional routine and gives it an extra spin with a real challenge. Because of that it forces your muscles to work in unfamiliar ways that make it totally challenging.

CODEX

DAREBEE WORKOUT © darebee.com

LEVEL I 3 sets **LEVEL II** 5 sets **LEVEL III** 7 sets **REST** up to 2 minutes

hands never off the ground

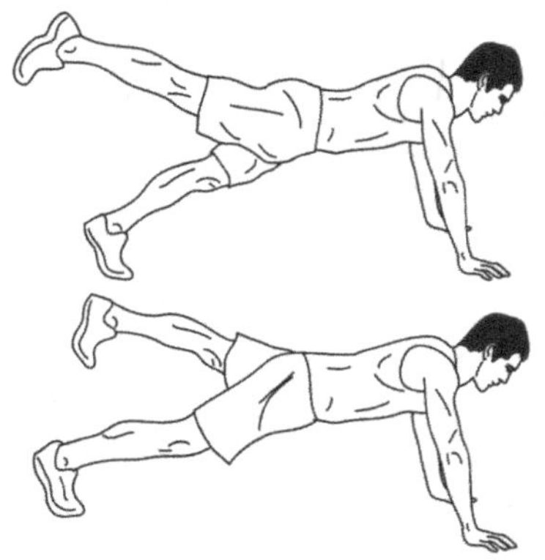

10 plank leg raises

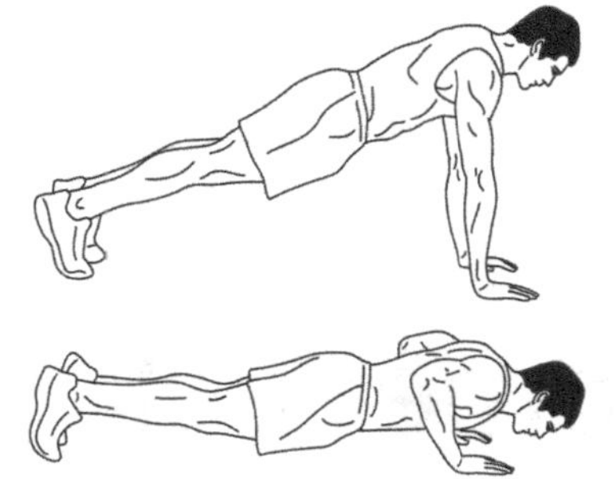

10 push-ups

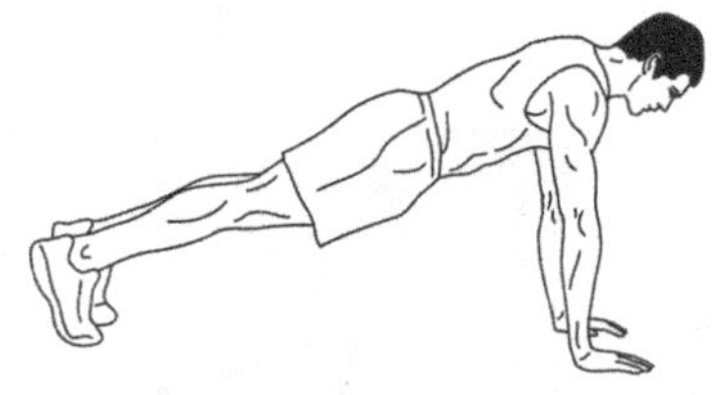

30sec plank

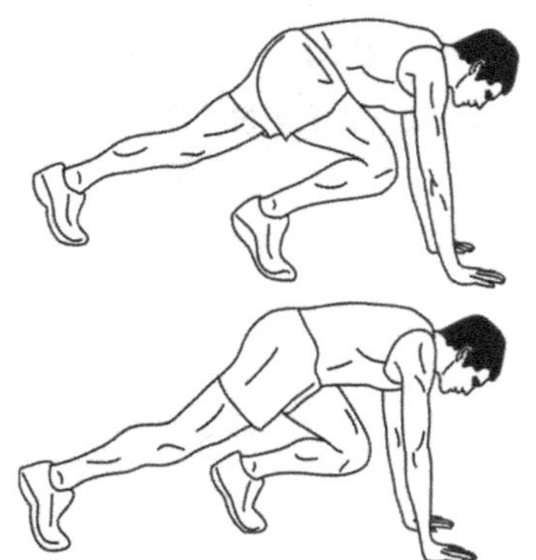

10 climbers

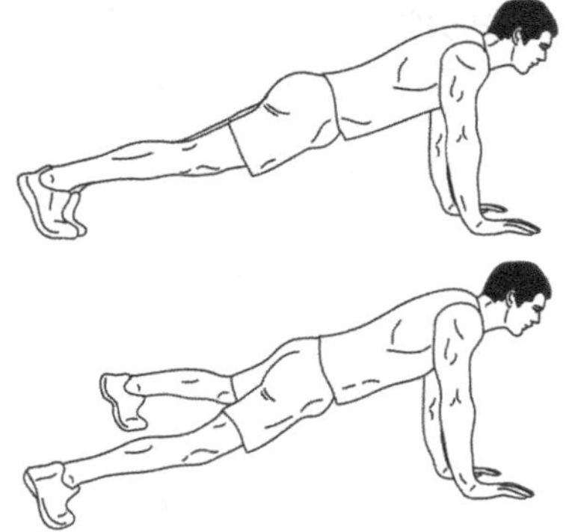

10 plank jacks

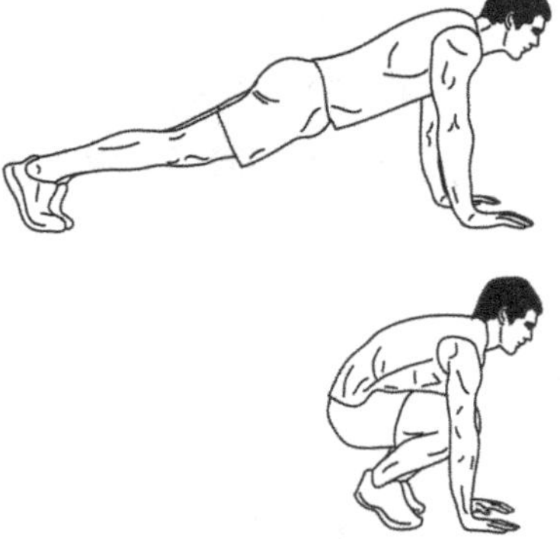

10 plank jump-ins

74 Comeback

The Comeback is a Level II workout which makes it perfect for those who want to find a workout to do on days when energy levels are low and time is short. This has an abs & core focus but it also works a whole lot of adjoining muscle groups, recruiting them in the transition from one exercise to another. Perform Jumping Jacks on the balls of your feet and bring your arms up all the way above your head. Perform each exercise with a focus on form but try to move as fast as you possibly can.

THE COMEBACK

DAREBEE WORKOUT © darebee.com

LEVEL I 3 sets **LEVEL II** 5 sets **LEVEL III** 7 sets **REST** up to 2 minutes

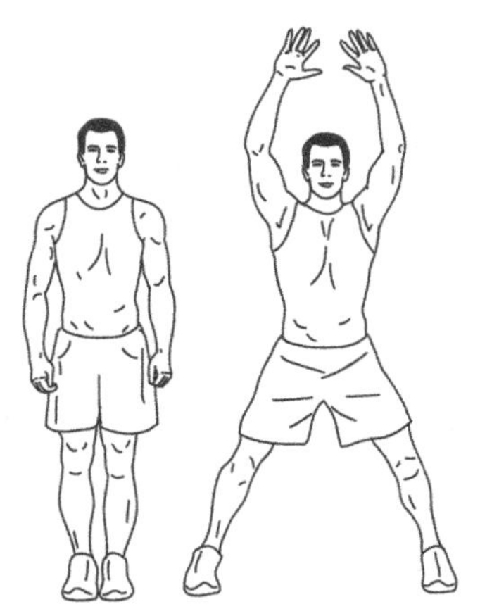

20 jumping jacks

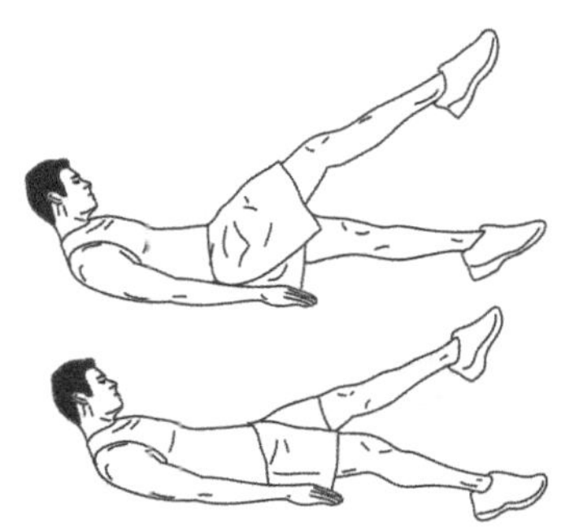

10 flutter kicks

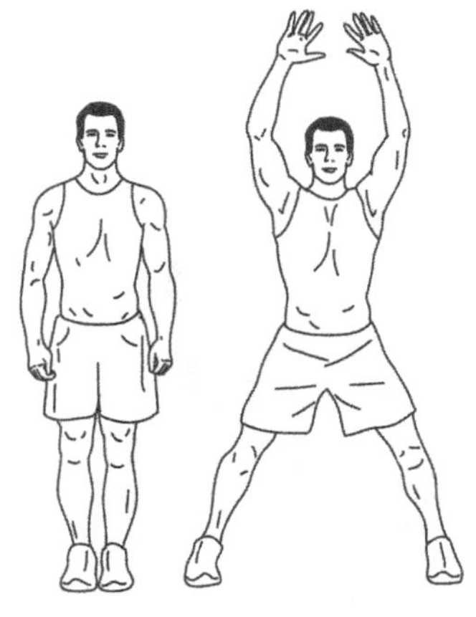

20 jumping jacks

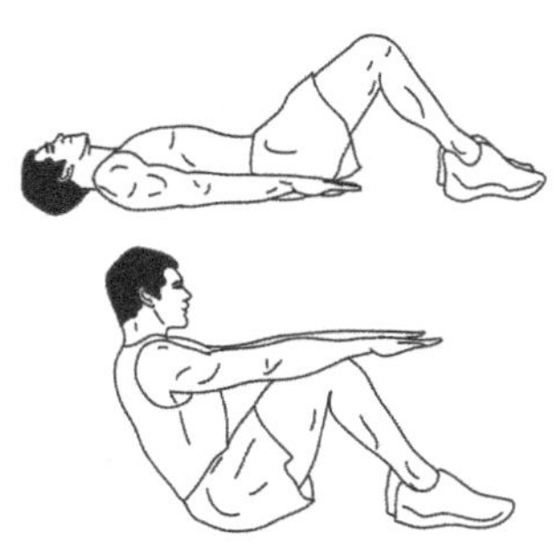

10 sit-ups

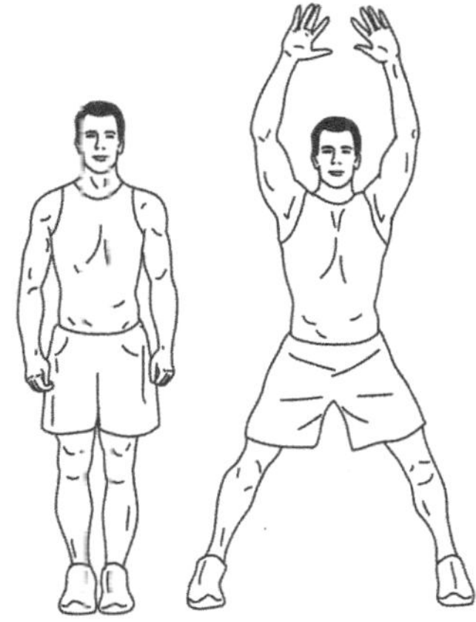

20 jumping jacks

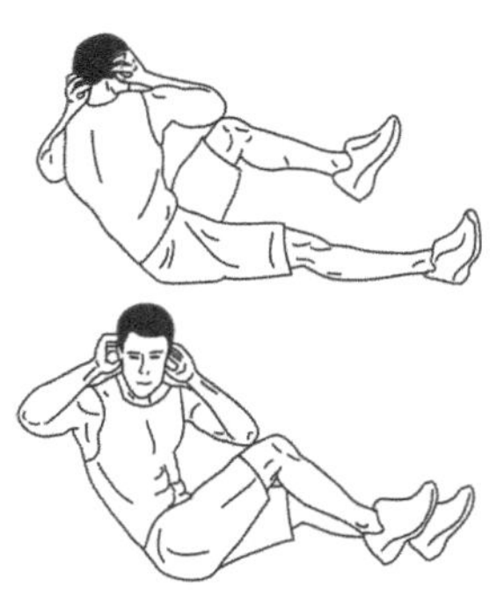

10 knee-to-elbow crunches

75 Core Burn

Core Burn demands perfect form when performing High Knees, which means your knees need to come to waist height each time and you only ever land on the ball of the foot. You pump your arms in synch to your legs. The rest of the exercises are not easy either but then again you're here to make your core and abs feel they've worked out. This will do it.

Core Burn

DAREBEE HIIT WORKOUT © darebee.com

Level I 3 sets **Level II** 5 sets **Level III** 7 sets

2 minutes rest between sets

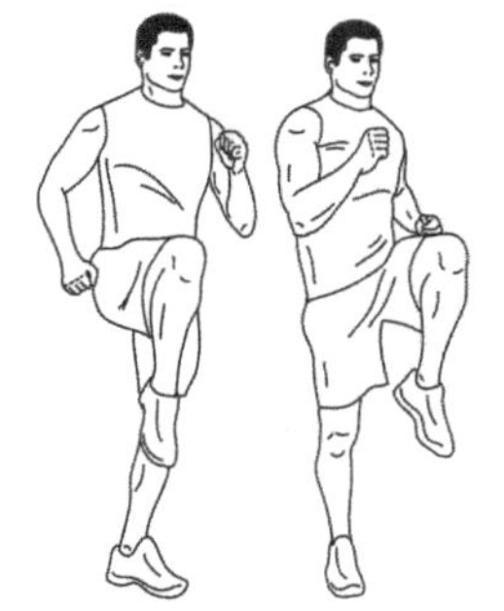

20sec high knees

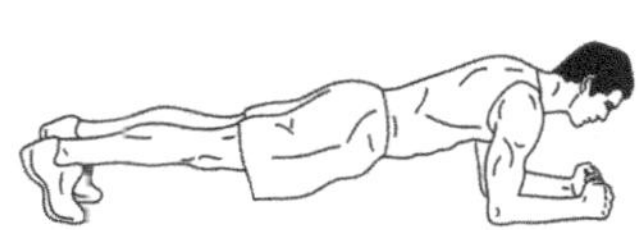

20sec elbow plank

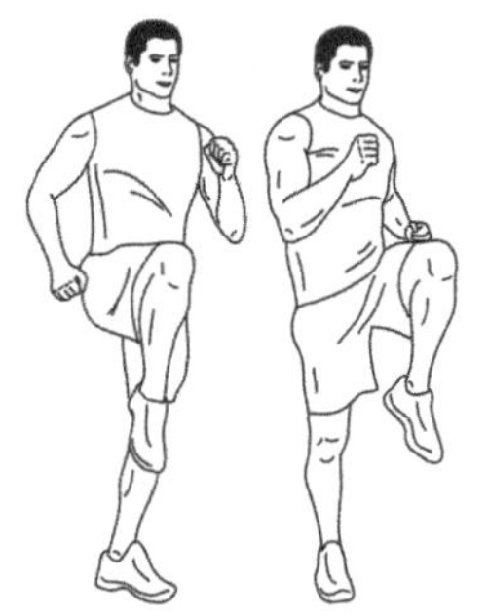

20sec high knees

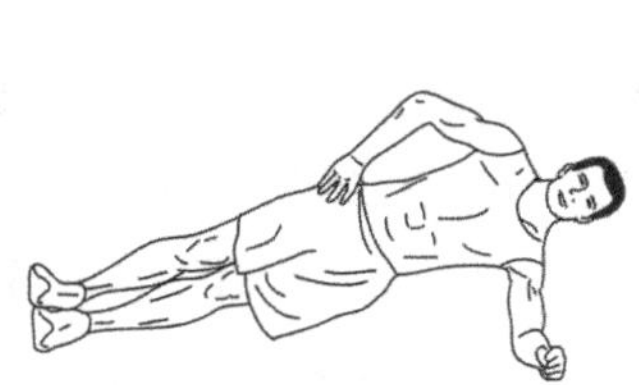

20sec side plank (left)

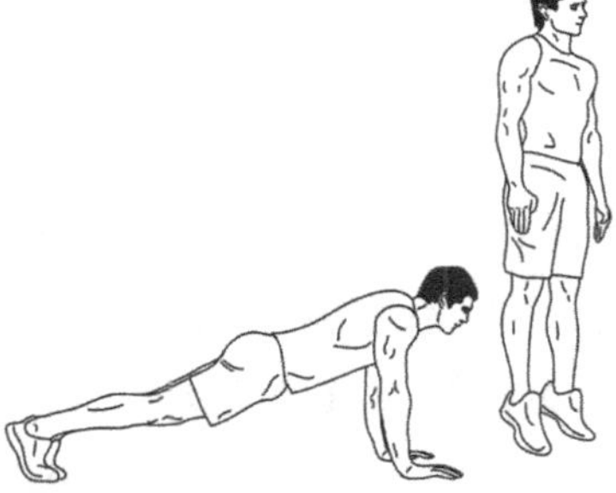

20sec basic burpees

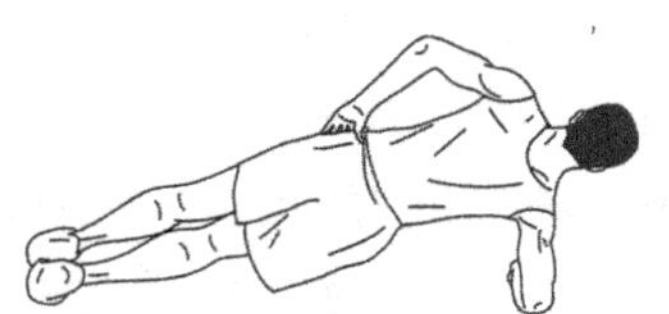

20sec side plank (right)

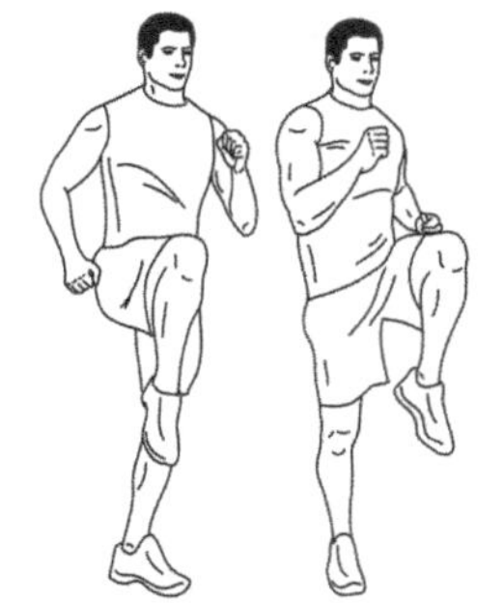

20sec high knees

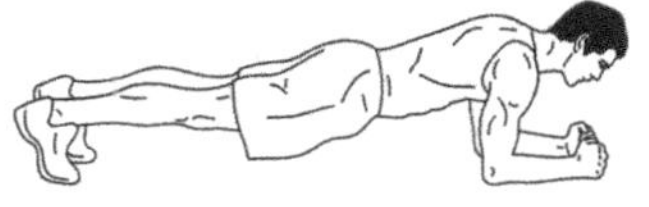

20sec elbow plank

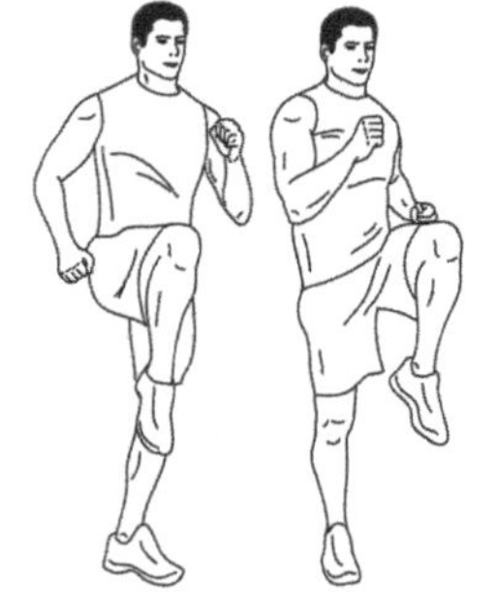

20sec high knees

76 Core Forge

Core Forge is a Level IV workout that will test your VO2 Max to the limit and push your quads against the very edge of their ability to perform. It focuses on lower body strength and core but it also works all the other abdominal muscle groups and, seeing how it is Burpees that power it, it manages to deliver a burn to your lower body muscles and a massive load to your lungs. Since it's time based speed of execution is key to maintain momentum and quality in the workout.

CORE FORGE

DAREBEE HIIT WORKOUT © darebee.com

Level I 3 sets **Level II** 5 sets **Level III** 7 sets

2 minutes rest between sets

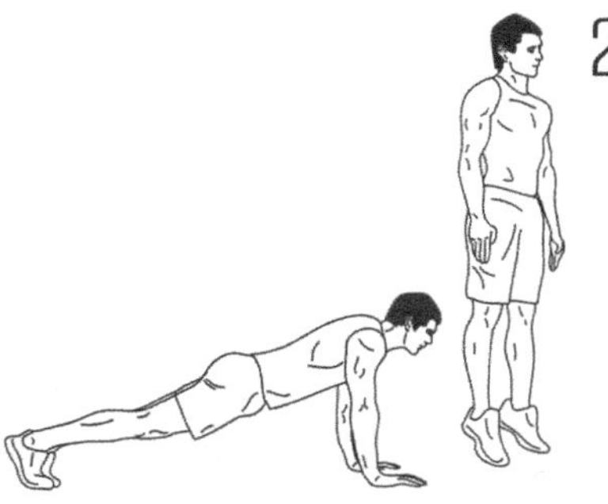

10sec basic burpees

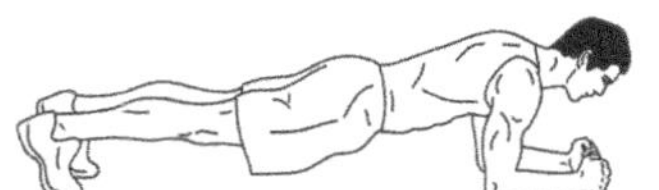

30sec elbow plank

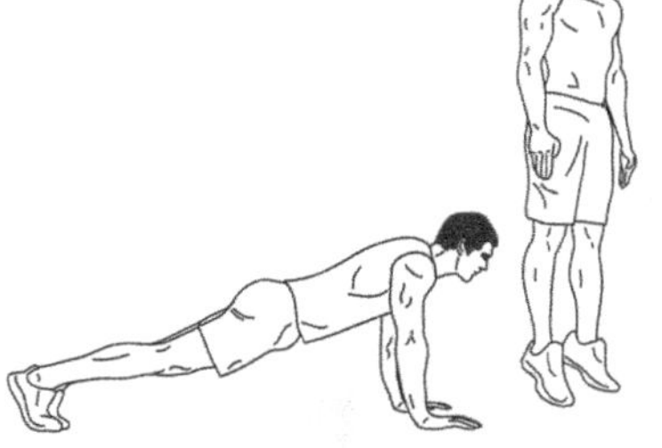

10sec basic burpees

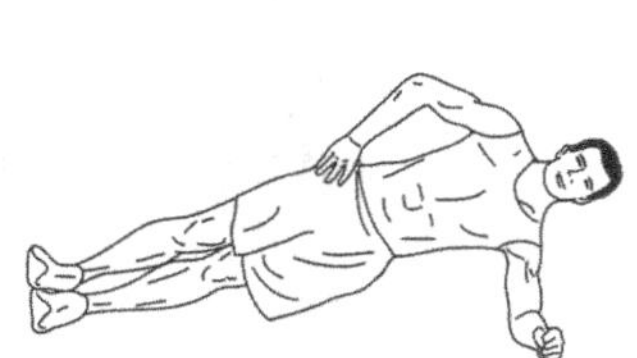

30sec side plank (left)

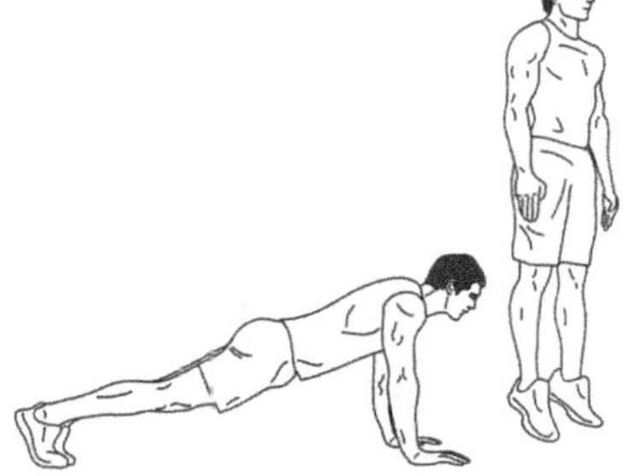

10sec basic burpees

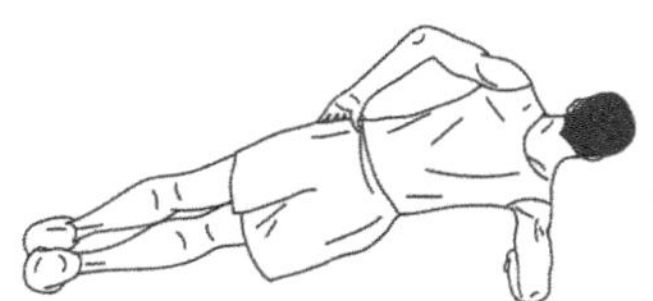

30sec side plank (right)

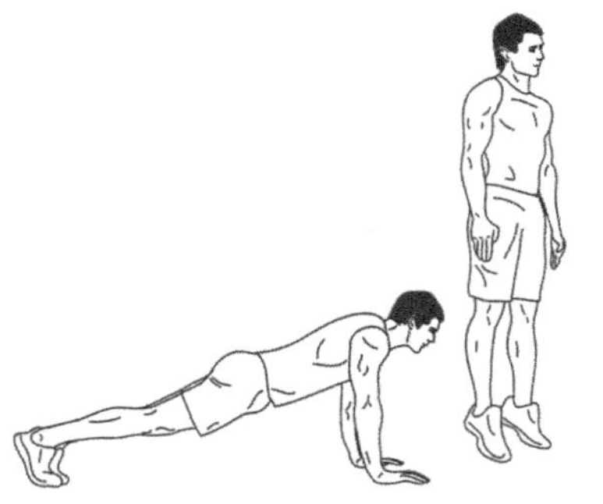

10sec basic burpees

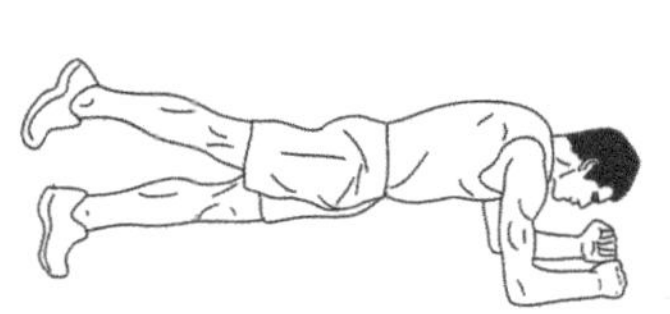

30sec raised leg plank

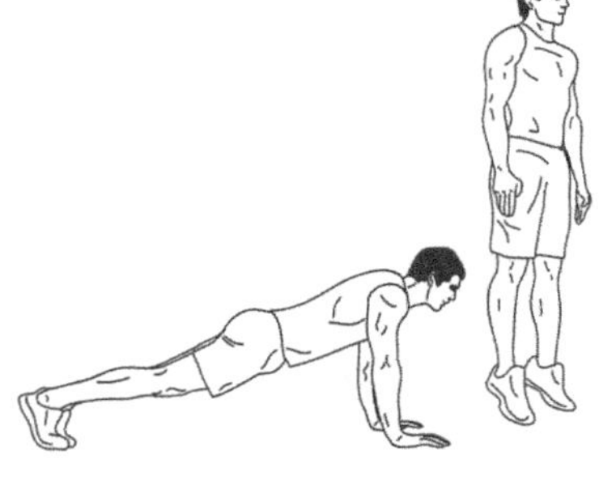

10sec basic burpees

77 Core Fusion

You know that your core is core to your physical fitness. Beyond stating the obvious what we do know is that core abdominals are hard to train, unless you happen to own a yacht and spend a lot of time walking around on deck in choppy seas. So, if no yacht, this is the next best thing.

core fusion

DAREBEE WORKOUT © darebee.com

LEVEL I 3 sets **LEVEL II** 4 sets **LEVEL III** 5 sets **REST** up to 2 minutes

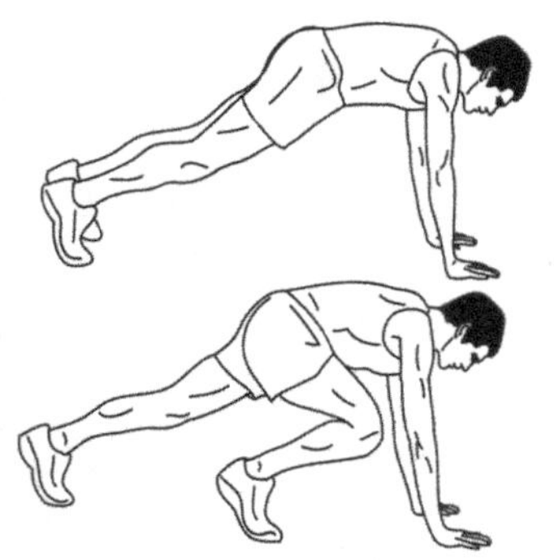

10 slow climbers

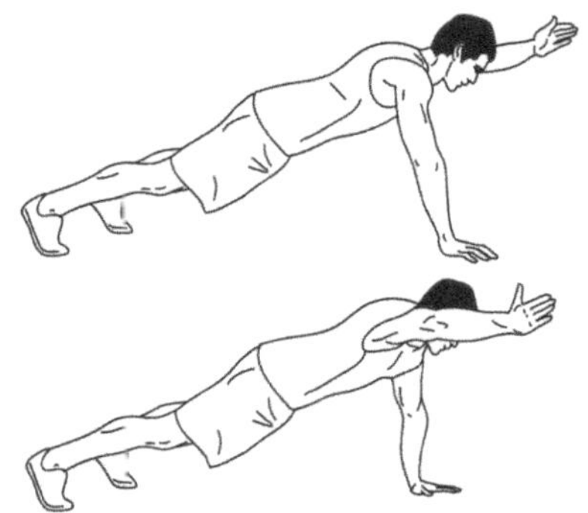

10 plank arm raises

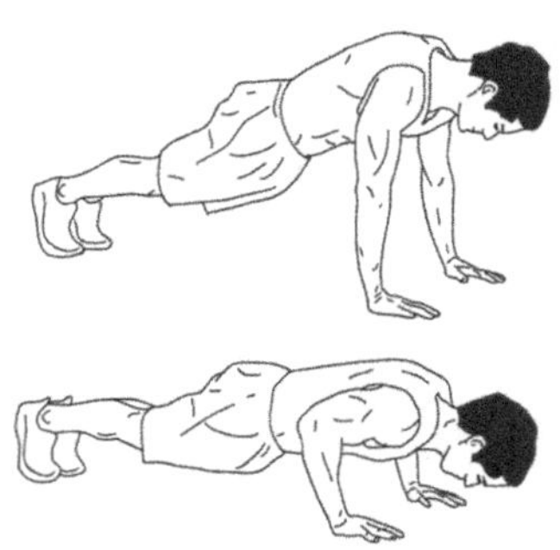

5 push-ups

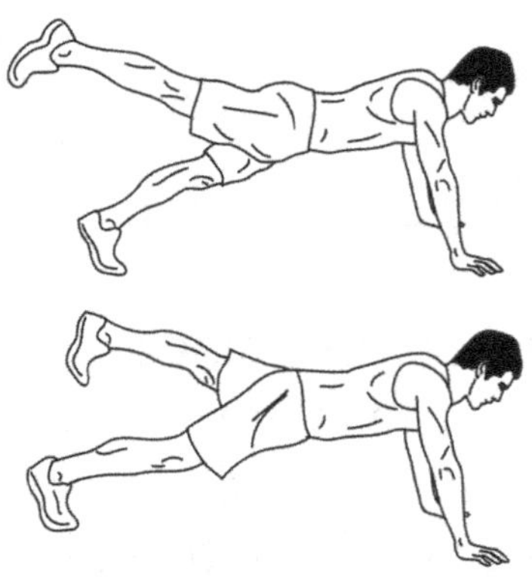

10 plank leg raises

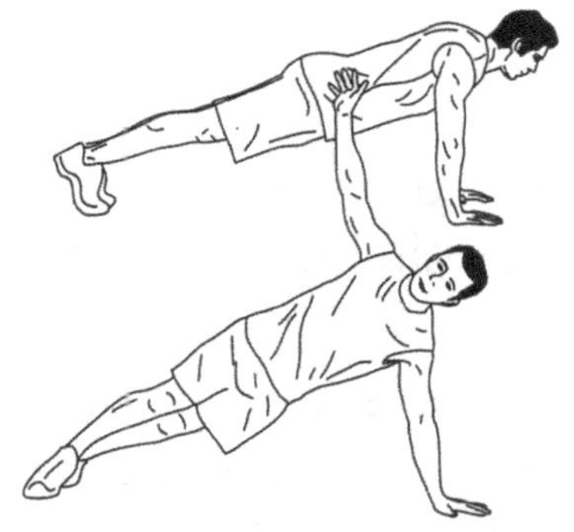

10 planks with rotations

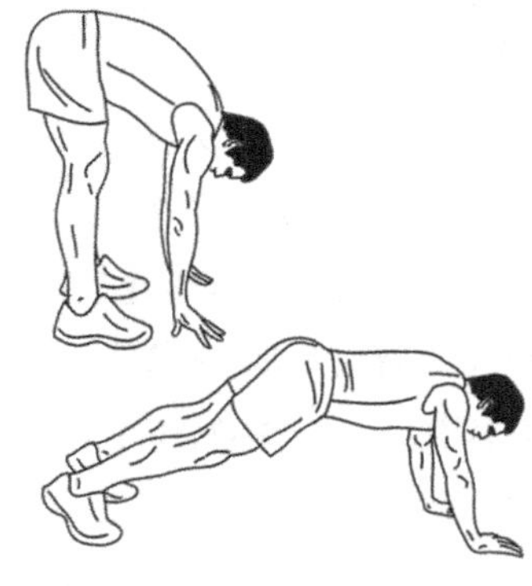

5 plank walk-outs

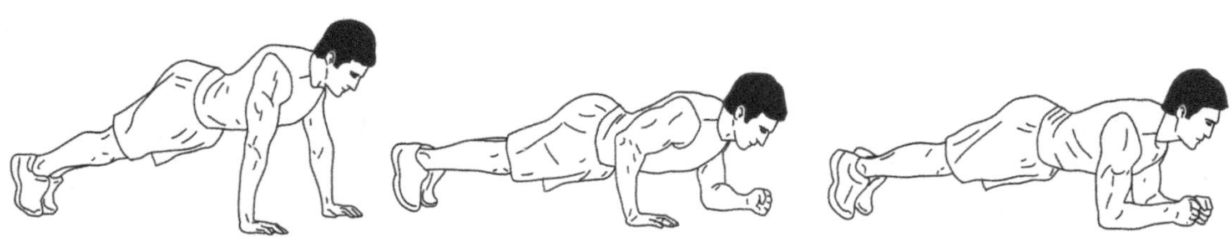

5 up and down planks

78 Core Sculpt

Core Sculpt uses High Knees and some basic core training exercises to raise your body temperature, challenge tendon strength and VO2 Max performance and work the main abdominal groups. The floor exercises provide a handy active recovery stage which means High Knees are performed at high intensity with lots of pumping of the arms and with the knees coming up to waist height, each time. Remember to land on the ball of your foot.

core sculpt

DAREBEE HIIT WORKOUT © darebee.com

Level I 3 sets **Level II** 5 sets **Level III** 7 sets

2 minutes rest between sets

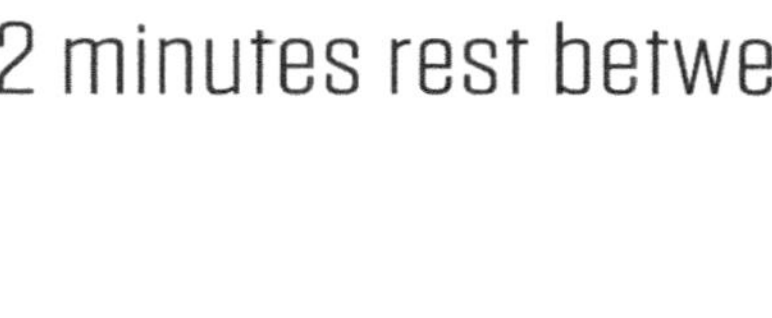

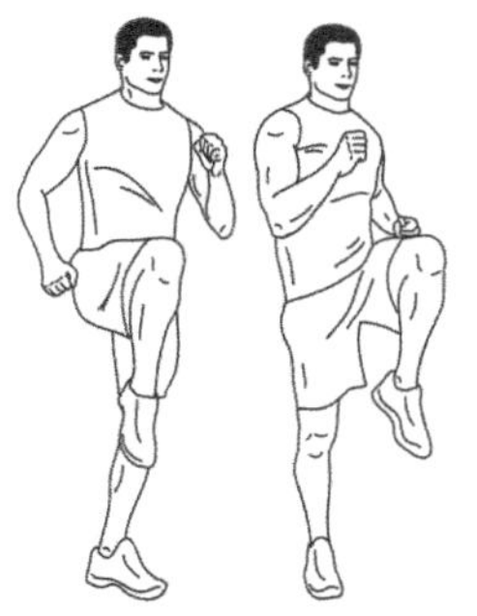

20sec high knees

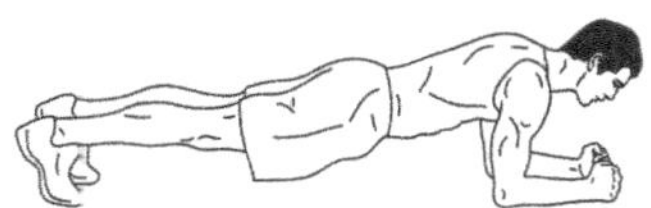

20sec elbow plank

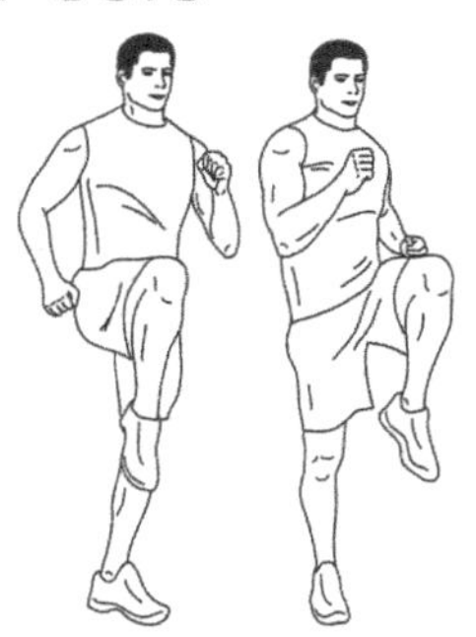

20sec high knees

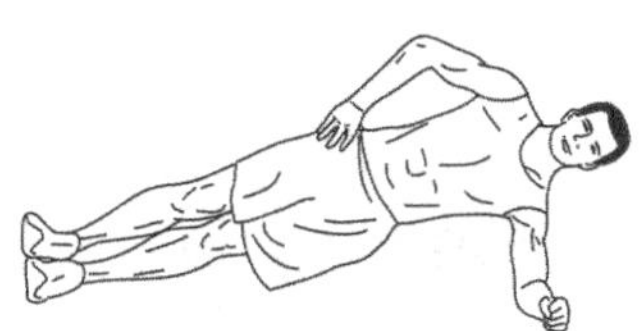

20sec side plank (left)

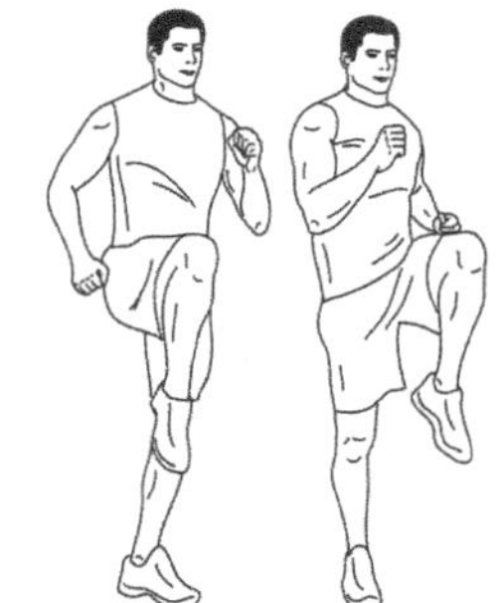

20sec high knees

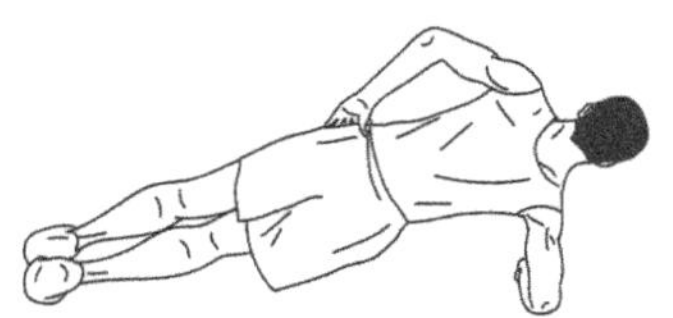

20sec side plank (right)

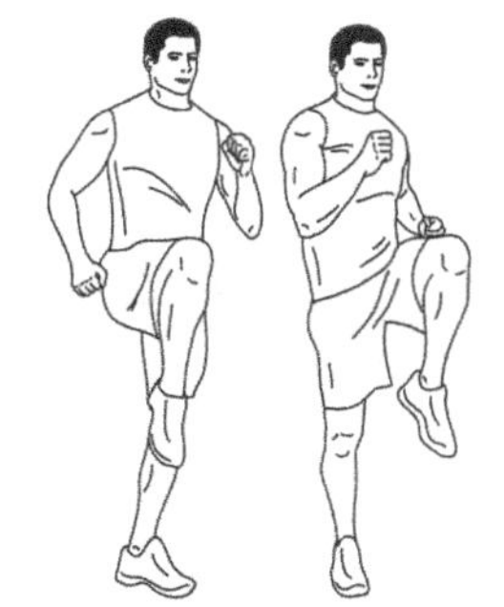

20sec high knees

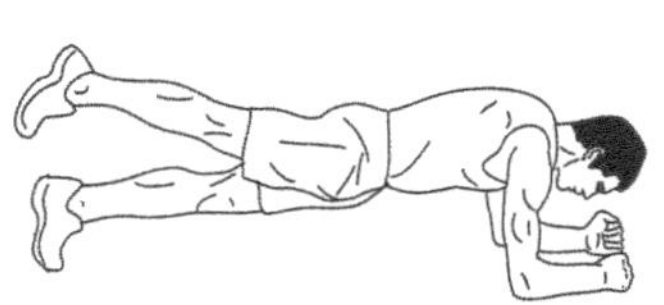

20sec raised leg elbow plank

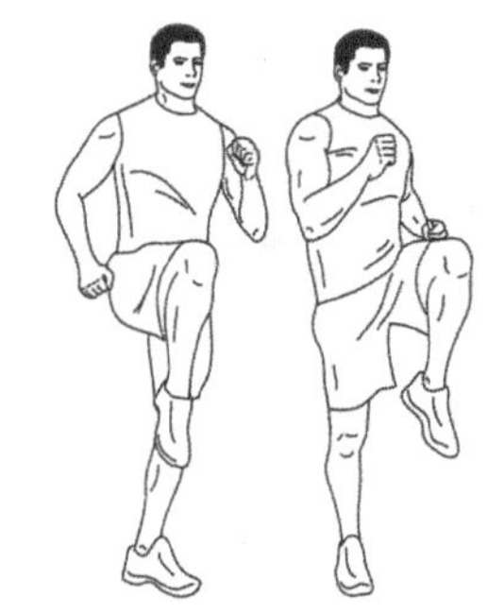

20sec high knees

79 Cycle Core

If you were looking for a workout that specifically targets abs and core and helps you develop that rock solid foundation then Cycle Core is just what you need. Over six, successive exercises it begins to load and work specific muscle groups designed to help you build a solid foundation for your athletic performance.

cycle core

DARBEBEE BACK WORKOUT © darebee.com

LEVEL I 3 sets **LEVEL II** 4 sets **LEVEL III** 5 sets **REST** up to 2 minutes

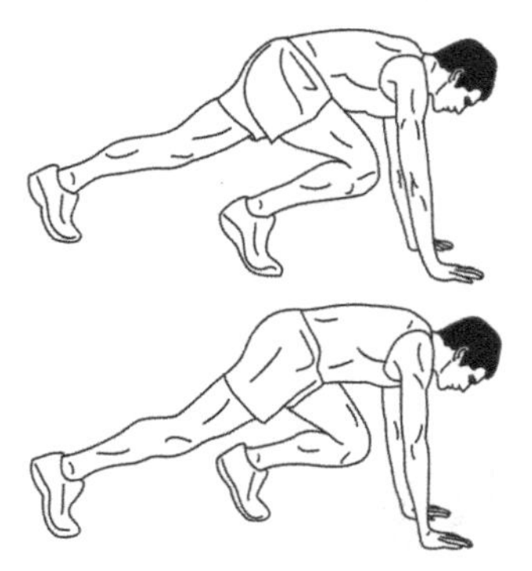

10 climbers

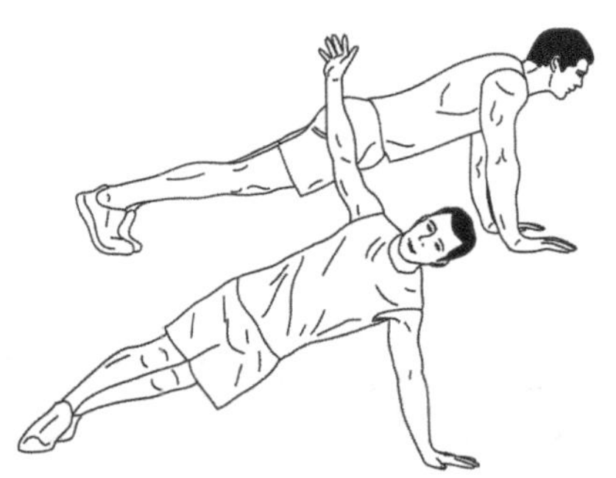

10 plank rotations

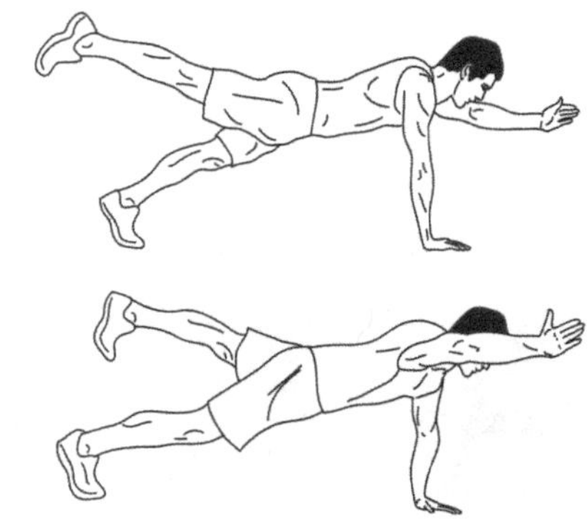

10 alt arm / leg raises

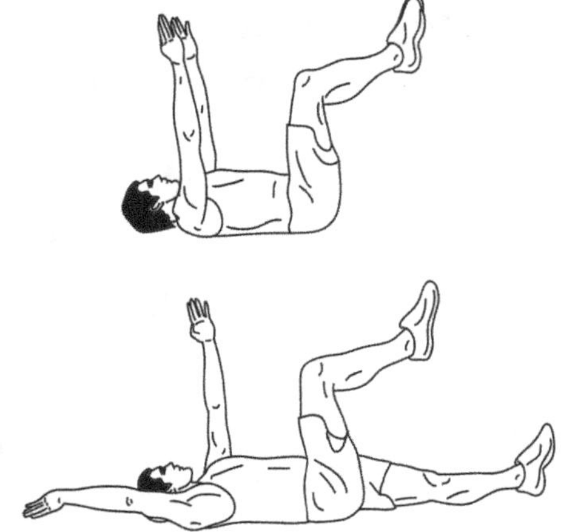

10 dead bug

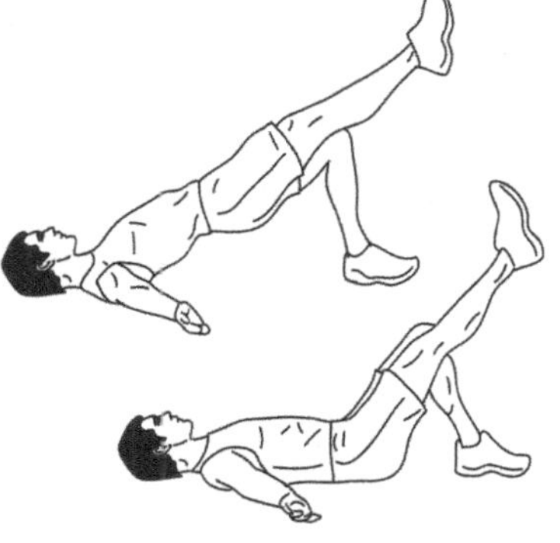

10 single leg bridges

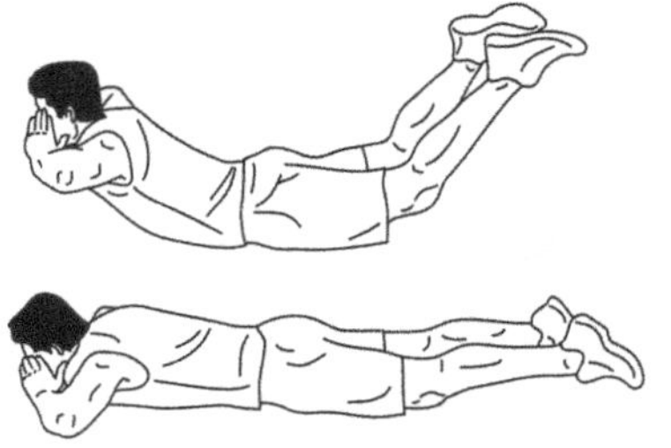

10 back extensions

80 Expedited Delivery

Expedited delivery is zippy and even the floor exercises are designed to put a load on muscles ans tendons that are used in the rest of the workout. That makes it a challenge to get through without a groan 9or two) which means it will work to bring up your body temperature and put you in the sweatzone, fast.

EXPEDITED DELIVERY

DAREBEE HIIT WORKOUT © darebee.com

Level I 3 sets **Level II** 5 sets **Level III** 7 sets | 2 minutes rest

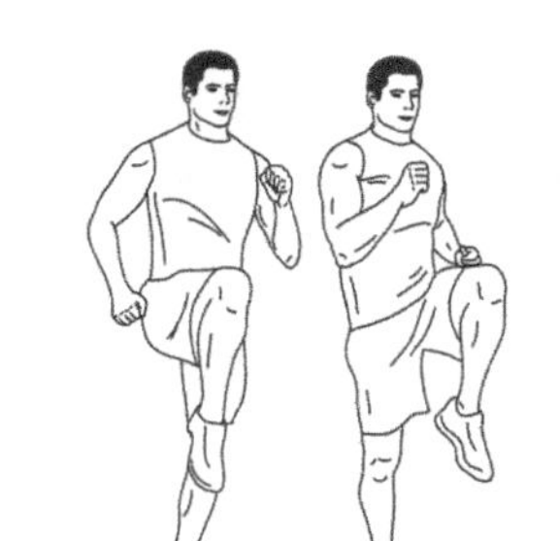

20sec high knees

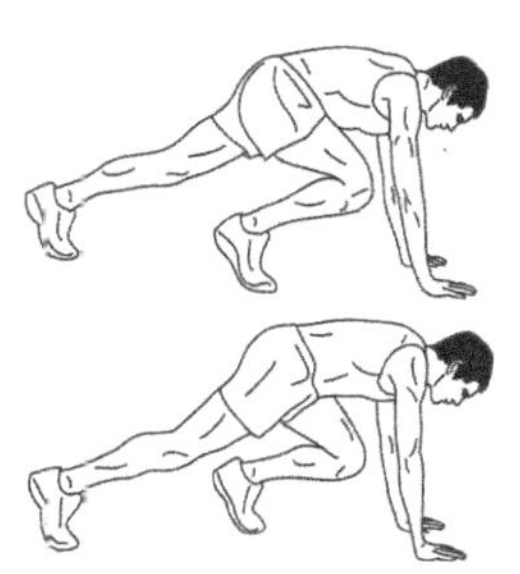

20sec climbers

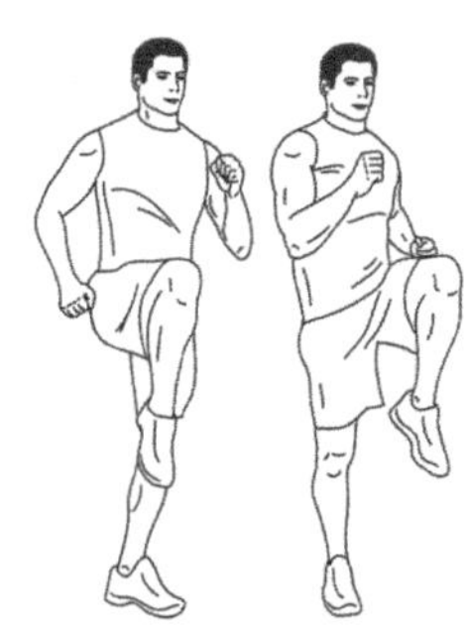

20sec high knees

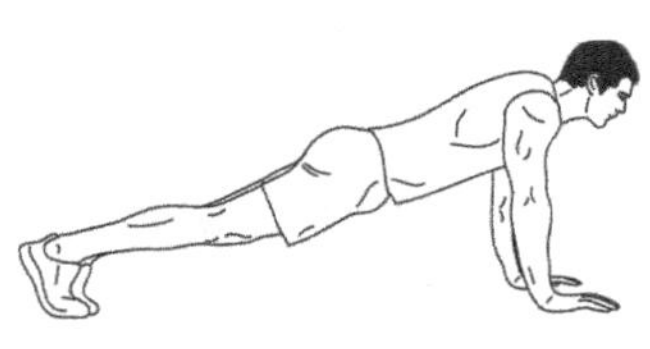

20sec plank hold

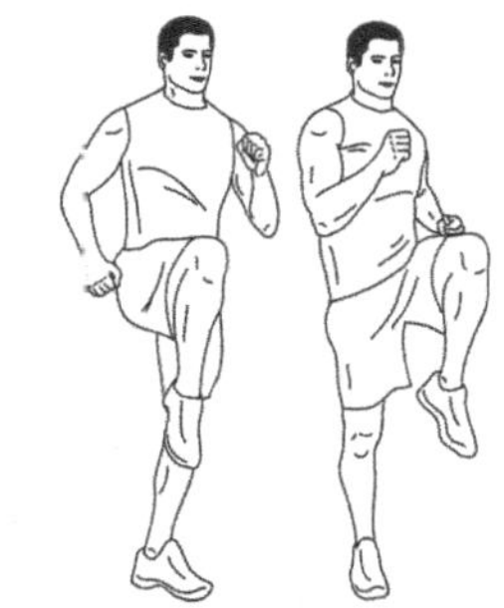

20sec high knees

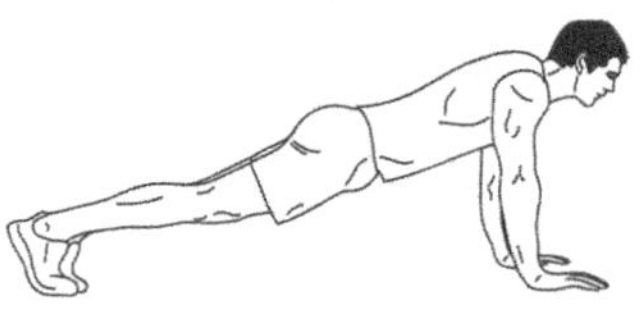

20sec plank hold

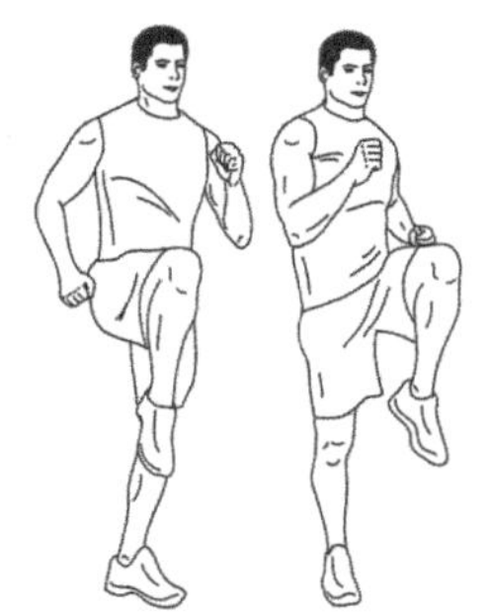

20sec high knees

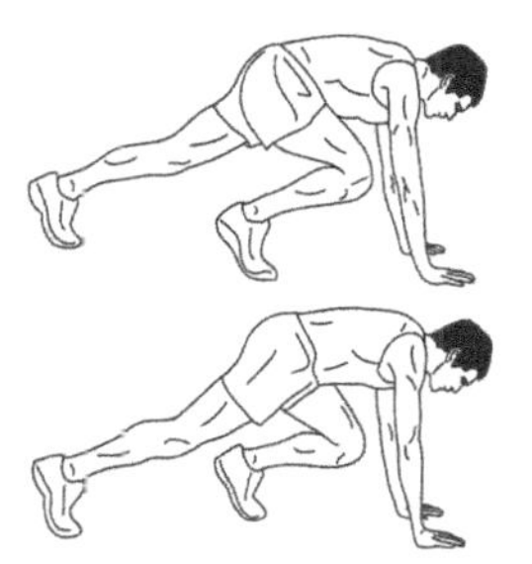

20sec climbers

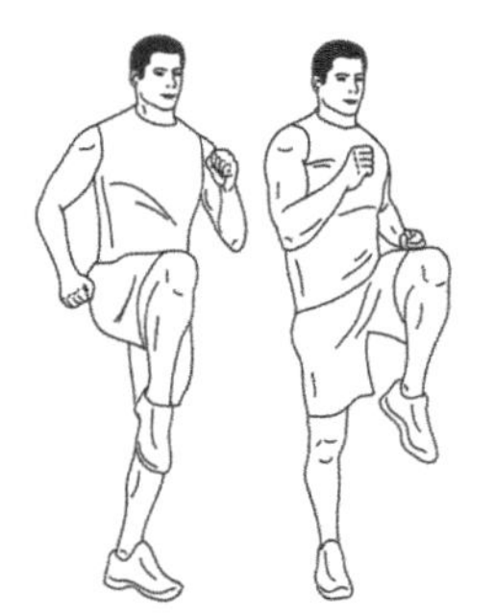

20sec high knees

81 Fab Abs

The abs and core are the junction at which lower body strength is translated into upper body power. But for that to happen you need strong abs and a strong core. Fab Abs works all of that in a dynamic and static fashion. The cross-mix delivers a potent abs workout that demands you raise your knees to waist height during High Knees and keep your body as absolutely straight as you possibly can during plank.

FAB ABS

DAREBEE HIIT WORKOUT © darebee.com

Level I 3 sets **Level II** 5 sets **Level III** 7 sets | 2 minutes rest

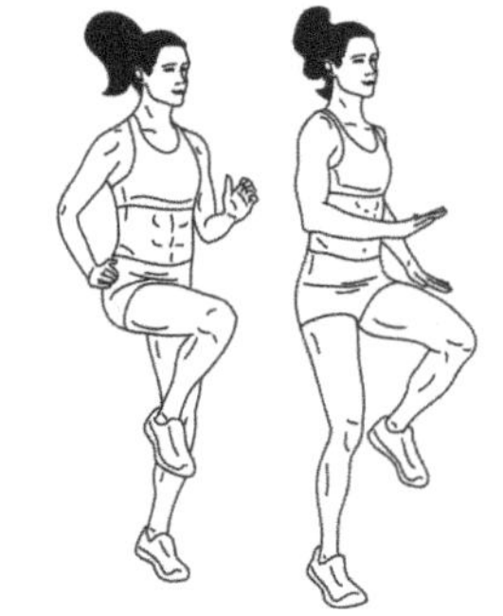

20sec high knees

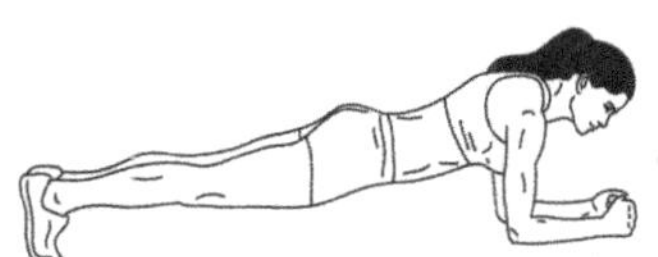

20sec elbow plank hold

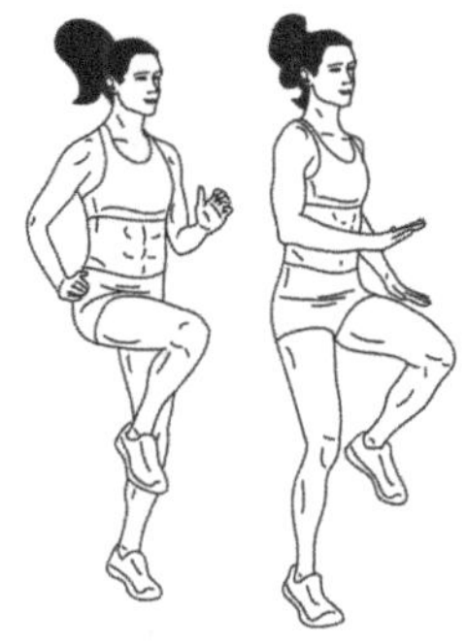

20sec high knees

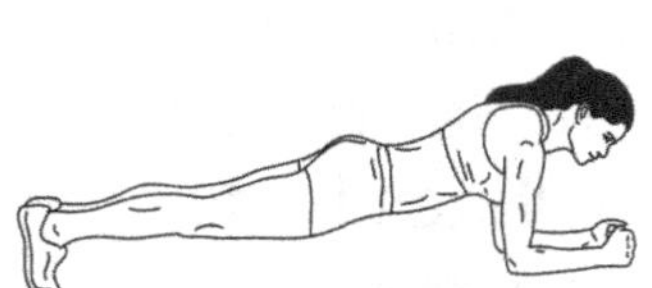

20sec elbow plank hold

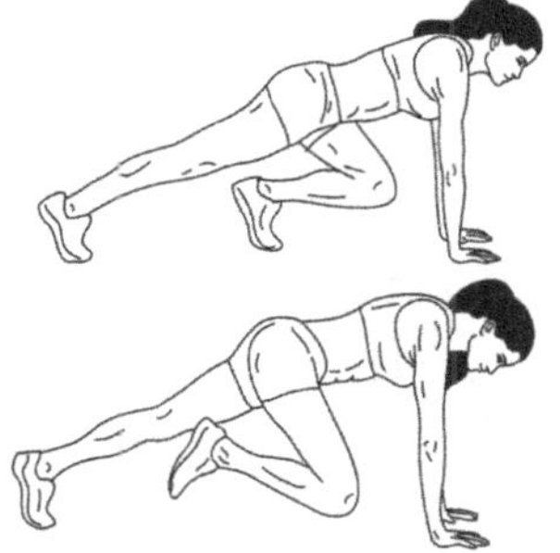

20sec climbers

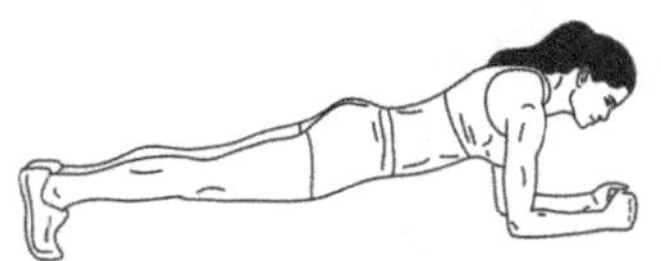

20sec elbow plank hold

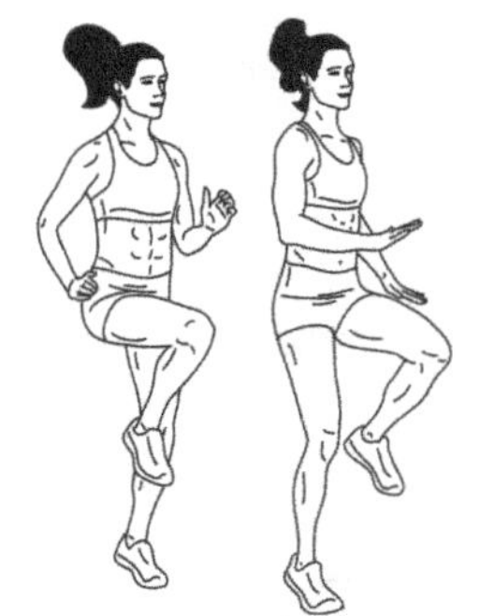

20sec high knees

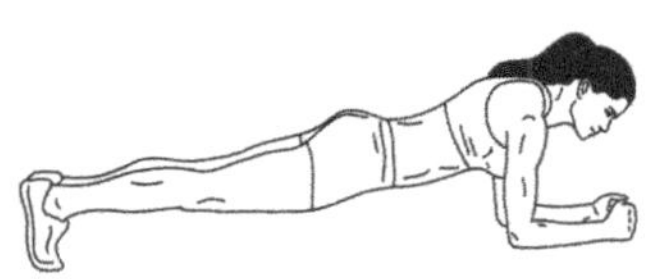

20sec elbow plank hold

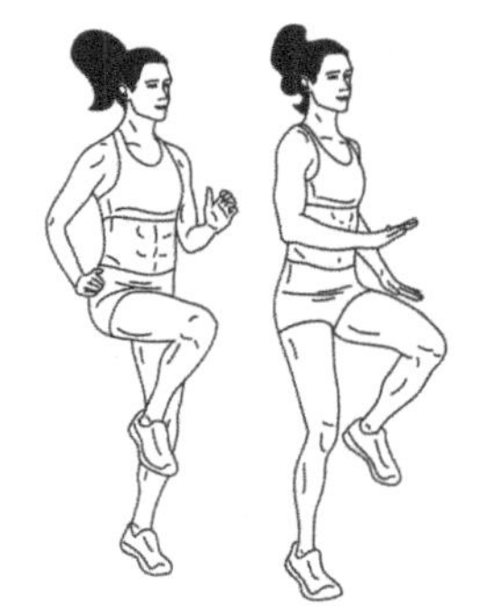

20sec high knees

82 Flat Stomach

The Flat Stomach workout targets all the muscle groups required for a strong, taut stomach but the workout does more than that. Seeing how you can't lose weight locally the Flat Stomach workout elevates body temperature, loads large muscle groups through specific exercises and helps the body become more streamlined which then helps with the desired goal.

FLAT STOMACH

DAREBEE WORKOUT © darebee.com

repeat 5 times in total | 2 minutes rest between sets

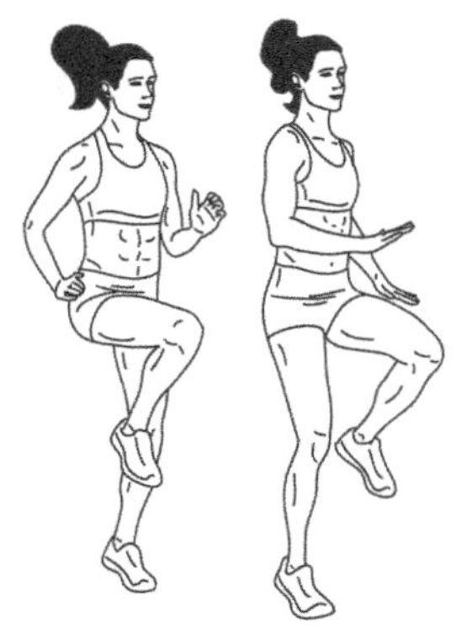

40 high knees

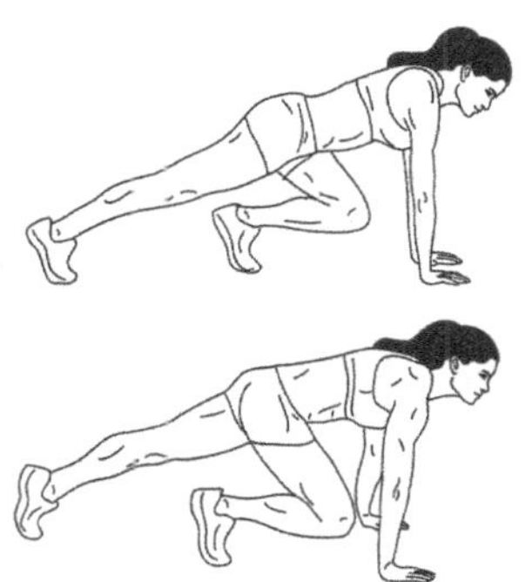

20 climbers

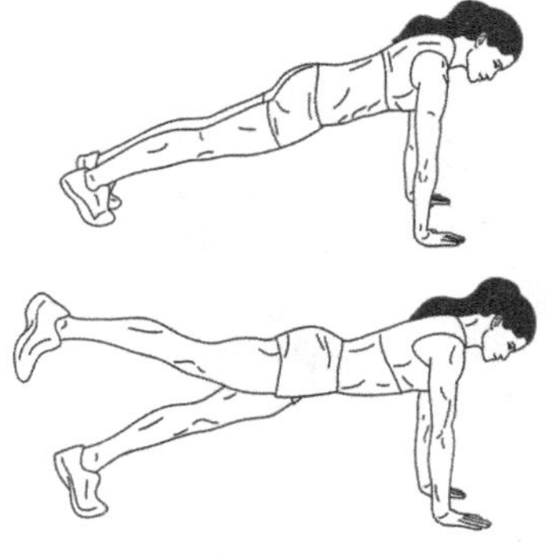

40 plank leg raises

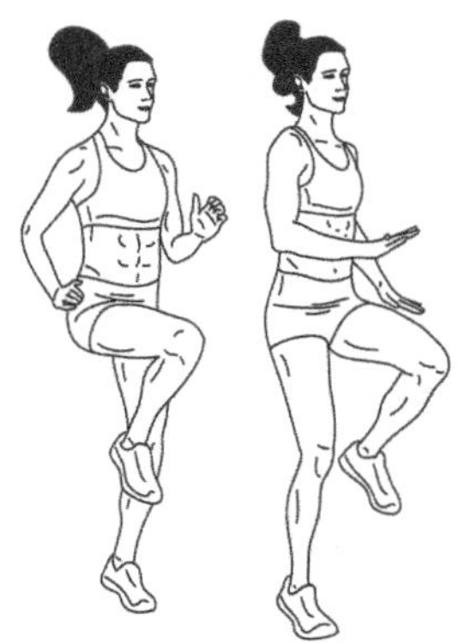

40 high knees

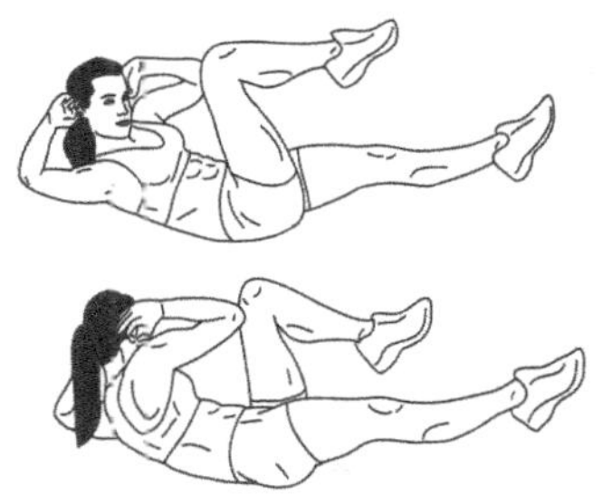

20 knee-to-elbow crunches

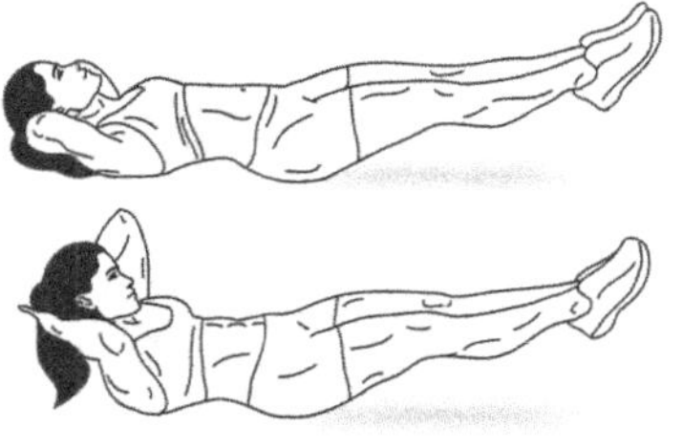

40 raised leg crunches

83 Gut Buster

A minute's worth of High Knees is approximately equivalent to running a mile provided you pump your arms back and forth properly and bring your knees to waist height each time. Gut Buster is a workout that raises your body's temperature and maintains it throughout the workout.

GUT BUSTER

DAREBEE WORKOUT

5 sets | 2 minutes rest between sets

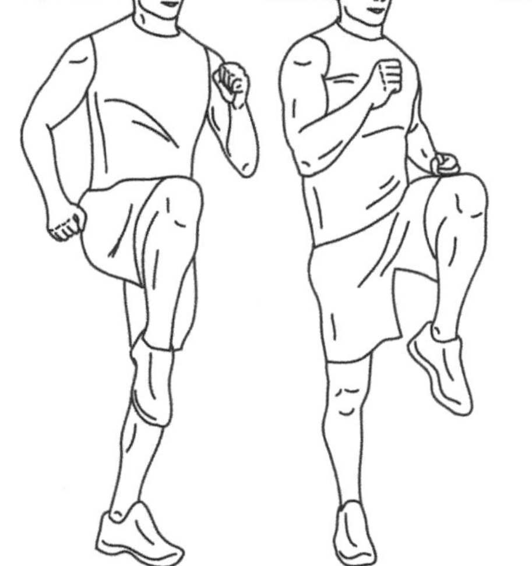

20 high knees

10 march steps (walk)

20 high knees

10 march steps (walk)

20 high knees

10 march steps (walk)

20 high knees

10 march steps (walk)

20 high knees

10 march steps (walk)

done

84 Hellraiser

It takes just 270 seconds to transport you from the Earthly plane to the special world of Hell Week and the Hellraiser workout is your ticket to that place. Stay on the balls of your feet when you perform High Knees, bring your knees to waist height each time and pump your arms as you run. The core and abs exercises also require perfect form.

HELLRAISER

DAREBEE **HIIT** WORKOUT © **darebee.com**

Level I 3 sets **Level II** 5 sets **Level III** 7 sets | 2 minutes rest

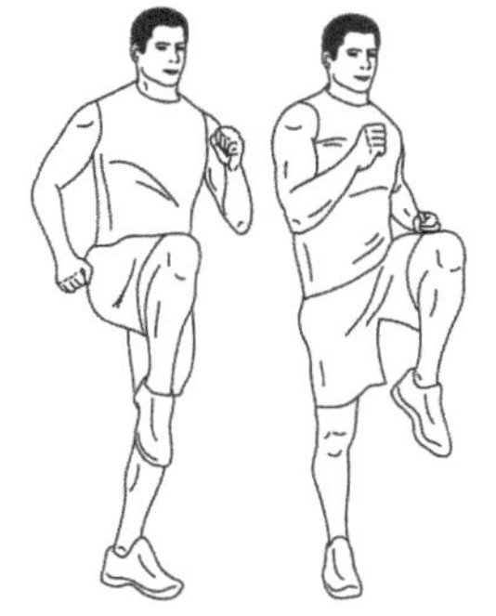

30sec high knees

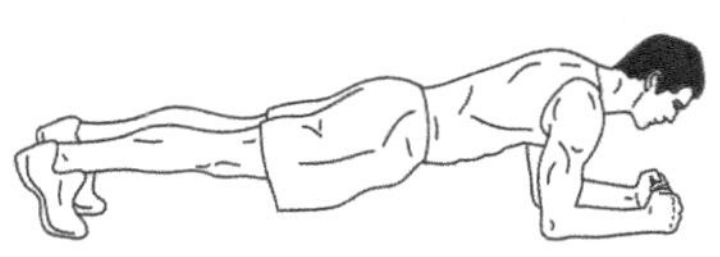

30sec elbow plank hold

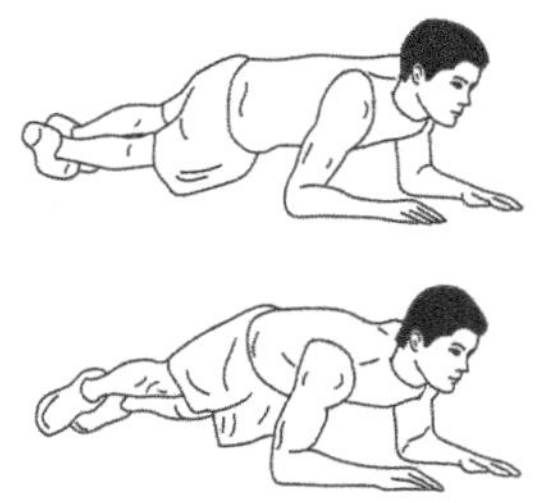

30sec plank rolls

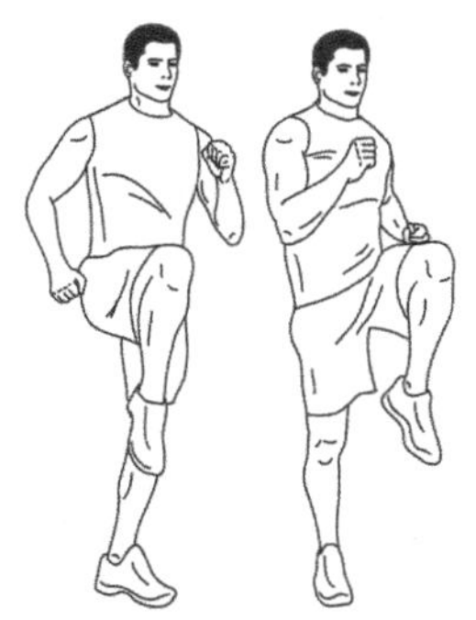

30sec high knees

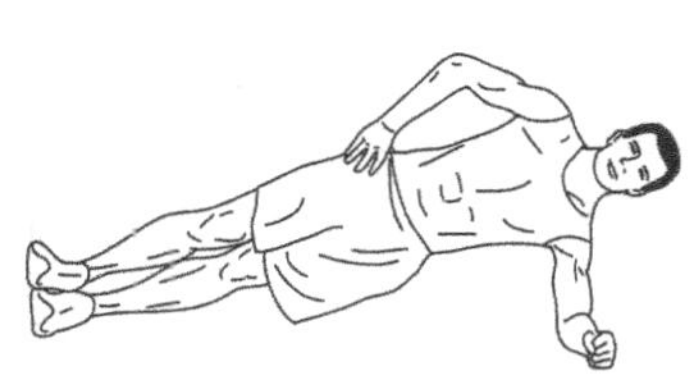

30sec side plank hold

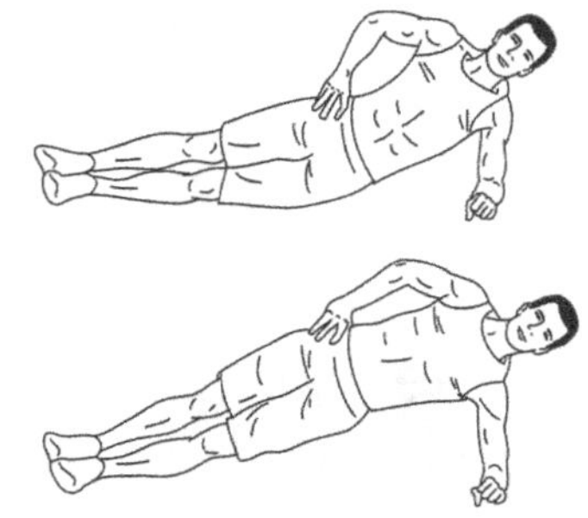

30sec side planks

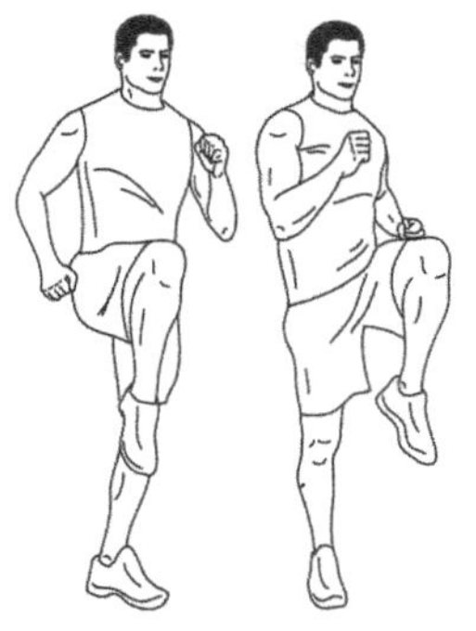

30sec high knees

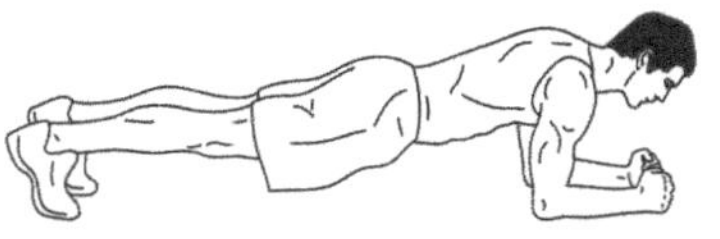

30sec elbow plank hold

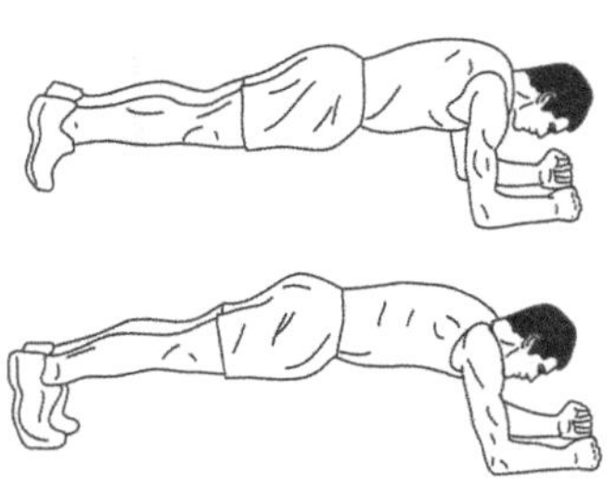

30sec bodysaw

85 Howler

Some workouts you are prepared for right from the moment you see them and others kinda sneak up on you and leave you feeling wasted on the floor, wondering why you did not see them coming. Howler is definitely one of the latter.

HOWLER

DAREBEE HIIT WORKOUT © darebee.com

LEVEL I 3 sets **LEVEL II** 5 sets **LEVEL III** 7 sets **REST** up to 2 minutes

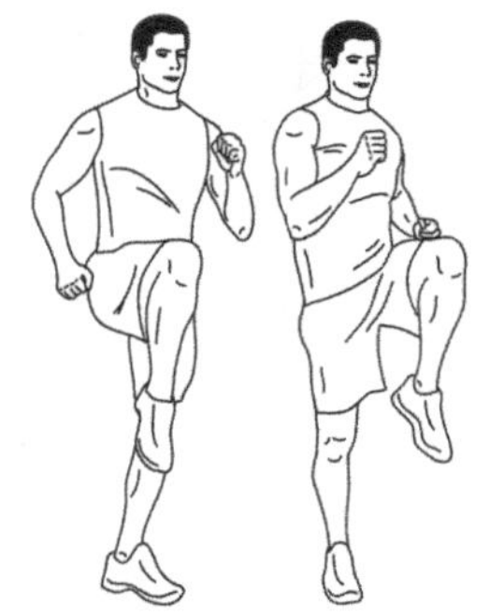

40sec high knees

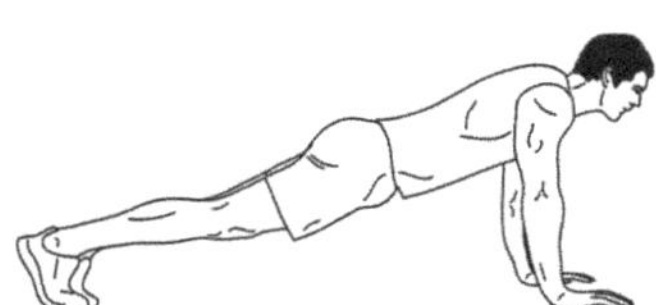

10sec plank

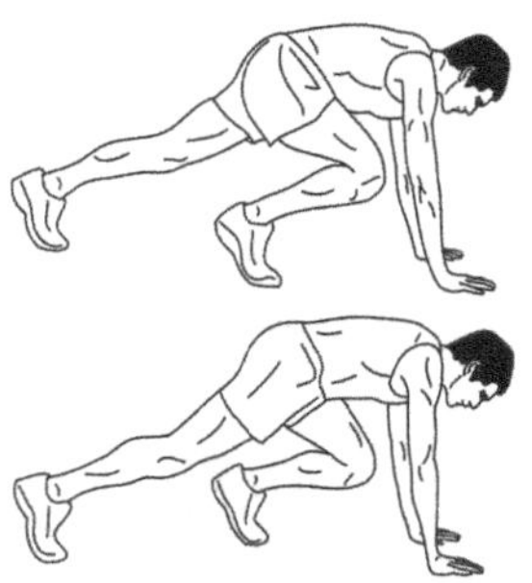

10sec climbers

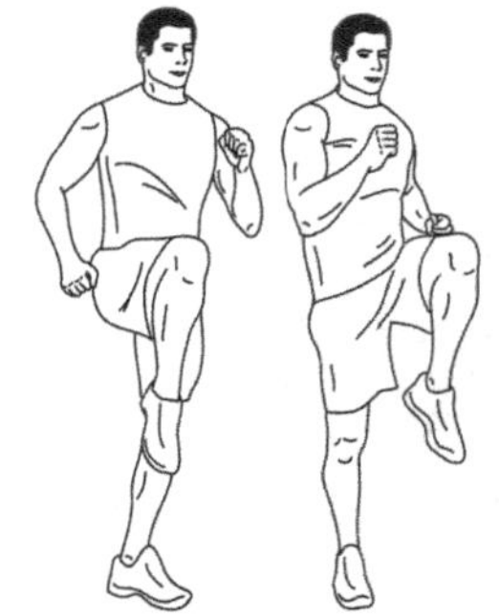

40sec high knees

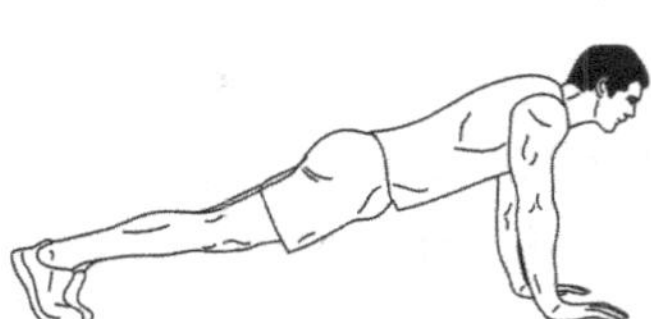

10sec plank

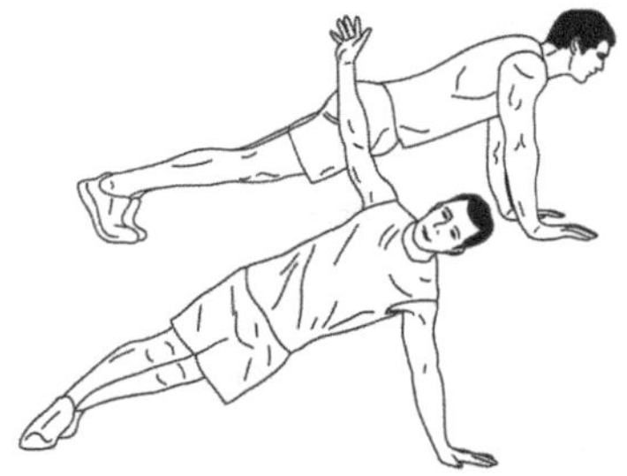

10sec plank rotations

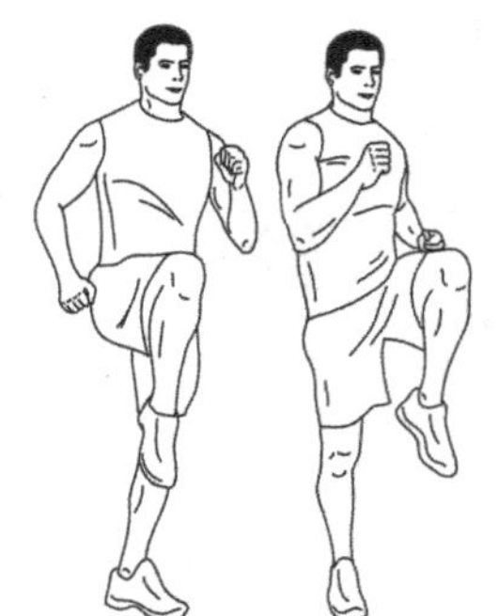

40sec high knees

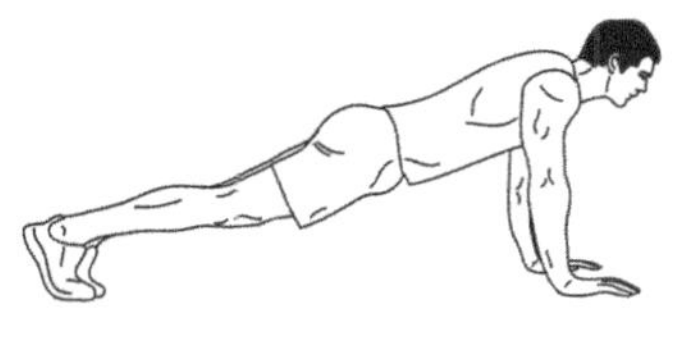

10sec plank

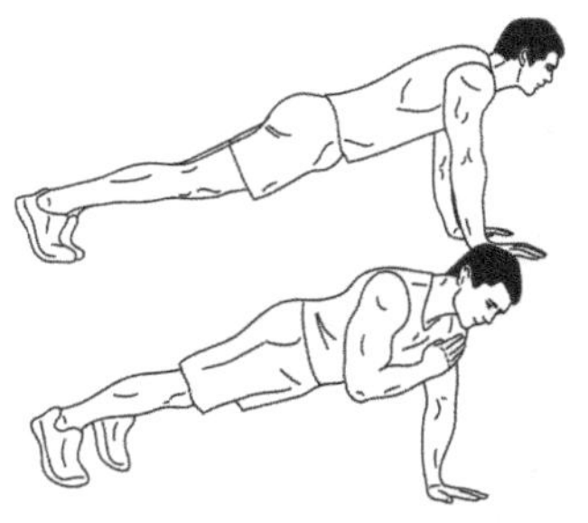

10sec shoulder taps

86 Lean & Mean

There are a few things you need to get lean: a high-burn workout that will work large muscle groups, force you to use up a lot of oxygen and get you into the sweatzone fast. Exercises that keep on applying a load to your muscles. And a combination that forces you to recruit a large number of muscle groups. Lean and Mean combines all that. You now just need to power through it. Maintain perfect form.

LEAN & MEAN

DARBEE WORKOUT © darebee.com

LEVEL I 3 sets **LEVEL II** 5 sets **LEVEL III** 7 sets **REST** up to 2 minutes

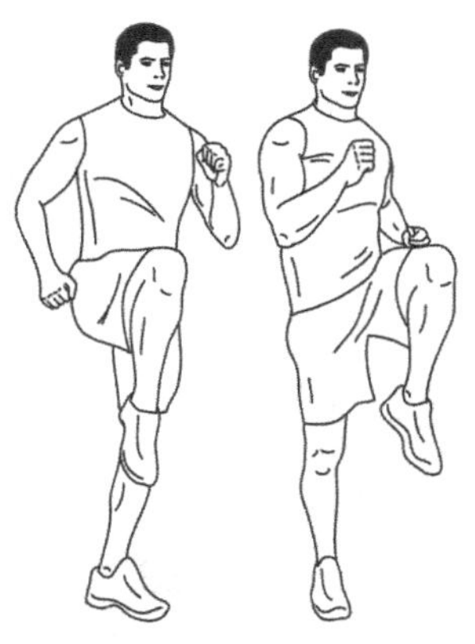

40 high knees

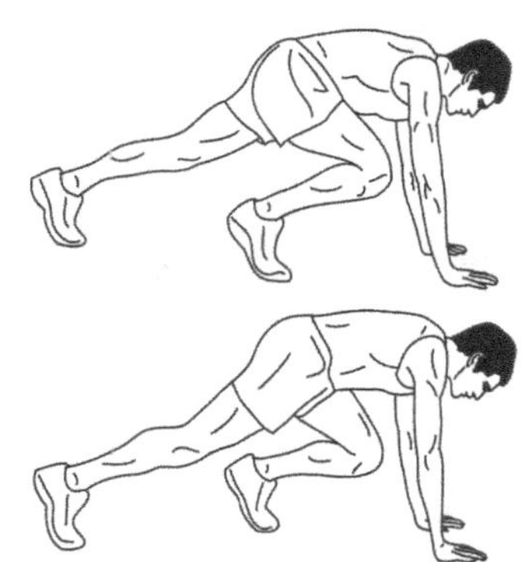

40 climbers

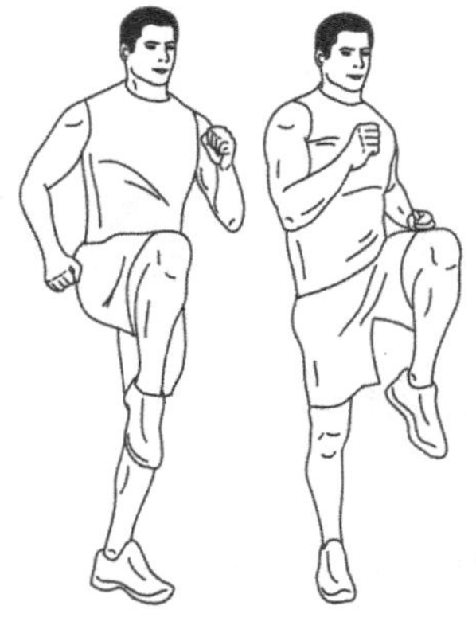

40 high knees

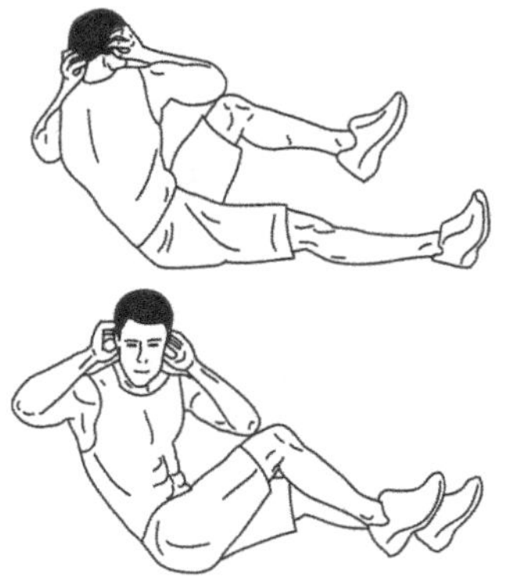

20 knee-to-elbows

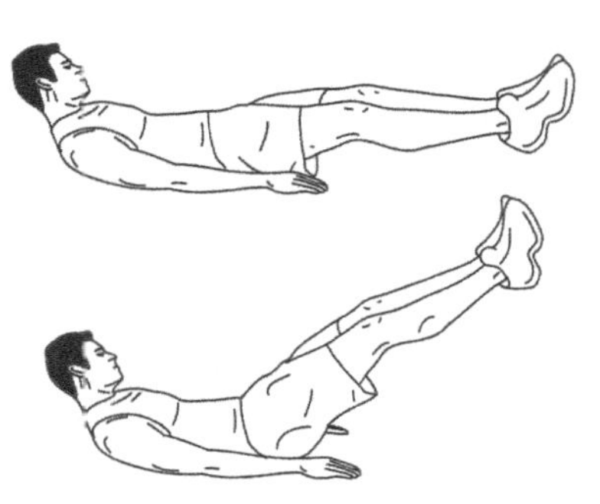

20 leg raises

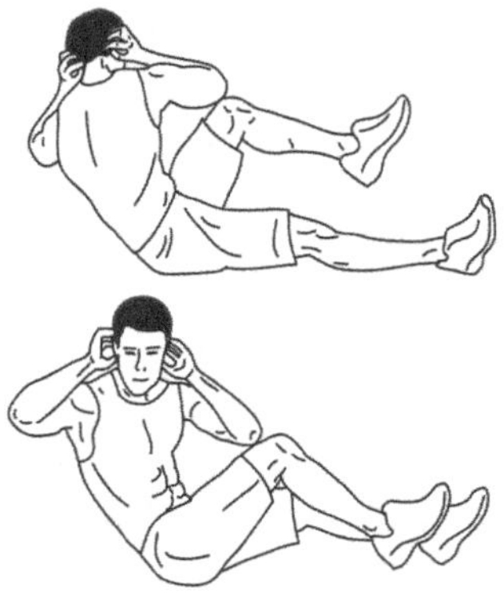

20 knee-to-elbows

87 Love Handles

Shape your body and tighten up your obliques with the Love Handles workout, designed to specifically work these areas. You work muscles designed to move the body in short, sharp moves which means the workout will get you into the sweatzone pretty fast and keep you there until you complete it.

Love Handles

DAREBEE WORKOUT © darebee.com

LEVEL I 3 sets **LEVEL II** 5 sets **LEVEL III** 7 sets **REST** up to 2 minutes

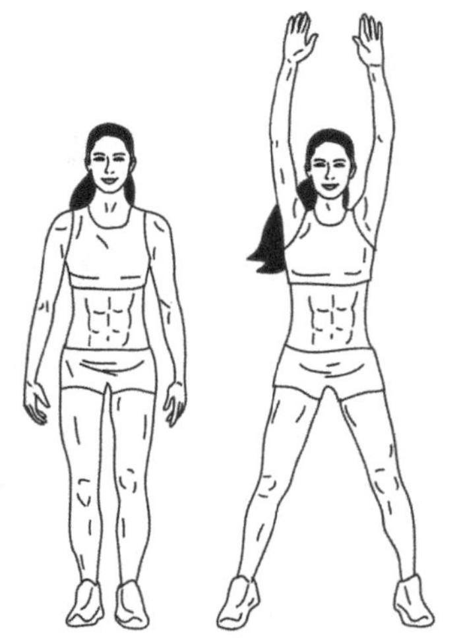

30 jumping jacks

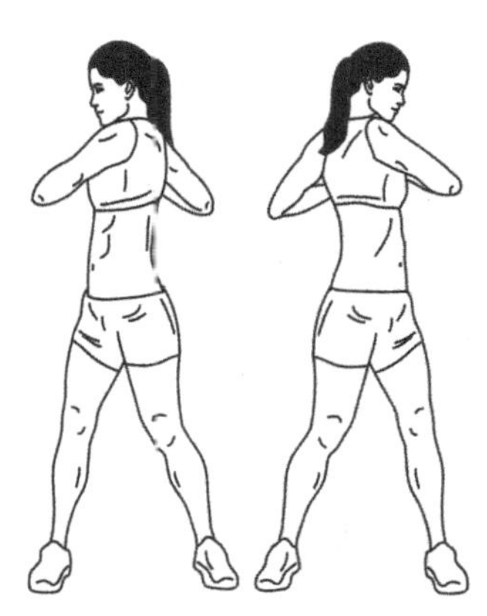

10 twists

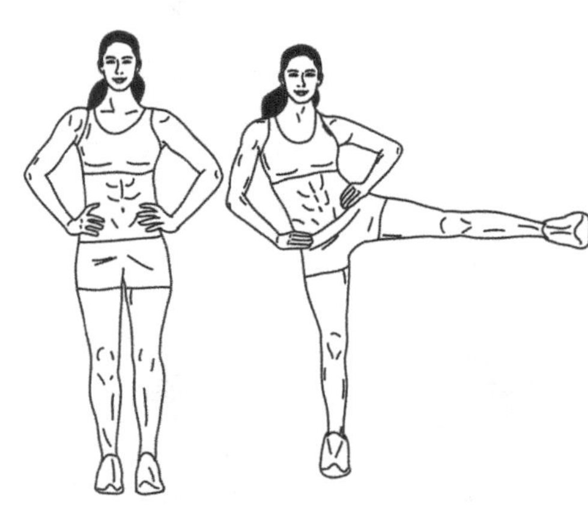

30 side leg raises

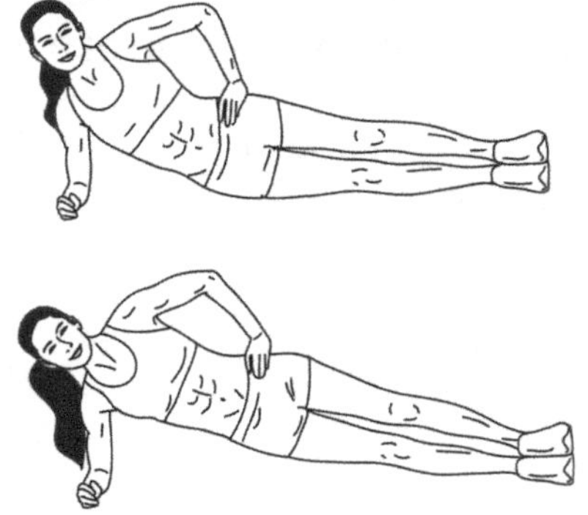

30 side bridges

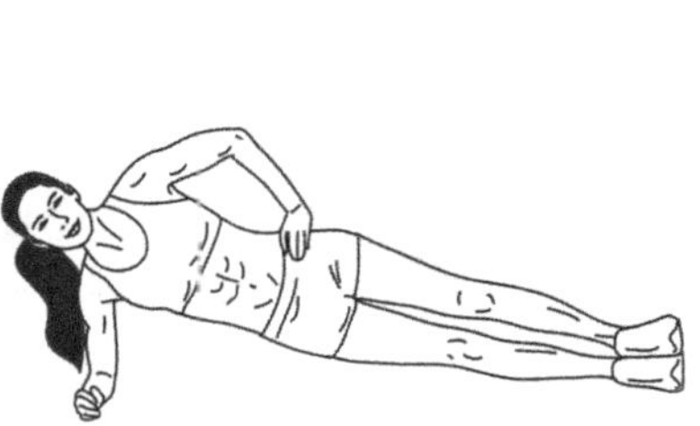

30sec side plank hold

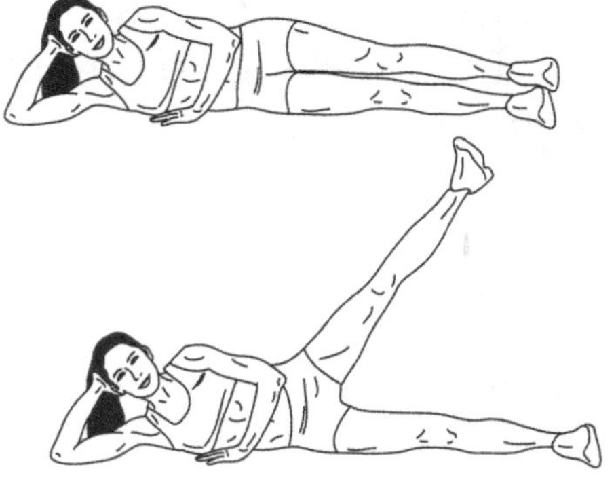

30 side leg raises

88 Melt Off

Melt Off uses large muscle groups under a heavy load to test your VO2 Max. Form and rep count are important here. Bring your knees to waist height during High Knees and work fast and hard with your Burpees to get in as many as you can in each 20 second time slot. Your active recovery is the Elbow Plank so breathe slow and deep during those times to oxygenate your muscles.

MELT OFF

DAREBEE **HIIT** WORKOUT © **darebee.com**

Level I 3 sets **Level II** 5 sets **Level III** 7 sets | 2 minutes rest

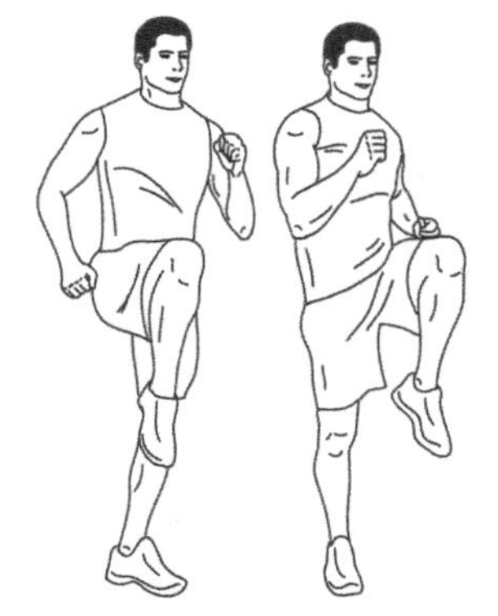

20sec high knees

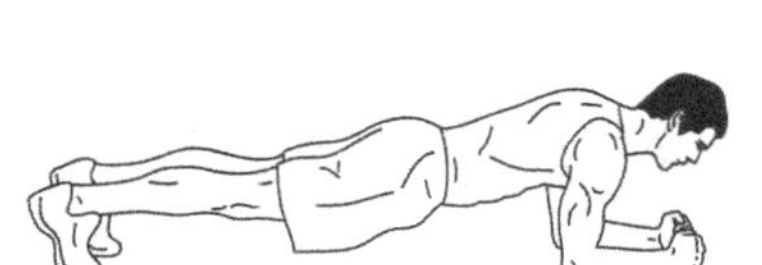

20sec elbow plank

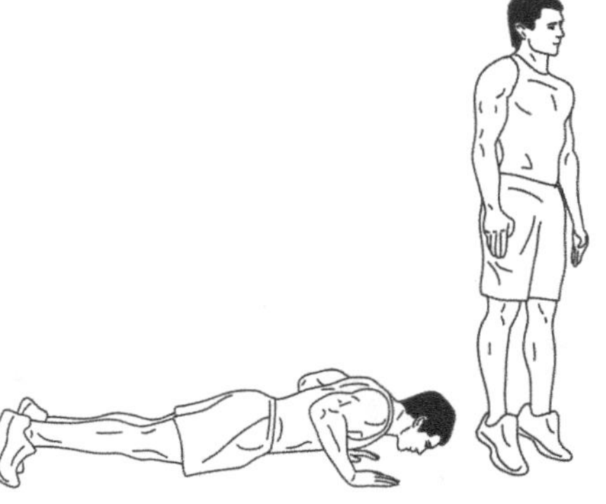

20sec burpees

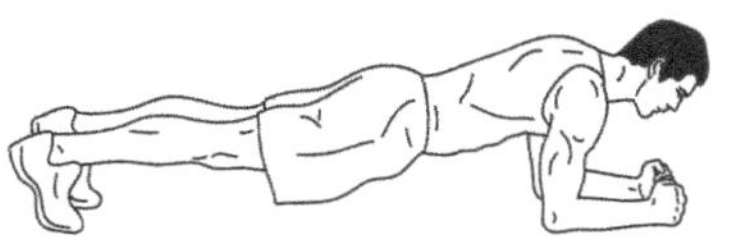

20sec elbow plank

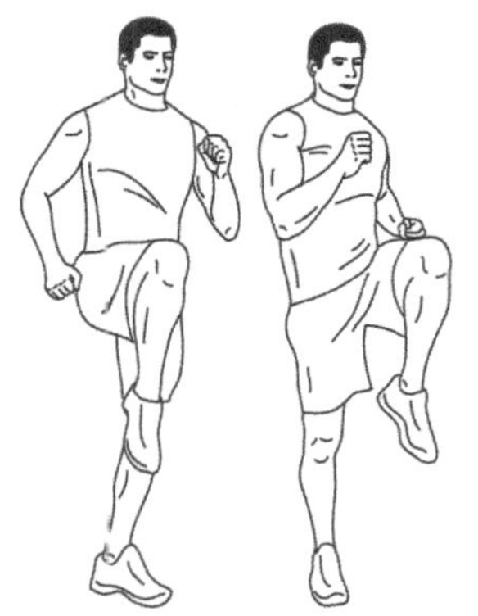

20sec high knees

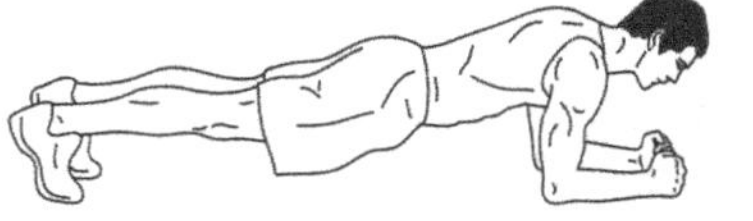

20sec elbow plank

89 Muffin Top

Every time you move large muscle groups at high intensity you incur quite a high oxygen debt that needs to be repaid. That repayment comes with a higher energy burn and an overall increased energy burn. Yes you will sweat and yes again, you will gasp for breath but you will also get to extend your endurance, test your VO2 Max and will get to work pretty hard.

muffin top

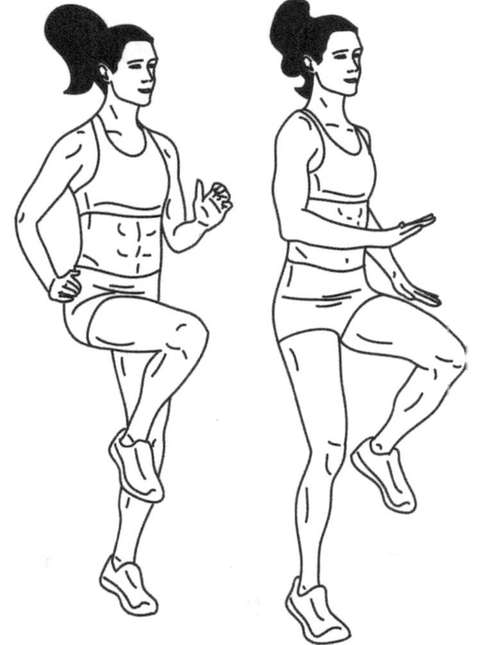

WORKOUT by © darebee.com

20 high knees

6 knee-to-elbow crunches

20 high knees

6 knee-to-elbow crunches

20 high knees

6 knee-to-elbow crunches

20 high knees

6 knee-to-elbow crunches

20 high knees

6 knee-to-elbow crunches

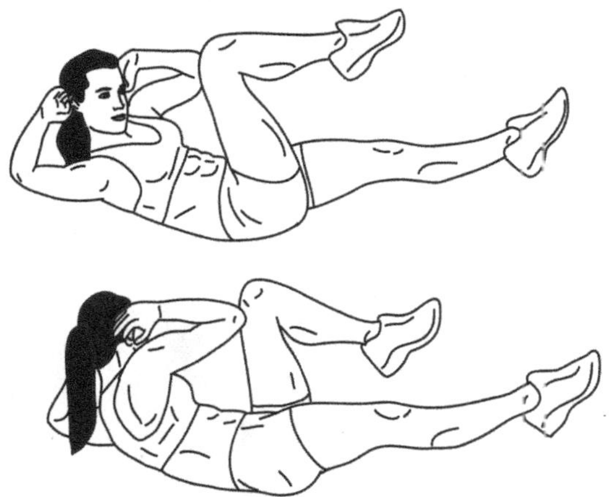

repeat 3 times

2 minutes rest in between

90 Outcast

Fascial fitness demands using your body like a spring and Outcast makes you use all the muscle groups and tendons that drive the fascial tissue throughout the body. The result is a high-burn streamlining workout that takes you one step closer to acquiring total control of your body.

outcast

DAREBEE WORKOUT © darebee.com

LEVEL I 3 sets **LEVEL II** 5 sets **LEVEL III** 7 sets **REST** up to 2 minutes

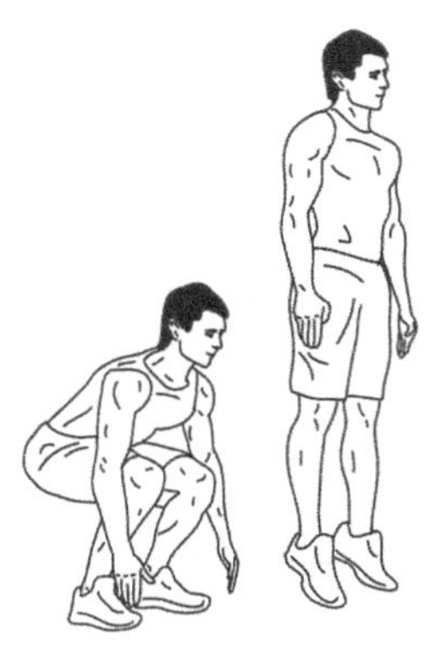

10 jump squats

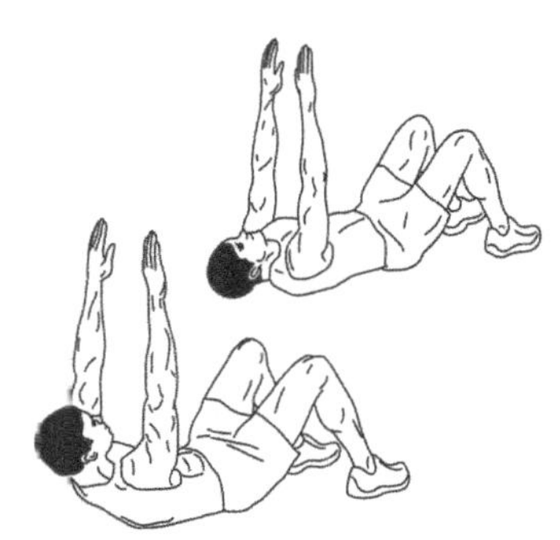

10 high crunches

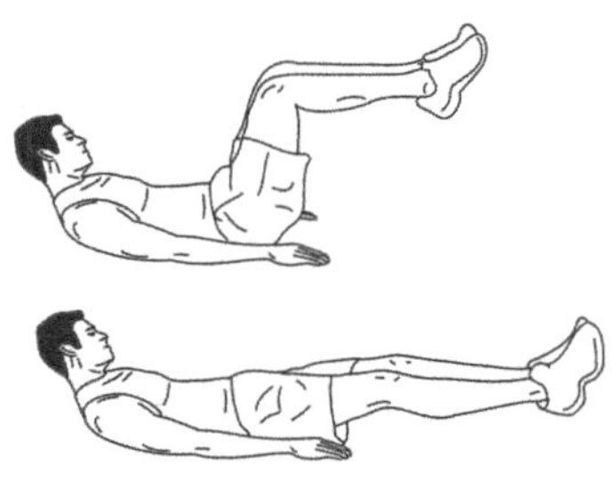

4 crunch kicks

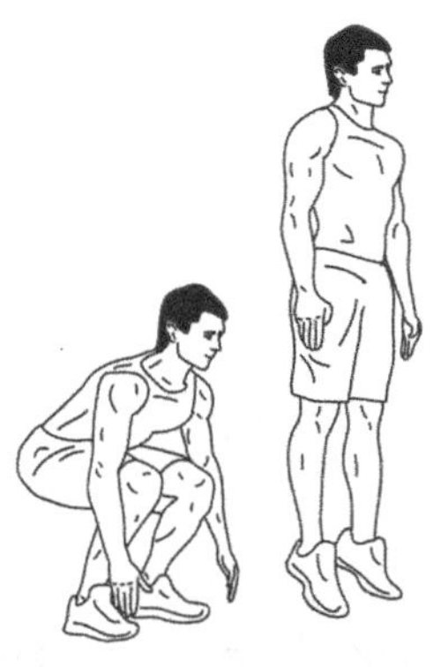

10 jump squats

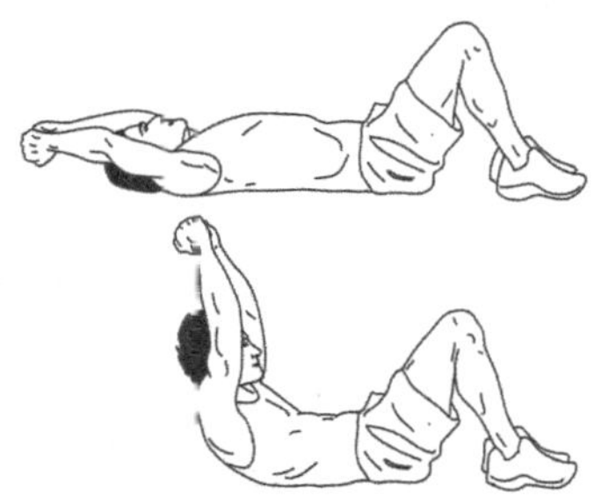

10 long arm crunches

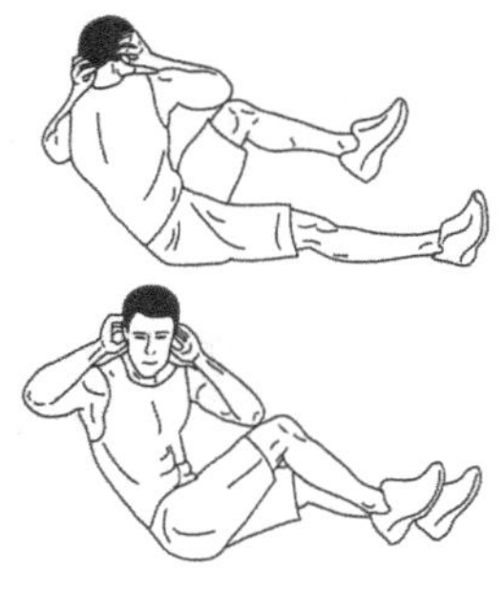

4 knee-to-elbow crunches

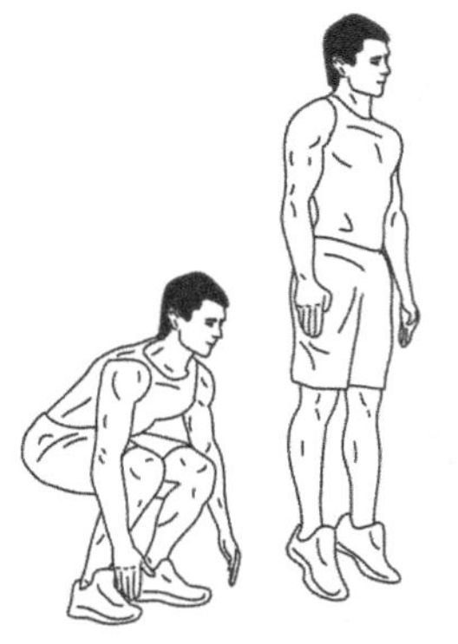

10 jump squats

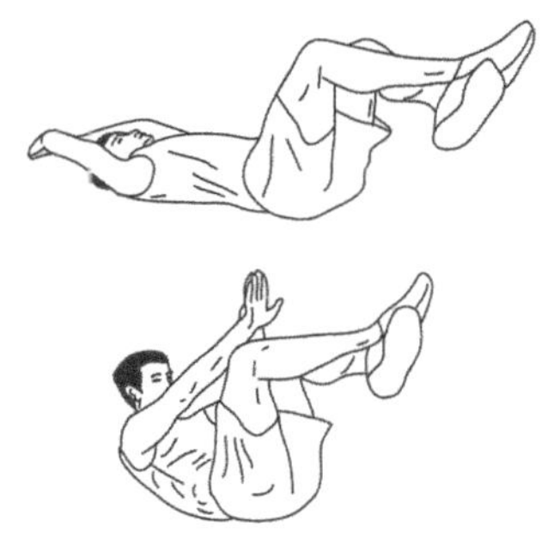

10 knee crunches

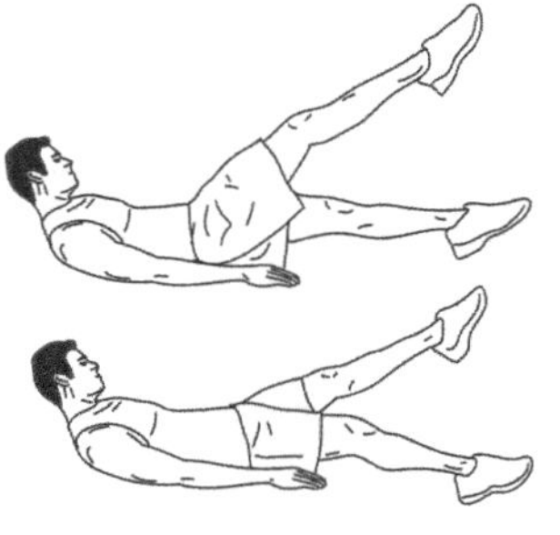

4 flutter kicks

91 Overhaul

Overhaul is a workout that targets tendons and muscles that power the lower body. It is used to build explosiveness and power. Make sure you bring your knee up to waist-height when performing March Steps and High Knees. Pump your arms in unison with your legs and bring the pace up that way. Try to work to the same count of reps or better each time, throughout each set.

OVERHAUL

DAREBEE HIIT WORKOUT © darebee.com

Level I 3 sets **Level II** 5 sets **Level III** 7 sets | 2 minutes rest

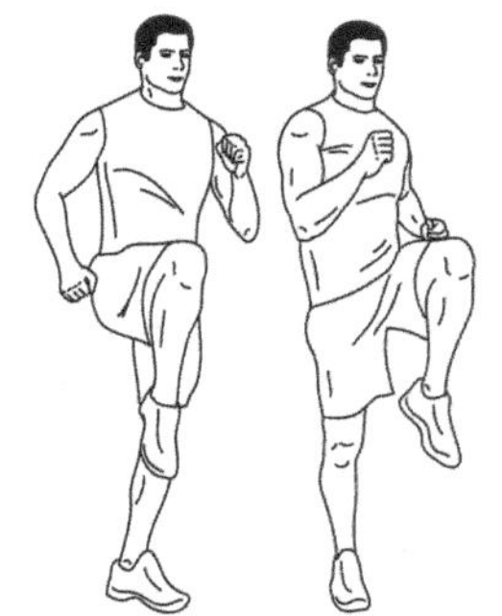

20sec high knees

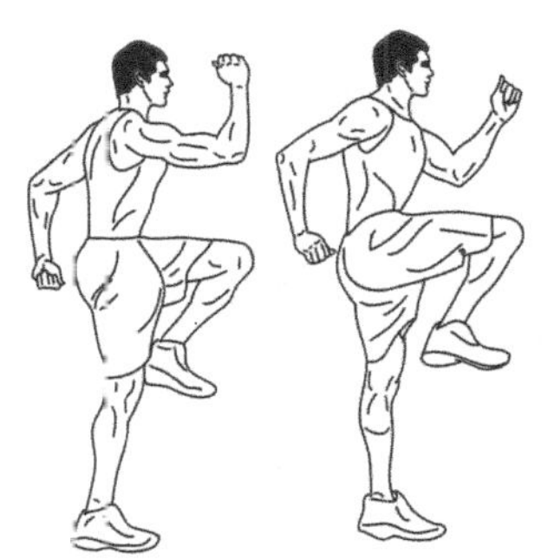

20sec march steps

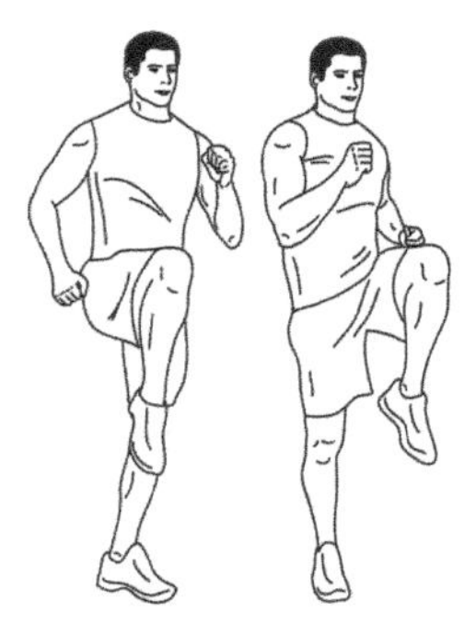

20sec high knees

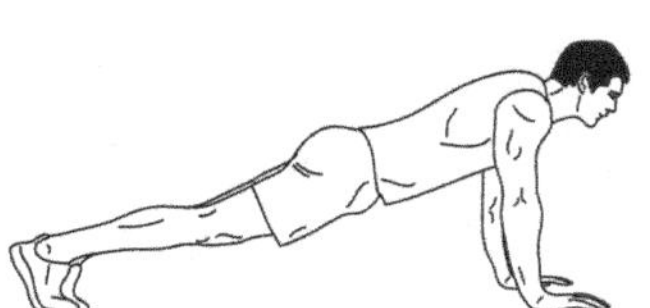

20sec plank hold

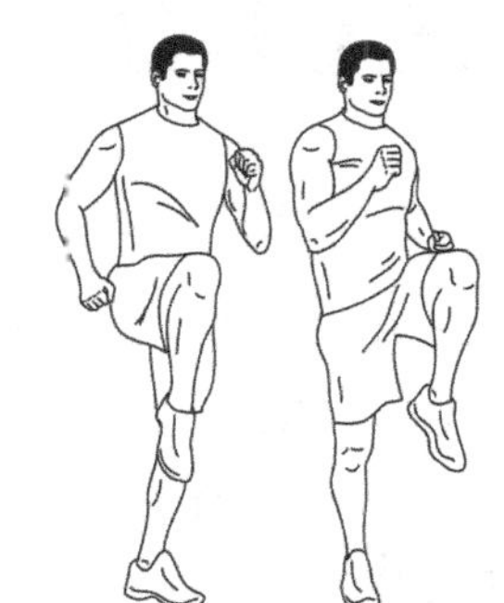

20sec high knees

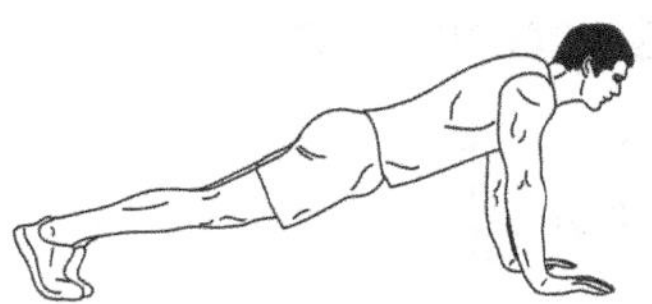

20sec plank hold

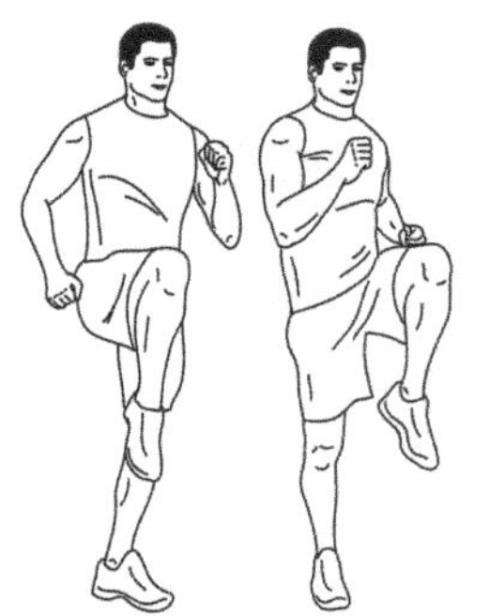

20sec high knees

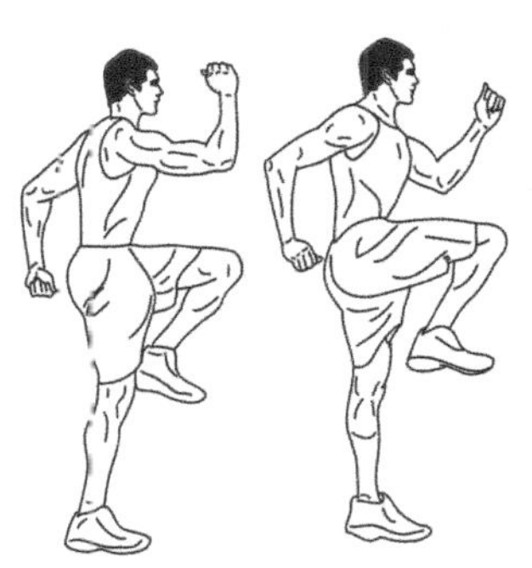

20sec march steps

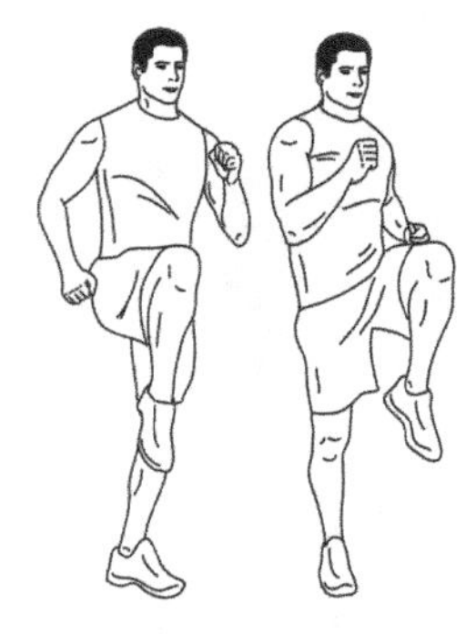

20sec high knees

92 Persephone

Persephone, in Greek mythology, spends half her time in the Underworld and the rest in the world above ground. The workout that bears her name however is all pure Hell Week. Two alternating exercises, performed to perfection, will push your muscles and lungs to the very edge of your capability. This is exactly what you want, right?

PERSEPHONE

DAREBEE HIIT WORKOUT © darebee.com

Level I 3 sets **Level II** 5 sets **Level III** 7 sets | 2 minutes rest

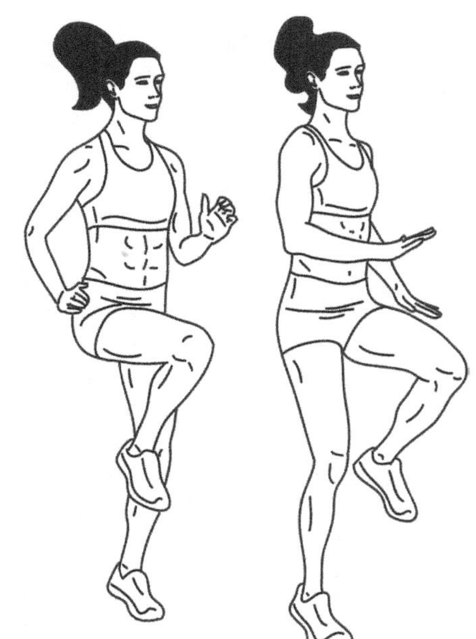

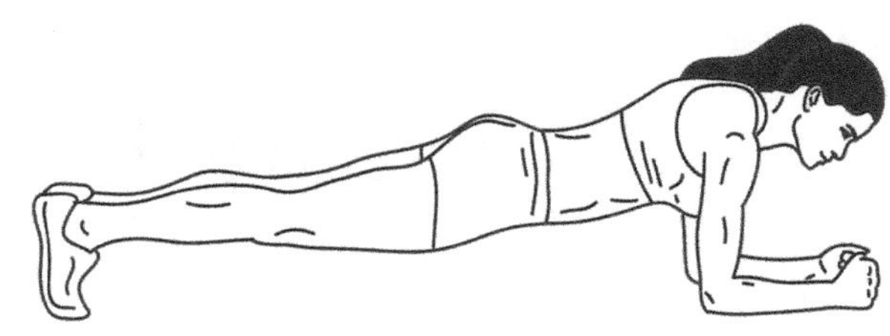

30sec high knees

30sec elbow plank

30sec high knees

30sec elbow plank

30sec high knees

30sec elbow plank

30sec high knees

30sec elbow plank

done

93 Pouncer

The Pouncer workout will work your abs but it won't neglect the rest of your body. It looks deceptively easy and with just two alternating, time-based exercises you'd be tempted to think it is. The Pouncer has a bite however that begins to make itself felt after the first set. Treat with care. Come back to it often.

POUNCER

DAREBEE HIIT WORKOUT © darebee.com

Level I 3 sets **Level II** 5 sets **Level III** 7 sets

2 minutes rest between sets

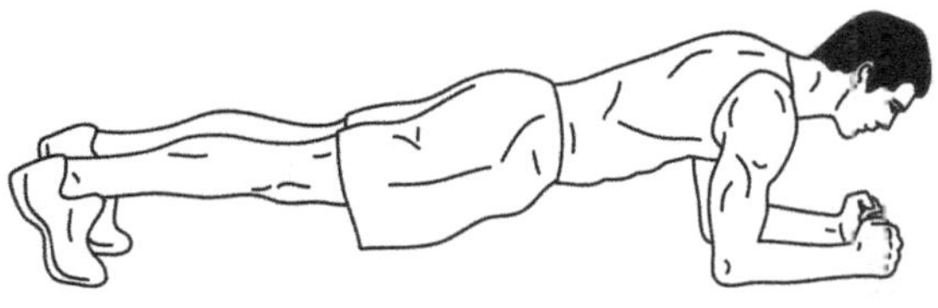

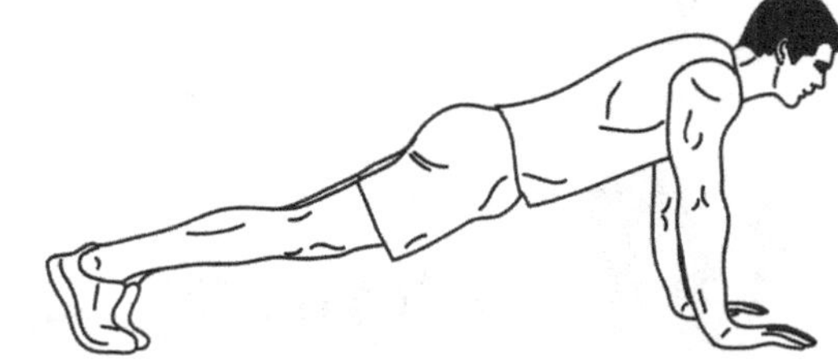

20sec elbow plank

10sec basic burpees

20sec elbow plank

10sec basic burpees

20sec elbow plank

10sec basic burpees

20sec elbow plank

10sec basic burpees

done

94 Power Abs

The abdominal muscle wall is made up of four, distinct muscle groups: obliques (interior and exterior), front abdominals (rectus abdominis), and core abdominals (transverse abdominis). The Power Abs workout uses exercises that activate all of those muscle groups helping your body develop a powerful abdominal wall that will take your physical ability to an entirely new level. Perfect for those looking for an abs workout that will use every ab wall muscle group, it is also useful for leveling up on physical performance by unlocking the body's full potential.

power abs

DAREBEE WORKOUT © darebee.com

LEVEL I 3 sets **LEVEL II** 4 sets **LEVEL III** 5 sets **REST** up to 2 minutes

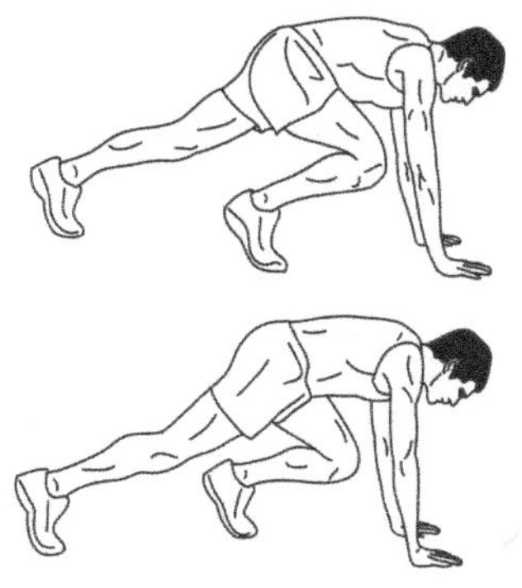

20 climbers

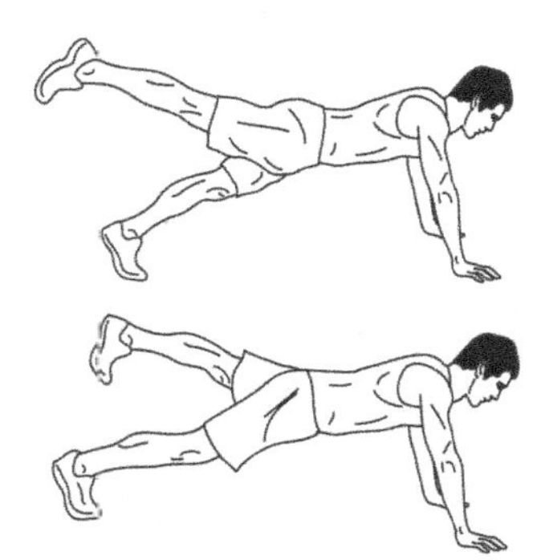

20 plank leg raises

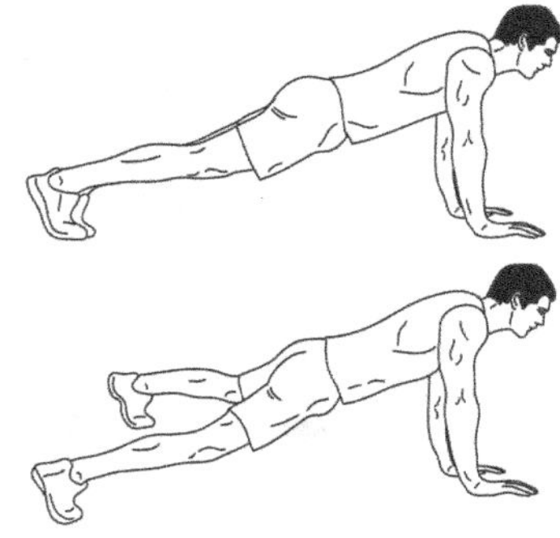

20 plank jacks

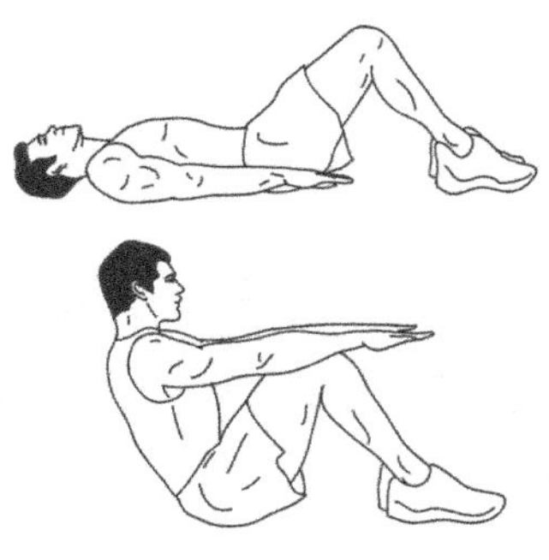

10 sit-ups

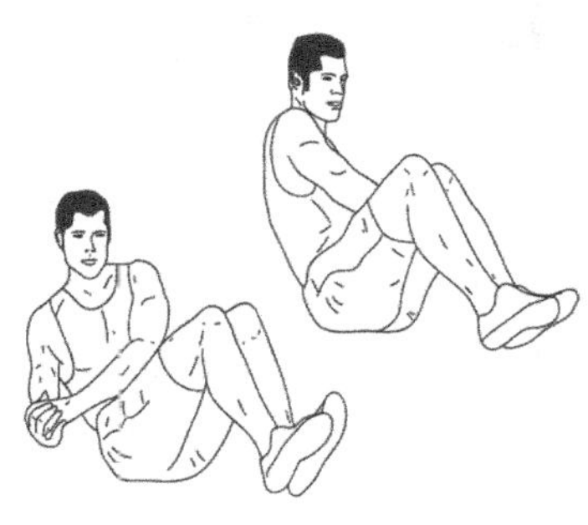

10 sitting twists

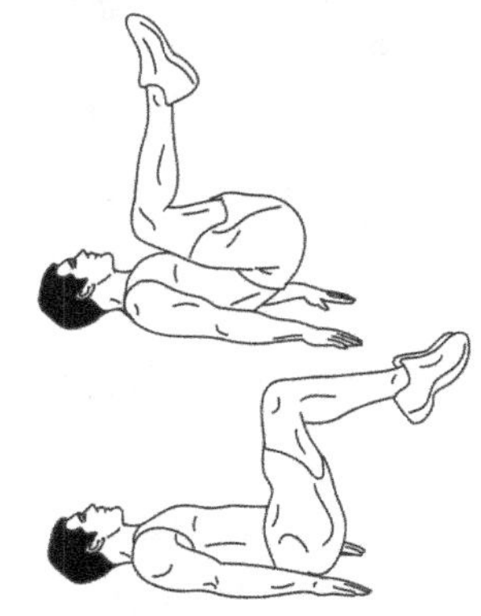

10 reverse crunches

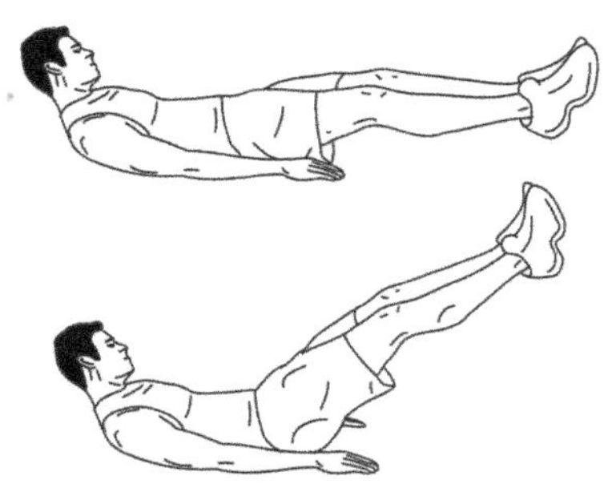

10 leg raises

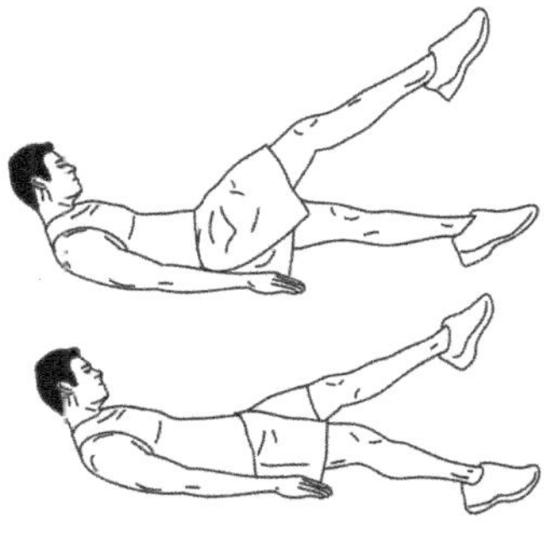

10 fluter kicks

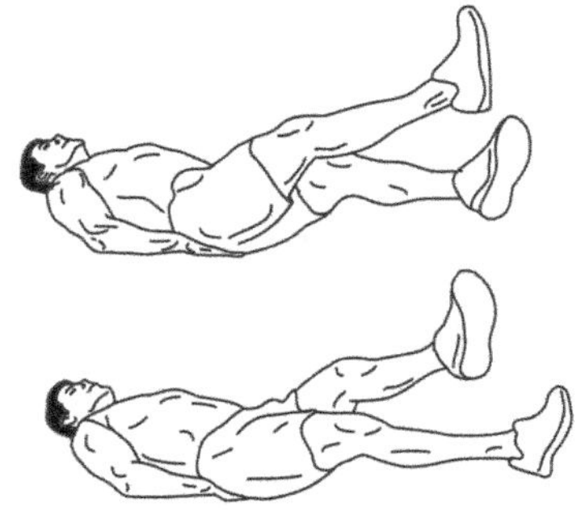

10 scissors

95 Rapid Fire

Rapid Fire is a fast-paced workout that targets core and abs and demands they work explosively to power the body as you transition from basic Burpees to ground work (Plank) and back again. There are a couple of things to watch out for here in order to get the most out of this workout. First make each transition as fast as possible. Second pack in as many reps as possible in your burpees by moving your legs out and back again to get in burpee jump positions as fast as you can.

Rapid Fire

DAREBEE HIIT WORKOUT © darebee.com

Level I 3 sets **Level II** 5 sets **Level III** 7 sets

2 minutes rest between sets

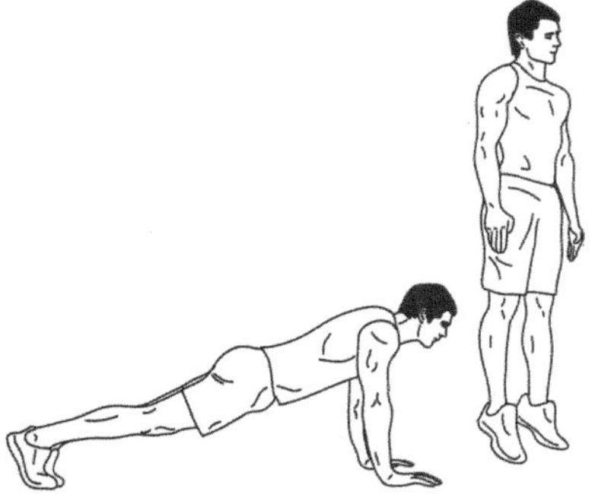

10sec basic burpees

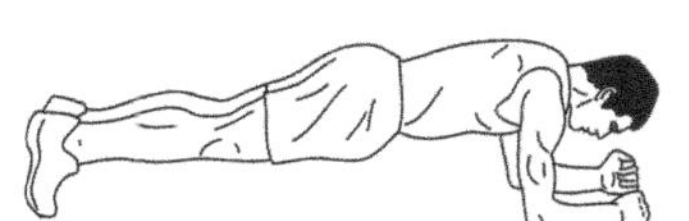

30sec elbow plank

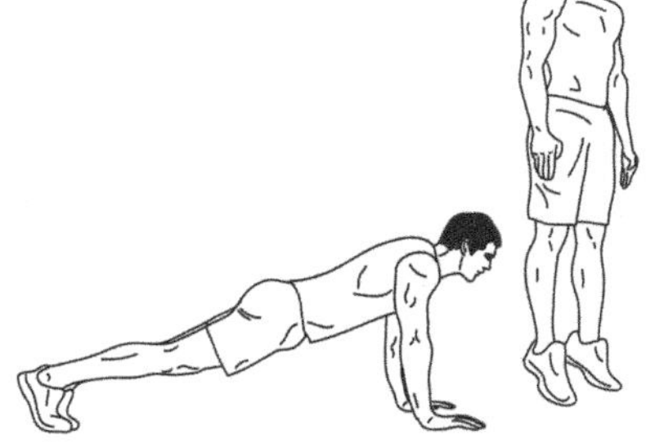

10sec basic burpees

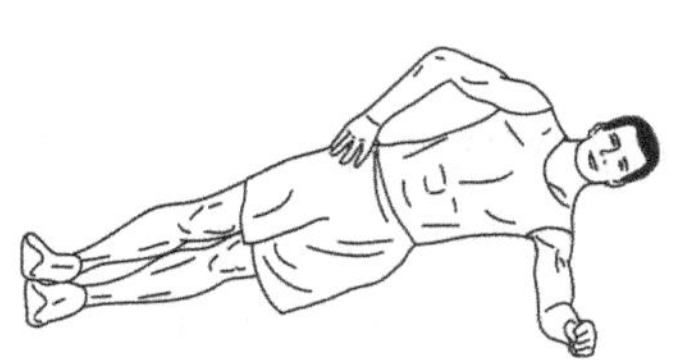

30sec side plank

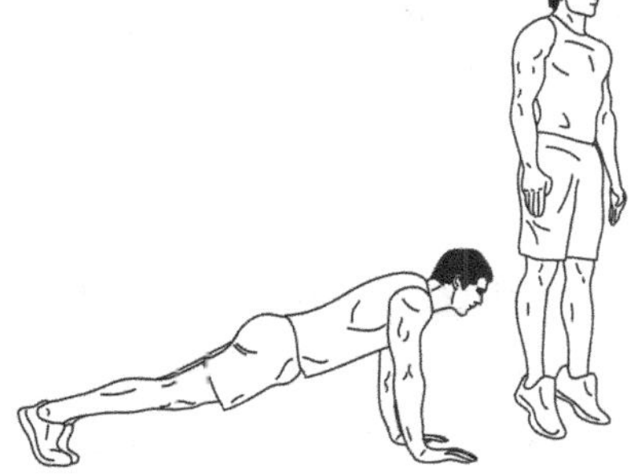

10sec basic burpees

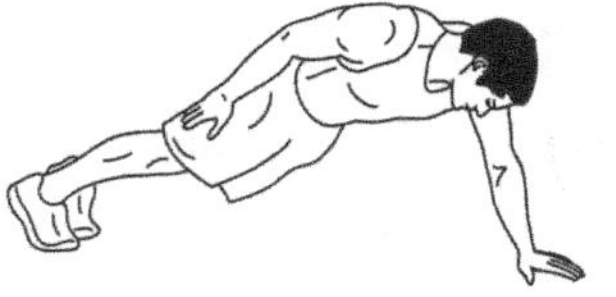

30sec one arm plank

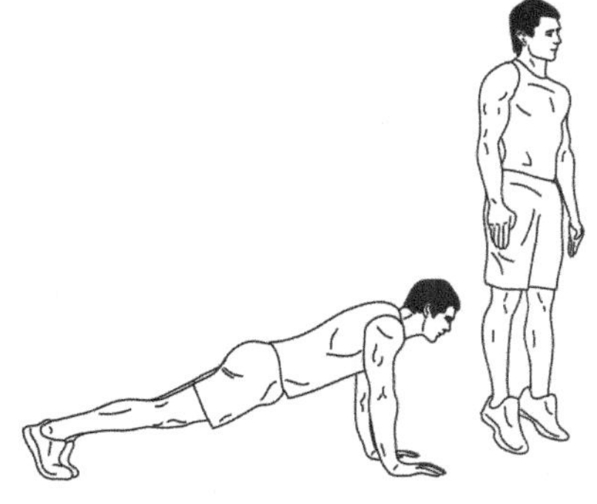

10sec basic burpees

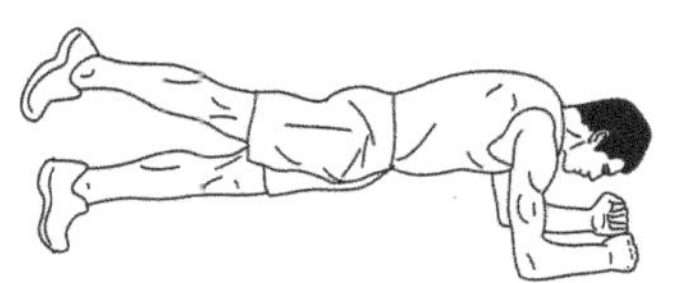

30sec raised leg plank

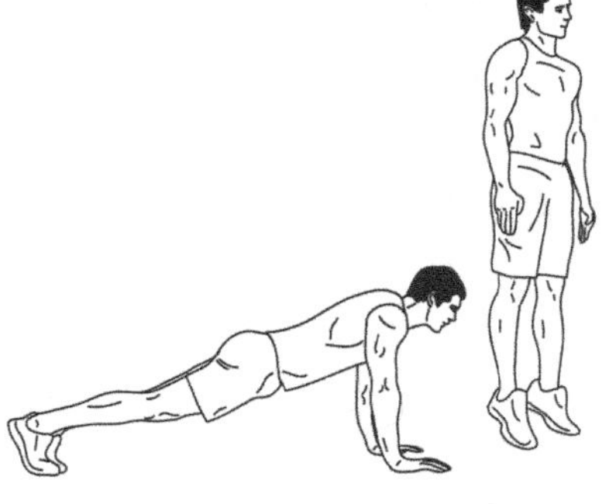

10sec basic burpees

96 Sizzler

The Sizzler is the kind of HIIT workout where you can increase the intensity by adding a little precision to your form. Stay on the balls of your feet throughout, for instance, and insist on bringing your arms down as fast as you send them up during Jumping Jacks and you get a pretty intense HIIT experience that will have you in the sweatzone from the very first set.

the sizzler

DAREBEE HIIT WORKOUT © darebee.com

Level I 3 sets **Level II** 5 sets **Level III** 7 sets

2 minutes rest between sets

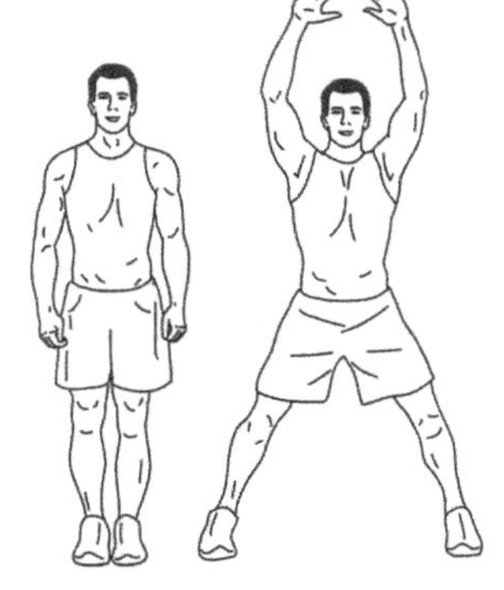

20sec jumping jacks

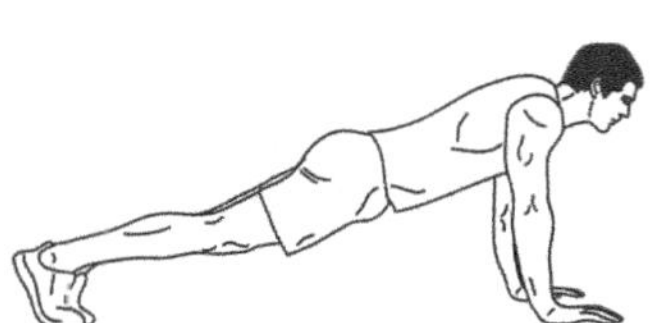

20sec plank hold

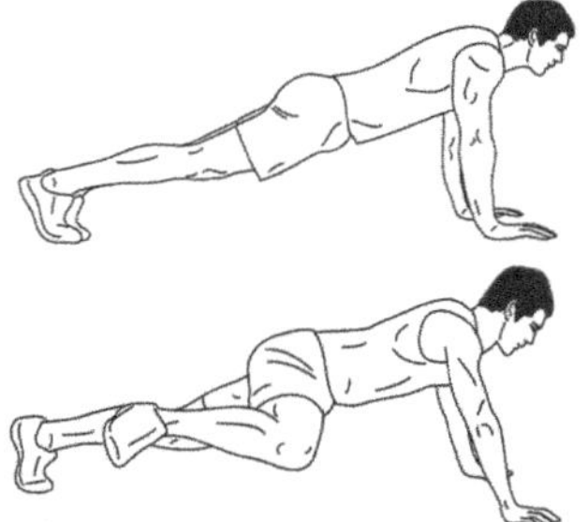

20sec side crunches

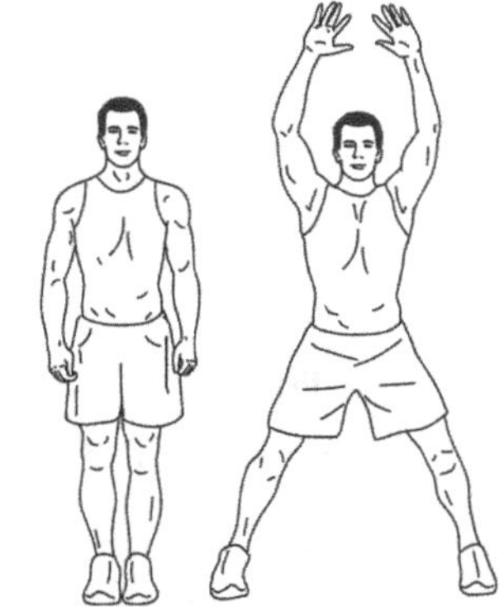

20sec jumping jacks

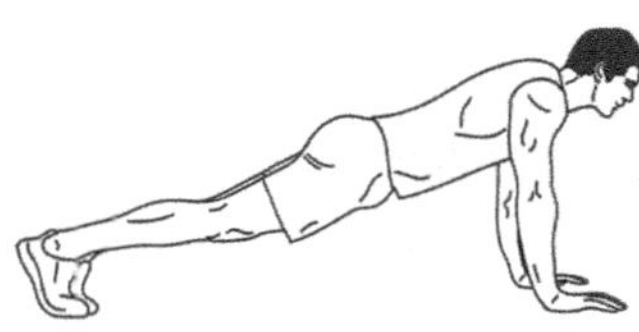

20sec plank hold

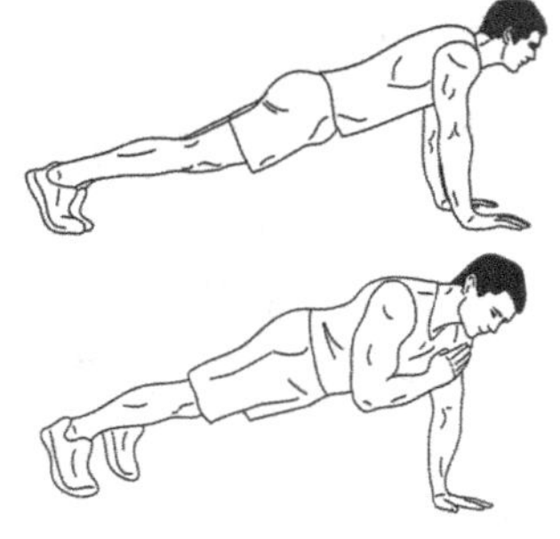

20sec shoulder taps

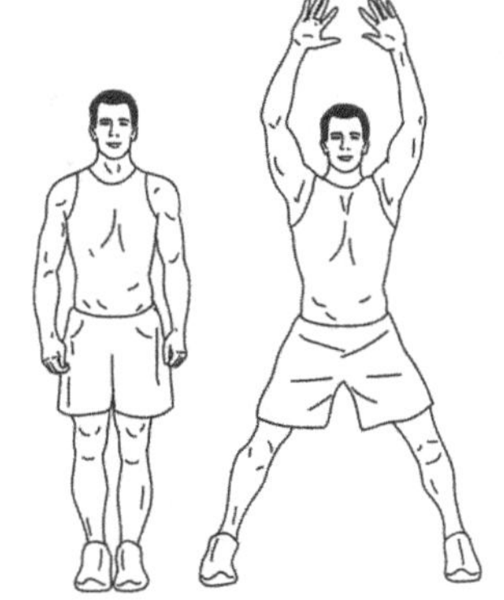

20sec jumping jacks

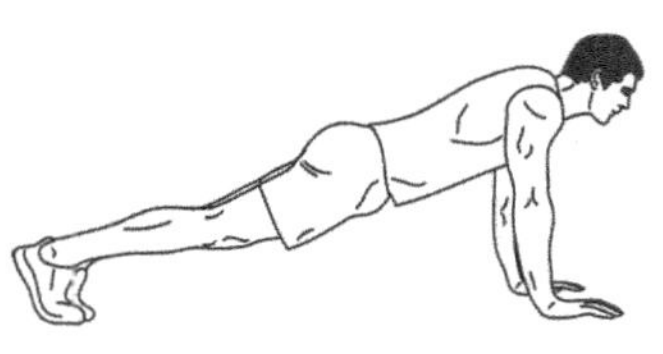

20sec plank hold

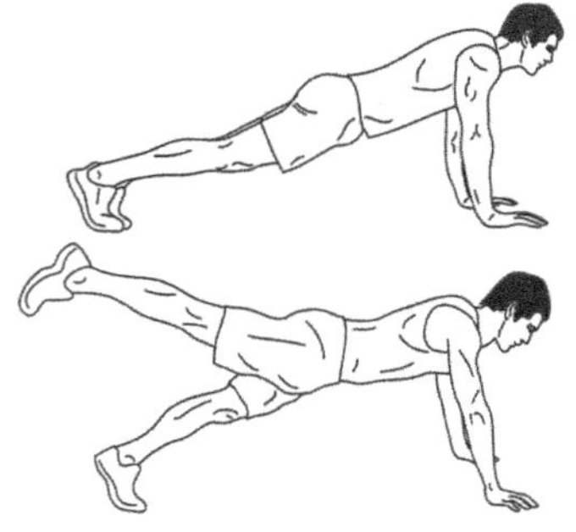

20sec leg raises

97 Speedster

For those of you looking to add an edge to your running and increase lower body tendon strength and explosiveness the Speedster workout is just what you need. A difficulty Level IV workout this is hard from set one and it simply gets no easier. But the results will astound you, plus feeling the burn is just how you know you've worked hard. Make sure your knees come to waist height during March Steps and High Knees. Land on the ball of the foot each time to offset the impact and work the calves.

SPEEDSTER

DAREBEE **HIIT** WORKOUT © **darebee.com**

Level I 3 sets **Level II** 5 sets **Level III** 7 sets | 2 minutes rest

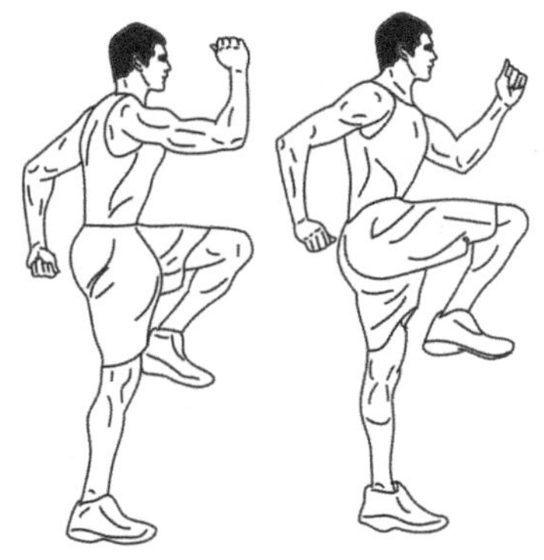
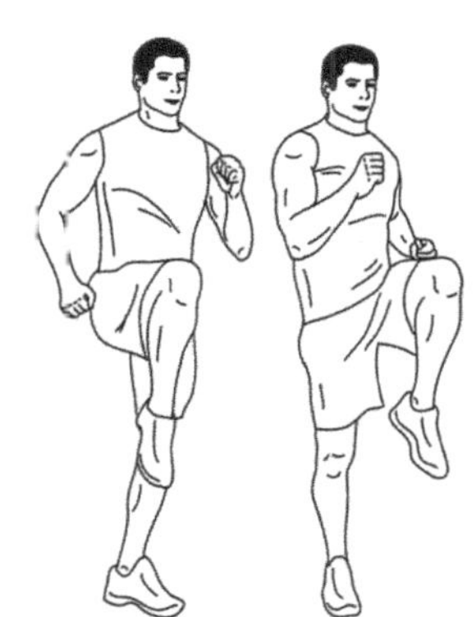

10sec march steps
10sec high knees
10sec march steps
10sec high knees
10sec march steps
10sec high knees

10sec plank hold
10sec climbers
10sec plank hold
10sec climbers
10sec plank hold
10sec climbers

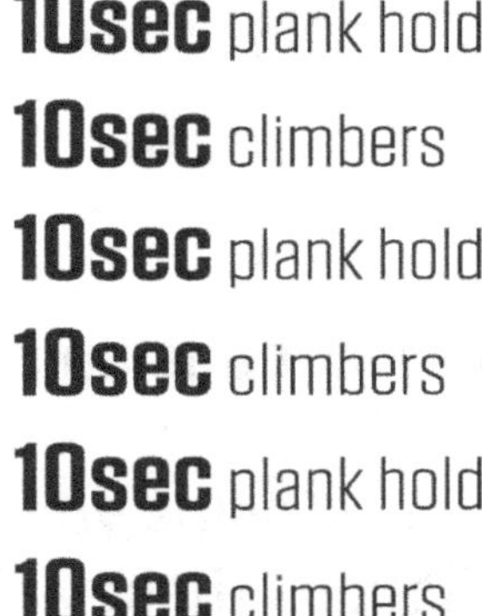
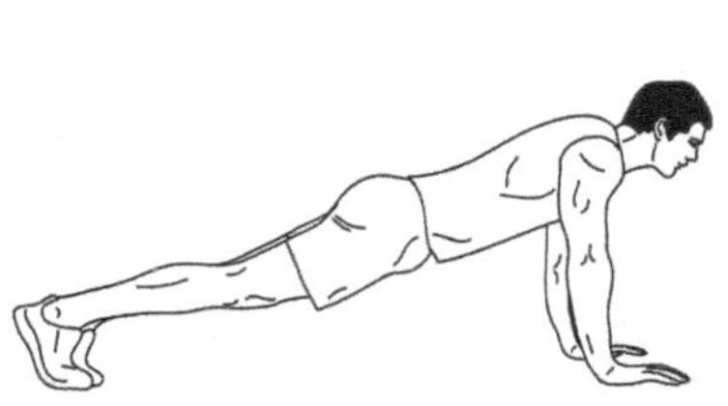
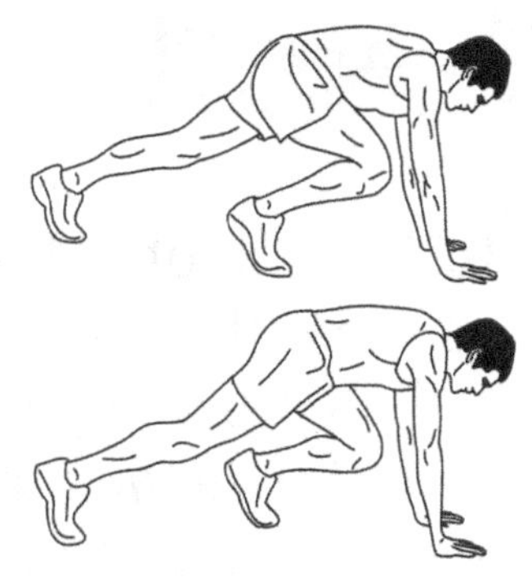

10sec hollow hold
10sec flutter kicks
10sec hollow hold
10sec flutter kicks
10sec hollow hold
10sec flutter kicks

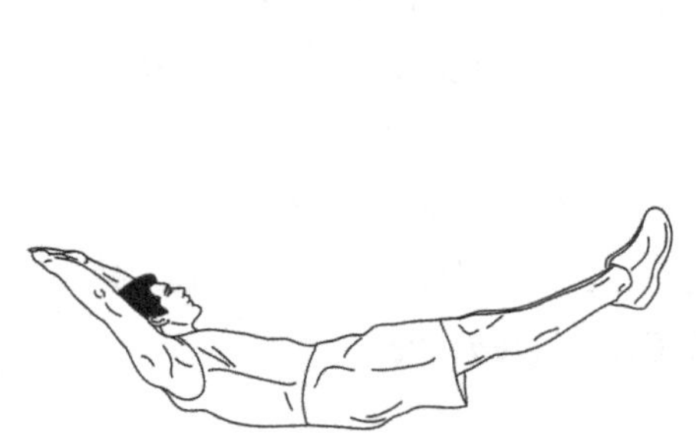
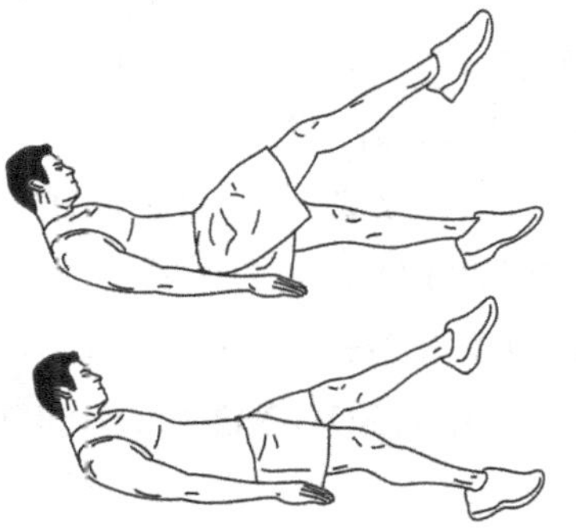

98 Standing Abs

DAREBEE Workout: What it Works
There is more than one way to train your abs. The ab wall is made up of four distinct muscle groups: Rectus Abdominis (the traditional six-pack you see in the movies and which every superhero sports) - it helps you move your lower and upper body, together. External Obliques - these are the muscles stretching over your ribs (the ones that really ache if you do a lot of push-ups, fast). They help you twist your body from side to side (and throw a punch or jump over obstacles). Internal Obliques - you do not really see them, but they help bring your body back into alignment every time you twist it in one direction or another. Finally there is the Transverse Abdominis - what we so popularly call "the core". These wrap around the spine and provide stability, keep us upright and make sure we don't get back pain from our upright posture. The standing abs workout targets all four muscle groups for a performance-enhancing experience.

standing **abs**

DAREBEE WORKOUT © **darebee.com**

repeat 3 times | up to 2 minute rest between sets

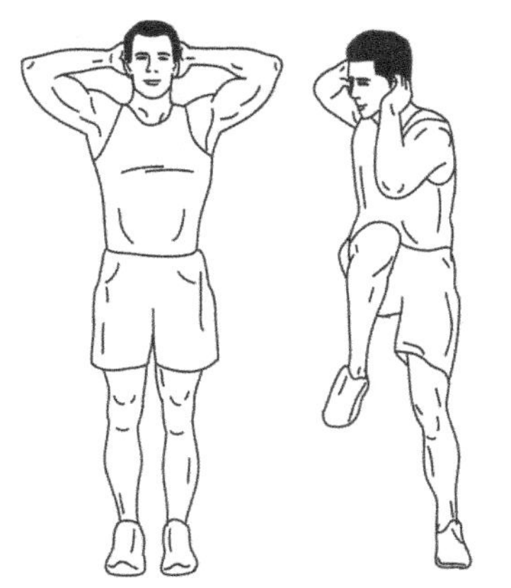

20 knee-to-elbows

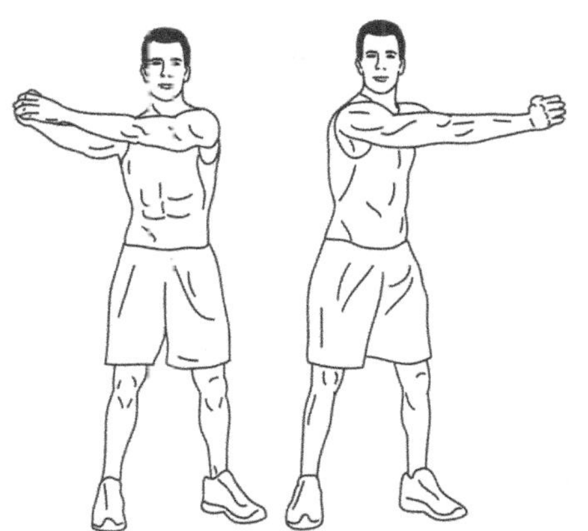

20 side-to-side chops

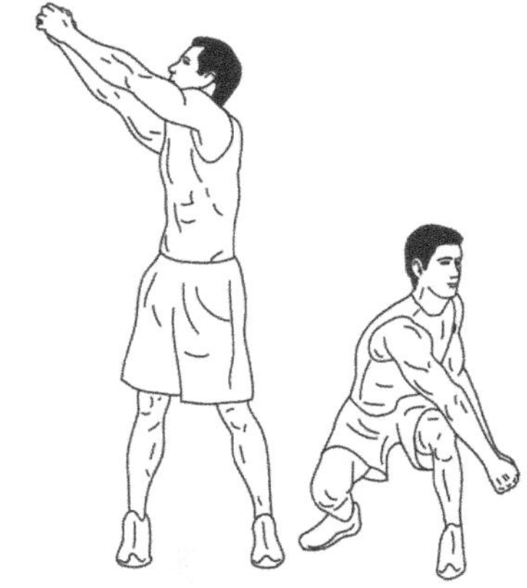

10 cross chops

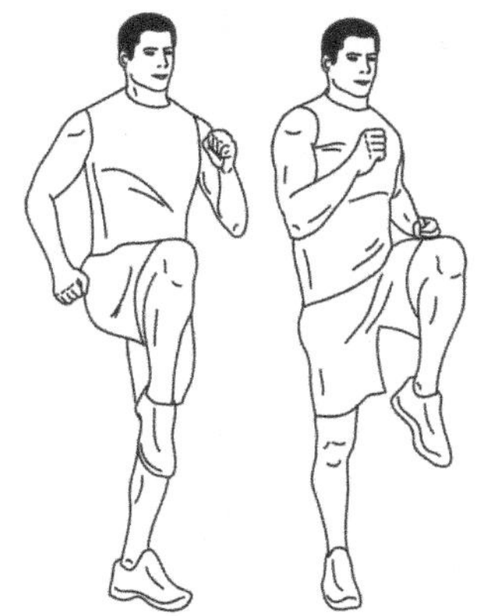

20 high knees

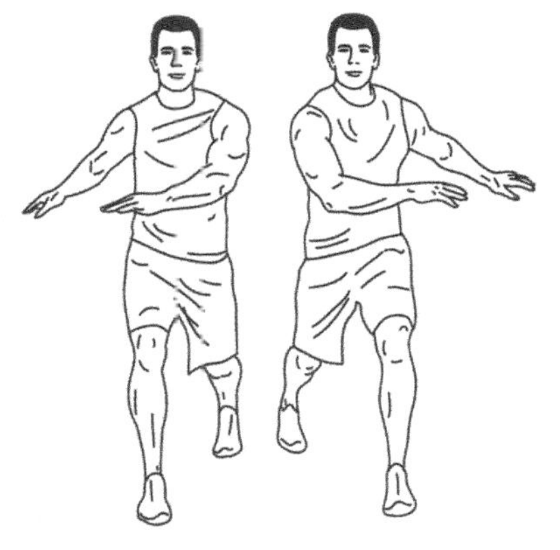

20 twist jacks

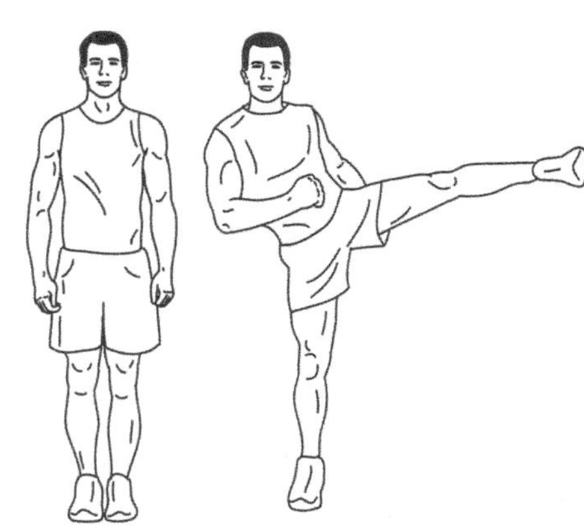

10 side leg raises

99 Total Core

Total Core is a high-burn, fast-paced workout designed to raise your body temperature and get you into the sweat zone from the very first set. Make sure your knees come up to waist height when performing High Knees, pump your arms and make sure you land on the ball of your foot. The exercises are designed to challenge your core and strengthen the ab muscle groups.

Total Core

DAREBEE WORKOUT © darebee.com

LEVEL I 3 sets **LEVEL II** 5 sets **LEVEL III** 7 sets **REST** up to 2 minutes

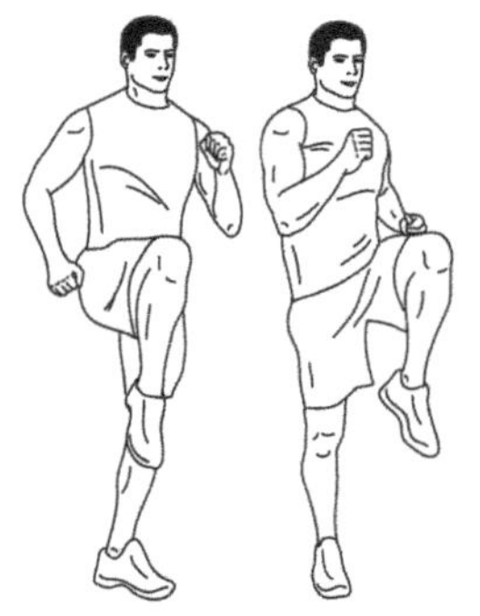

30 high knees

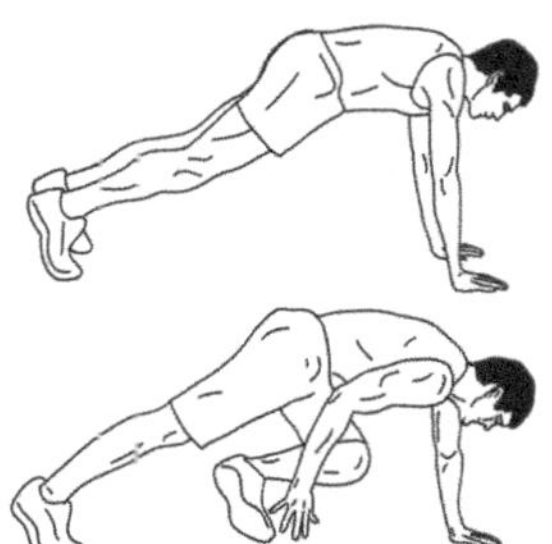

10 climber taps

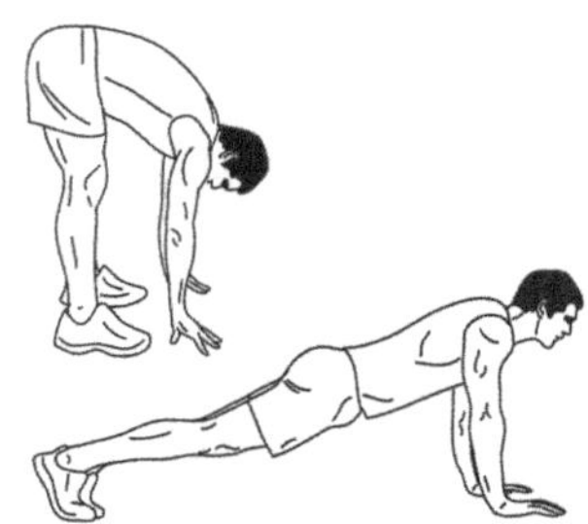

10 plank walk-outs

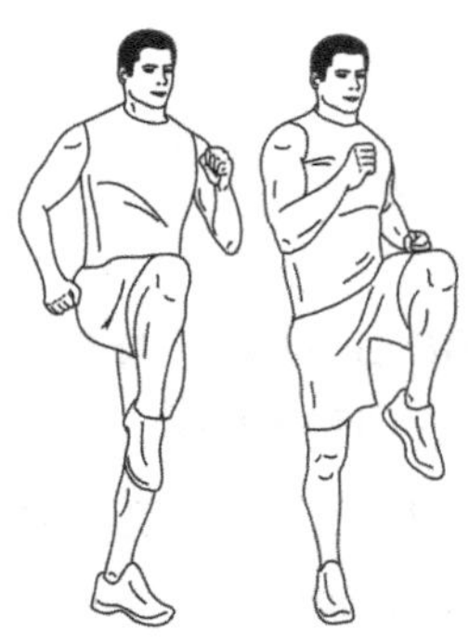

30 high knees

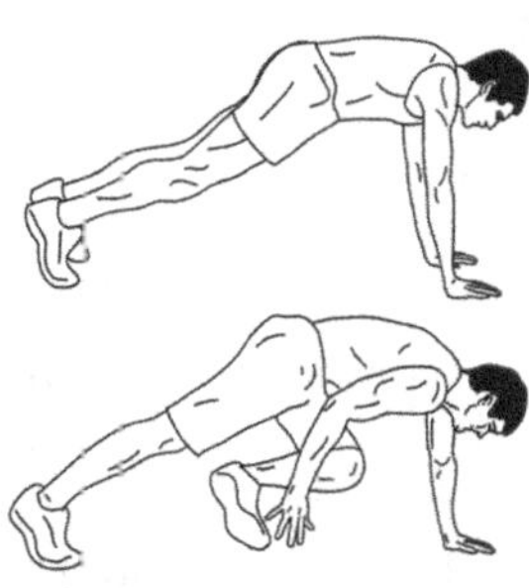

10 climber taps

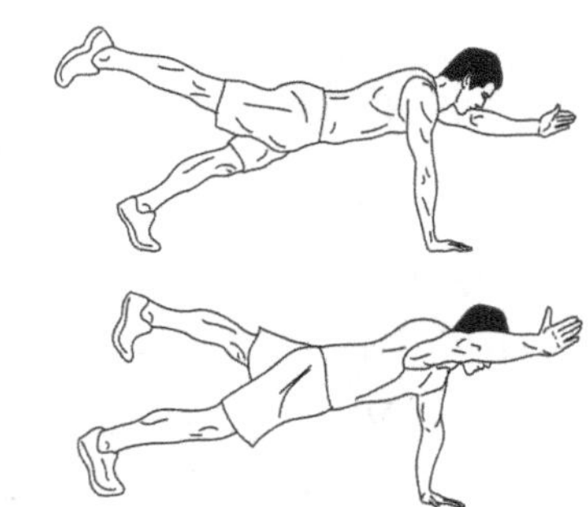

10 alt arm/ leg raises

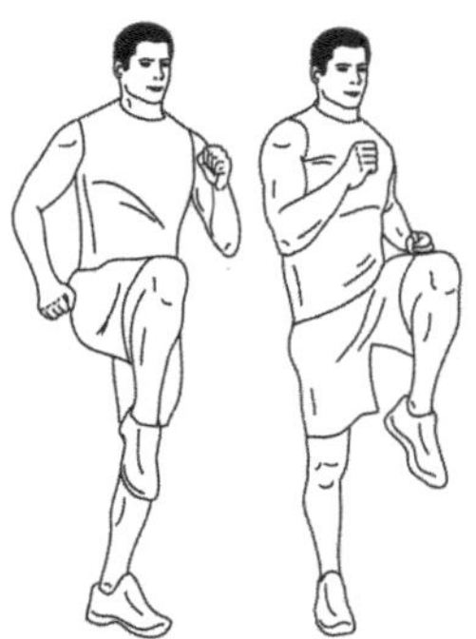

30 high knees

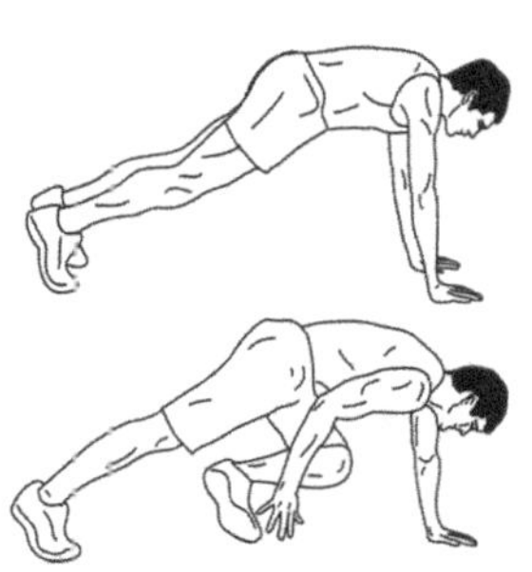

10 climber taps

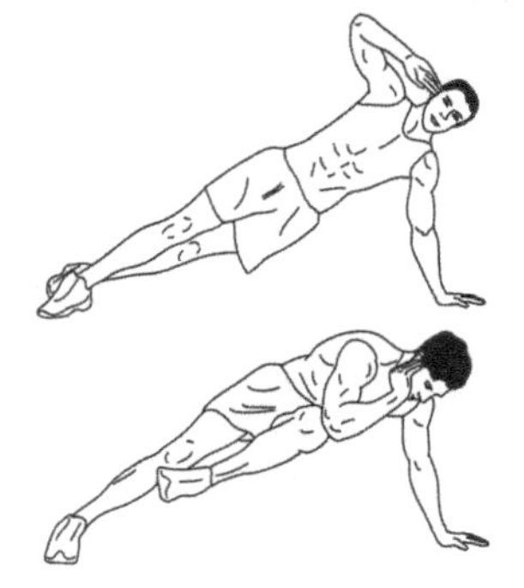

10 side plank crunches

100 Tune Up

Tune Up is a deceptive-looking workout that promises to be a walk in the park and turns out to be quite the battle, especially if you do the right thing and bring your knees up to waist height when doing High Knees (and make sure you land on the ball of the foot as you bring your feet down). It works the core, abs and lower body plus your lungs (of course). You think you're taking a little bit of a break when you're on the ground but you will soon know differently.

tune up

DARECEE HIIT WORKOUT © darebee.com

LEVEL I 3 sets **LEVEL II** 5 sets **LEVEL III** 7 sets **REST** up to 2 minutes

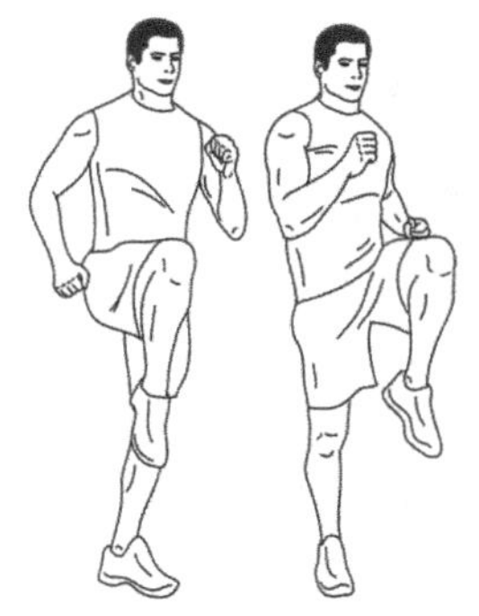

30sec high knees

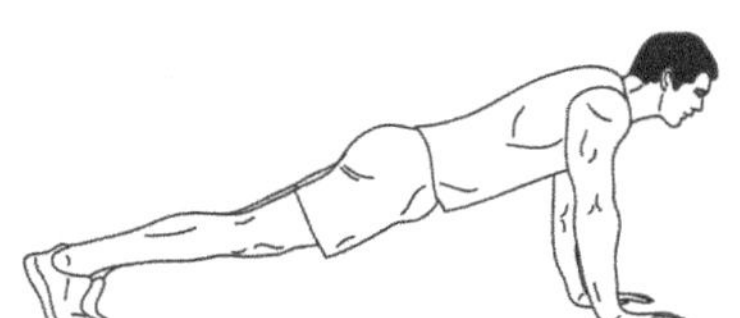

10sec plank

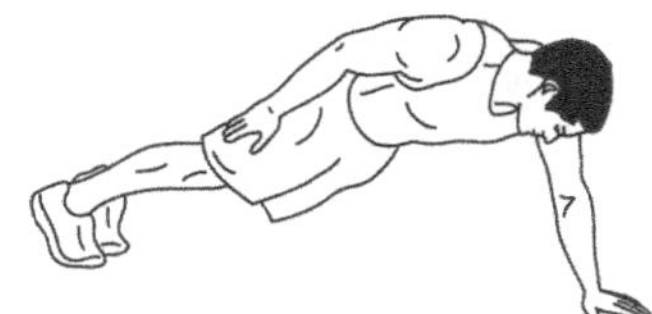

20sec one-arm plank

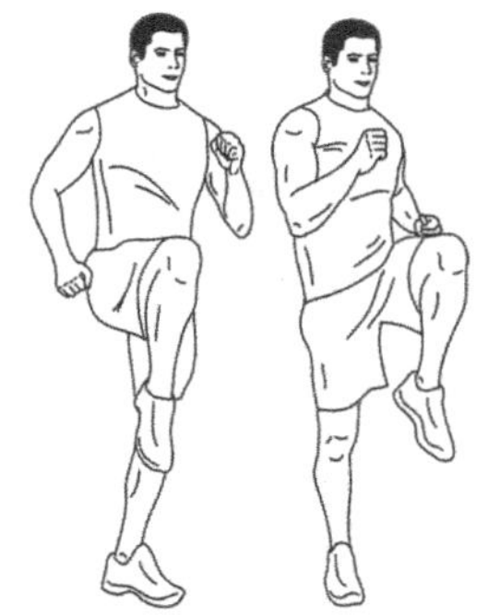

30sec high knees

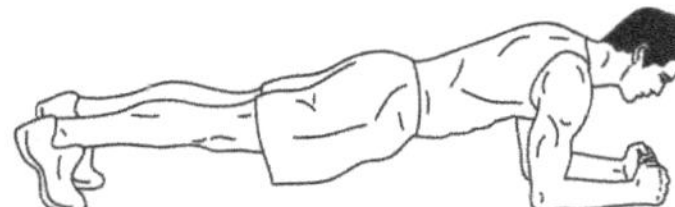

10sec elbow plank

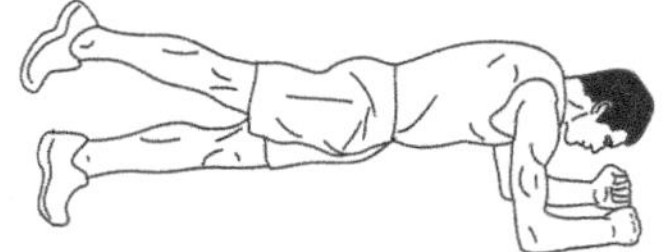

20sec raised leg plank

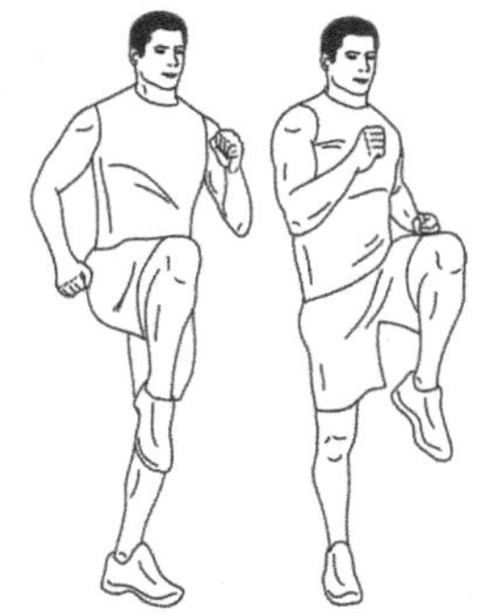

30sec high knees

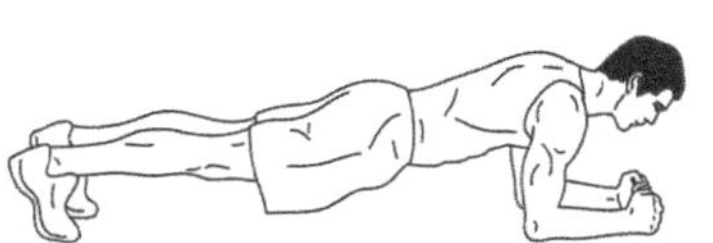

10sec elbow plank

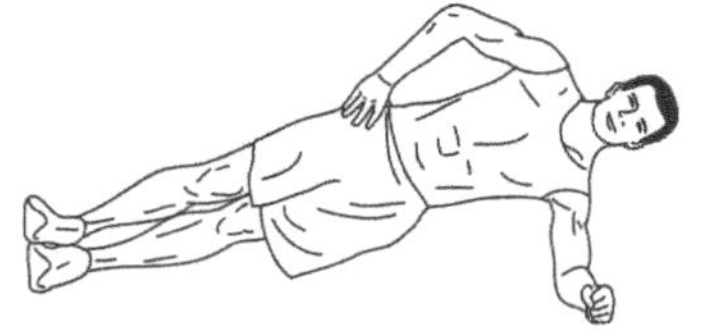

20sec side elbow plank

CPSIA information can be obtained
at www.ICGtesting.com
Printed in the USA
LVHW060016201020
669248LV00014B/421

9 781844 810093